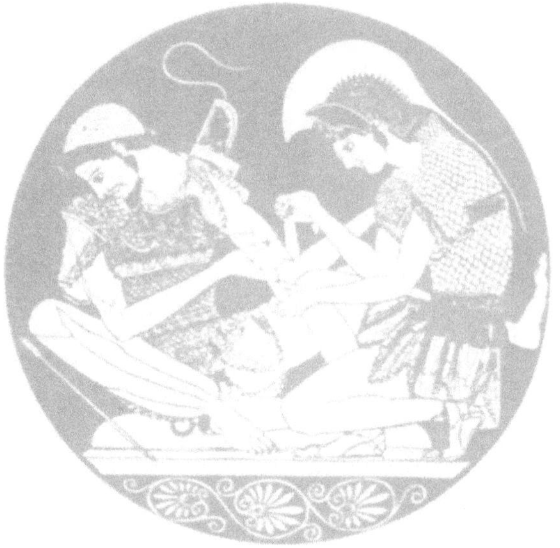

To Luciana
Marco
Roberto

Franco Postacchini

Lumbar Spinal Stenosis

With a Contribution
by Wolfgang Rauschning
on the Anatomy and Pathomorphology

Foreword: Lamberto Perugia

Drawings: Attilio Mancini

Springer-Verlag
Wien New York

Aulo Gaggi Editore
Bologna

Franco Postacchini, M.D.
Associate Professor of Orthopaedic Surgery,
«La Sapienza» University, Rome, Italy

Wolfgang Rauschning, M.D., Ph.D.
Associate Teaching Professor, Department of Orthopaedic Surgery,
University Hospital, Uppsala, Sweden

Lamberto Perugia, M.D.
Professor of Orthopaedic Surgery,
Director of the Orthopaedic Clinic,
«La Sapienza» University, Rome, Italy

Attilio Mancini, M.D.
Associate Professor of Orthopaedic Surgery,
«La Sapienza» University, Rome, Italy

Translation from the Italian edition
Le stenosi lombari

Softcover reprint of the hardcover 1st edition 1989

Sole distribution rights: Springer-Verlag Wien - New York

With 176 partly coloured Figures

Library of Congress Cataloging-in-Publication Data: Postacchini, Franco, 1944-. [Stenosi lombari. English.] Lumbar spinal stenosis / Franco Postacchini ; with a contribution by Wolfgang Rauschning on the anatomy and pathomorphology; foreword, Lamberto Perugia ; drawings, Attilio Mancini. p. cm. Translation of: Le stenosi lombari. Includes bibliographies and index. ISBN-13: 978-3-7091-9023-4
1. Spinal canal - Stenosis. 2. Spinal canal - Stenosis - Surgery. 3. Vertebrae. Lumbar - Surgery. I. Rauschning, Wolfgang. II. Title. [DNLM: 1. Spinal Stenosis. WE 750 P8568s.] RD771.S74P6713. 1989. 617'.375-dc19. 89-4333.

ISBN-13: 978-3-7091-9023-4 e-ISBN-13: 978-3-7091-9021-0
DOI: 10.1007/978-3-7091-9021-0

FOREWORD

Up until two decades ago, clinical interest in the etiopathogenetic interpretation of lumbo-radicular syndromes was prevalently concentrated on the pathology of the intervertebral disc. This vision gradually changed and grew as a result of the affirmation of the concept of pathological narrowing of the osteoligamentous vertebral canal as a cause of compression of the lumbar nervous structures. Finally, in the last ten years, lumbar stenosis has become more and more a subject of current interest not only as a result of problems related to nosography, diagnosis, and therapy, but also as a result of the increasing frequency with which vertebral canal or nerve root canal stenosis syndromes are recognized and treated. At the same time there was a tendency to include in stenotic pathology other pathological conditions responsible for lumbo-radicular syndromes. This led to dilation of the concept of stenosis, which perhaps no longer responded to reality, and which was not useful from a practical point of view. The need to define stenotic pathology and to correctly locate it within the vast field of lumbar pathology inspired the writing of this volume.

This monograph gathers many diagnostic and therapeutic concepts matured at our Institution over the years. Some of these concepts have already been defined in scientific meetings or in publications. Others are widely dealt with in this text, the main merit of which is that of having gathered in a single body the most diverse aspects of a condition which is still not well-known or properly defined.

Four chapters particularly deserve to be mentioned: the anatomy of the vertebral canal, pathomorphology, diagnostic investigations and treatment. The anatomy of the vertebral canal is described in great detail, particularly as regards the distinction between its various parts and the relationship between the walls and the spinal nervous structures; this chapter is enriched by cryomicrotomic images, which provide an extremely accurate and suggestive view of the various anatomical structures. Images obtained with the same method are found in the carefully analytical description of the pathomorphology of the stenotic spinal canal. The chapter on diagnostic investigations provides a rigorous and exhaustive analysis of the capacities and limits of old and new methods of imaging; the concept that is emphasised is that each method may provide only a partial view of the pathological reality, and that an accurate diagnosis may only result from an integration of clinical data with the information provided by several diagnostic methods. The chapter on treatment deals with the importance of making a careful distinction between symptomatic and asymptomatic stenosis, accurate surgical planning, the correct execution of surgery in order to adequately decompress the nervous structures without causing a secondary pathology.

The qualities that make a volume attractive are the scientific and practical interest of the subject, the completeness of its analysis, the clarity of its organization and of the language used, and the richness of the illustrations. These are qualities which I found to be fully satisfied in this text, which is complete but not wordy, which analyzes the vast subject of lumbar stenosis supported by rich and accurate illustrations. For this reason it is my belief that the monograph may interest anyone, whether an orthopaedist or not, who studies or actively deals with the problems of vertebral pathology. In particular, it is my hope that this text may help to better understand the problems related to a diagnostic definition of the pathology and to the determination of the treatment of the various types of lumbar stenosis.

I wish Franco Postacchini's work the success which, much better than my words, may constitute a well-deserved acknowledgement of the commitment and the scientific rigor expressed in each chapter of this monograph.

LAMBERTO PERUGIA

PREFACE

Lumbar spinal stenosis constitutes a relatively new chapter in vertebral pathology as only during recent years have the multiple anatomical and clinical features of this clinical condition been identified. The term lumbar stenosis itself is of recent introduction, becoming of current use only at the beginning of the seventies. As often happens for new pathological conditions, initially some did not recognize the existence of stenotic pathology, while others tended to identify as stenosis most of the pathological conditions of the lumbar spine, particularly those difficult to define clinically or of uncertain diagnosis. Several factors contributed to this nosological confusion: the vast meaning of the term stenosis; the multiformity of the clinical picture of stenotic pathology, often less astounding and elementary than that typical of herniated disc; the frequent difficulty in identifying by myelography the discal or osteoligamentous genesis of compression of the lumbar neural structures. This difficulty was considerably overcome with the advent of transaxial tomographic investigations which greatly contributed to our knowledge of the pathomorphology of the stenotic spinal canal, at the same time often resulting in an incorrect diagnosis of stenosis, at least according to the clinical meaning of the term. This particularly occurred at the onset of the tomodensitometric era. In recent years, parallel to progress in instrumental technical means, we have arrived at a clearer and more uniform vision of stenotic pathology. Nevertheless, there are still many obscure aspects of the pathology as well as differences of opinion as to the concept of stenosis, the accuracy of diagnostic investigations, and the treatment of the various forms of stenosis.

This monograph is the product of many years of scientific interest in vertebral lumbar pathology at our Institution. It originated from the desire to define the concept of lumbar stenosis, and to determine its pathomorphological and clinical aspects, to analyze the capacities and limits of clinical investigations in the diagnosis of this pathological condition, and, finally, to delineate the conservative and surgical treatment of the various types of lumbar stenosis in light of the experience obtained over recent years.

In a time of rapid scientific and technological progress, any text is destined to become outdated by the acquisition of further knowledge. This awareness does not eliminate the hope that this text may represent, particularly for young people, an effective aid for a better comprehension of a difficult area of vertebral pathology. Encouraged in this sense, I attempted to make as complete an analysis as possible of stenotic pathology, expressing the concepts that I believe to be valid in light of current experience. It is my hope that these concepts will remain valid ones, for myself and for others, in the future, as well. In the meantime, nonetheless, I hope that they may be further defined and enriched, the result of a continuous growth in the knowledge produced by scientific research and experience.

FRANCO POSTACCHINI

ACKNOWLEDGEMENT

I wish to express my sincerest gratitude to Prof. Lamberto Perugia, who encouraged me to write this monograph, gave me much precious advice during its preparation, and allowed me to use the data from the Institute of Orthopaedic Surgery and Traumatology at "La Sapienza" University of Rome on which the text is based. I also wish to express my profound gratitude to Prof. Attilio Mancini who is responsible for the illustrations in the text and who demonstrated great ability in uniting technique with the clear anatomical vision of the expert surgeon.

Without the collaboration and availability of Dr. Wolfgang Rauschning, to whom I am deeply grateful, the iconography would not have contained the excellent images of anatomical sections obtained with cryomicrotomy, which are included in the chapters on the anatomy of the vertebral canal and the pathomorphology of stenosis.

Thanks also go to Dr. Henry Crock who kindly provided images of anatomical specimens illustrating the arterial and venous circulation of the cauda equina, and to Dr. Richard Porter who provided the ultrasound scans. Acknowledgement must also go to Prof. Cesare De Martino and Dr. Marinella Bellocci for their help in obtaining the histological and ultrastructural pictures.

I am grateful to many people — Dr. Maurizio Ripani, Dr. Cosimo Tudisco, Dr. Giovanni Battista Morace, Mr. Mario Termine, Mr. Massimo Risi, Mrs. Maria Schiavoncini, Miss Laura Vassallo — who varyingly contributed to the realization of this monograph, which Aulo Gaggi published with great care and commitment.

My sincerest thanks go to the Centro Studi di Patologia Vertebrale of Rome, which provided the funding which made it possible to publish this text.

CONTENTS

Chapter I
HISTORICAL REVIEW ... pag. 15

Chapter II
ANATOMY OF THE VERTEBRAL CANAL AND THE NEURAL STRUCTURES IN THE LUMBAR SPINE (F. Postacchini, W. Rauschning) ... » 21
Vertebral foramen ... » 21
Morphology ... » 21
Dimensions ... » 26
Width of the lateral recesses ... » 29
Vertebral canal ... » 31
Nerve root canal ... » 32
Intervertebral foramen ... » 35
Neural structures in the vertebral canal ... » 37
Spinal cord and cauda equina ... » 37
Extradural course of the spinal nerver roots ... » 39
Functional changes of the vertebral canal and nerve roots ... » 42
Blood supply ... » 43
Vascular pattern of the spinal cord and cauda equina ... » 43
Intrinsic vasculature of the caudal nerve roots ... » 47

Chapter III
DEFINITION AND CLASSIFICATION ... » 49
Stenosis and pseudostenosis ... » 49
Previous definitions of lumbar stenosis ... » 49
The concept of stenosis ... » 50
Pseudostenosis ... » 53
Classification ... » 55
Spinal canal stenosis ... » 59
Primary stenosis ... » 61
Secondary stenosis ... » 64
Combined stenosis ... » 64
Mixed stenosis ... » 65
Isolated stenosis of the nerve root canal ... » 65
Stenosis of the intervertebral foramen ... » 65

Chapter IV
EPIDEMIOLOGY ... » 67
Incidence ... » 67
Sex ... » 67
Age ... » 68
Physical characteristics ... » 68
Occupation ... » 68
Familiarity ... » 69
Cases observed by the author ... » 69
Case reports ... » 69
Conclusions ... » 73

Chapter V
AETIOPATHOGENESIS ... » 75
Aetiopathogenetic factors ... » 75

Achondroplasia ... pag. 75
Developmental narrowing of the spinal canal ... » 75
Spondylotic changes ... » 76
Intervertebral disc ... » 76
Facet joints ... » 77
Vertebral body ... » 78
Degenerative spondylolisthesis ... » 78
Traumas ... » 83
Pathogenetic mechanisms ... » 84
Primary forms of stenosis ... » 84
Degenerative stenosis ... » 84

Chapter VI
PATHOMORPHOLOGY (F. Postacchini, W. Rauschning) ... » 87
Introduction ... » 87
Vertebral canal and intervertebral foramen ... » 87
Primary stenosis ... » 87
Degenerative stenosis ... » 89
Disc degeneration and osteophytosis of the vertebral body ... » 89
Osteoarthrotic changes of the facet joints ... » 89
Thickening of the laminae ... » 93
Changes of the ligamenta flava ... » 93
Dynamic stenosis ... » 94
Degenerative spondylolisthesis ... » 94
Epidural tissue ... » 97
Spinal nervous structures ... » 98
Dural sac ... » 98
Spinal nerve roots in the intrathecal course ... » 98
Spinal nerve roots in the extrathecal course ... » 99

Chapter VII
CLINICAL FEATURES ... » 101
Clinical syndromes ... » 101
Continuous radicular syndrome ... » 101
Intermittent radicular syndrome ... » 102
Combined radicular syndrome ... » 102
Illustrative case reports ... » 102
Incidence of the different types of syndrome ... » 110
Differential diagnosis with disc prolapse ... » 110
Lumbo-radicular intermittent claudication ... » 111
Pathogenesis ... » 111
Differential diagnosis with other types of claudication and pseudoclaudication ... » 113
Medullary intermittent claudication ... » 113
Vascular intermittent claudication ... » 113
Pseudoclaudication due to joint disorders in the lower limb ... » 115

Chapter VIII
DIAGNOSTIC INVESTIGATIONS ... » 117
Introduction ... » 117
Plain radiography ... » 117
Anteroposterior projection ... » 117
Length of the laminae and interlaminar angle ... » 117
Interapophysolaminar space ... » 117
Articular space of facet joints ... » 119
Degenerative changes of the facet joints ... » 119
Lateral projection ... » 120
Length of the pedicles ... » 120
Vertebral bodies ... » 121
Intervertebral foramina ... » 121
Oblique projections ... » 123
Measurements of vertebral canal dimensions ... » 123
Interpedicular distance ... » 123
Midsagittal diameter ... » 124

Jones and Thomson's spinal index ... pag. 124
Conventional tomography ... » 125
Electrodiagnostic investigations ... » 125
Electromyography ... » 125
H reflex ... » 126
Somatosensory evoked potentials ... » 126
Ultrasonography ... » 127
Myelography ... » 128
Technical details ... » 128
Elementary signs of stenosis ... » 129
Uniform narrowing of the dural sac ... » 129
Deformations of the dural sac ... » 130
Indentations ... » 130
Hour-glass deformations ... » 131
Block images ... » 132
Intrasaccular abnormalities ... » 133
Translucencies of the caudal nerve roots in the intrathecal course ... » 133
Dyshomogenous distribution of the contrast medium ... » 135
Redundancy of spinal nerve roots ... » 135
Abnormalities of the nerve root sheaths ... » 135
Longitudinal extension of stenosis ... » 137
Single level stenosis ... » 137
Multilevel stenosis ... » 137
Functional myelography ... » 138
Myelographic patterns in the various types of stenosis ... » 140
Spinal canal stenosis ... » 140
Nerve root canal stenosis ... » 143
Stenosis of the intervertebral foramen ... » 146
Discography ... » 148
Computerized tomography ... » 154
Spinal canal stenosis ... » 154
Vertebral canal ... » 154
Midsagittal diameter ... » 154
Articular processes ... » 154
Intervertebral disc and vertebral body osteophytes ... » 155
Ligamenta flava ... » 155
Dural sac ... » 155
Midsagittal and transverse dimensions ... » 155
Area ... » 155
Morphology ... » 156
Nerve root canal stenosis ... » 156
Stenosis of the intervertebral foramen ... » 162
Diagnostic accuracy of CT scan ... » 163
Myelo-CT ... » 169
Magnetic resonance imaging ... » 171

Chapter IX
TREATMENT ... » 173
Introduction ... » 173
Conservative treatment ... » 173
Drug therapy ... » 173
Physiotherapy ... » 174
Bracing ... » 174
Surgical treatment ... » 174
Indications and contraindications ... » 174
Planning of surgery ... » 175
Spinal canal stenosis ... » 175
Number of levels to decompress ... » 175
Mono- or bilateral decompression ... » 177
Type of decompression ... » 177
Longitudinal and transverse extent of decompression ... » 180
Vertebral fusion ... » 181
Effects of laminectomy on vertebral stability ... » 181

Indications to fusion .... pag. 183
Planning of surgery in degenerative spondylolisthesis .... » 187
Isolated stenosis of the nerve root canal .... » 189
Anaesthesia .... » 189
Hypotensive anaesthesia .... » 191
Patient positioning .... » 191
Preoperative identification of spinal levels .... » 194
Surgical technique .... » 198
Bilateral laminectomy .... » 198
Skin incision and superficial haemostasis .... » 198
Disinsertion of paraspinal muscles .... » 199
Opening of spinal canal .... » 202
Exploration of intervertebral discs and spinal nerve roots .... » 205
Excision of posterior osteophytes of the vertebral body .... » 206
Control of deep haemorrhage .... » 206
Opening of dural sac .... » 207
Prevention of epidural scar formation .... » 207
Wound closure .... » 208
Spinal fusion .... » 208
Laminotomy .... » 209
Microsurgery .... » 211
Postoperative treatment .... » 212
Complications .... » 212
Vertebral complications .... » 212
Extravertebral complications .... » 214

Chapter X
RESULTS OF TREATMENT .... » 217
Natural history .... » 217
Conservative treatment .... » 218
Surgical treatment .... » 219
Review of the literature .... » 219
Spinal canal stenosis .... » 219
Degenerative spondylolisthesis .... » 220
Nerve root canal stenosis .... » 221
Author's series .... » 221
Material .... » 221
Evaluation of the results .... » 223
Spinal canal stenosis .... » 223
Overall results .... » 223
Analytical results .... » 224
Nerve root canal stenosis .... » 228
Overall results .... » 228
Analytical results .... » 230
Isolated stenosis of the intervertebral foramen .... » 230
Clinical symptoms and signs after surgery .... » 231
Spinal canal stenosis .... » 231
Nerve root canal stenosis .... » 231
Conclusions .... » 231

Subject Index .... » 235

Chapter I

Historical review

The first description of spinal canal stenosis is attributed to Portal (1803), who at autopsy observed narrowing of the lumbar or thoraco-lumbar vertebral canal in three subjects suffering from rickets, syphilis, or both. All three, in addition to the compression of the neural structures at the stenotic vertebral levels, showed marked muscular atrophy in the lower limbs, associated in one subject with a history of paralysis, which had developed after an initial period of severe pain. Portal reports that similar cases had been described by Morgagni in «De sedibus et causis morborum» and also adds that he had observed subjects with a markedly narrow spinal canal and no clinical evidence of weakness, atrophy or paralysis in the lower limbs. Over the same period Ollivier (1824) reported on narrowing of the spinal canal in subjects with rickets.

Approximately a century later, Sachs and Fraenkel (1900) reported the case of a 48-year old patient suspected to be suffering from ryzomelic spondylitis, who had complained for the last two years of lumbosacral pain associated with weakness and tremor in the lower limbs and increasing difficulty in walking. The patient had also progressively developed a posture characterized by forward flexion of the trunk. The rapid increase in pain and the absence of the left knee reflex led to the suspicion of neoplastic disease or compression of the spinal nerve roots by an «exudate». At surgery — which consisted of a T_{11}-T_{12} laminectomy — the laminae were found to be unusually thick and «an enormously thickened lining membrane» was excised. Following surgery the pain and weakness decreased and the left knee reflex returned.

In 1910 Sumita described the first cases of narrowing of the spinal canal in achondroplastic dwarfs.

A year later, Bailey and Casamajor (1911) reported on a series of five patients with symptoms and signs of compression of the spinal cord or cauda equina, associated with radiographic evidence of spondylosis. The degenerative changes reported by these authors consisted mainly of lateral and anterior osteophytes, but they conceived that osteoarthritic changes of the apophyseal joints and thickening of the ligamenta flava might narrow the spinal canal and the intervertebral foramina and so could be responsible for a clinically relevant compression of the neural structures. The only patient treated conservatively, in their series of five, was a 40-year old man with back and bilateral leg pain, who had developed a standing posture with the trunk bent forward and who could walk only for a very limited distance. The operation, which was performed by Elsberg with a preliminary diagnosis of neoplastic disease, revealed a marked thickening of the laminae and the spinous process of T_{12}. Histology was reported as showing «osteochondritic» vertebral changes, together with new bone formation. On the basis of these observations the authors were the first to include lumbar spondylosis among the conditions that might cause compression of the spinal cord and cauda equina. This, however, was not Elsberg's opinion. In the following years he submitted to laminectomy a number of patients with similar clinical presentation to the case previously described, but continued to believe that at least the majority of them were suffering from a not-well-defined inflammatory disease of the spinal nerve roots. Most of these patients, as reported by Cramer (1943) had lumbar spondylosis and all of those who had

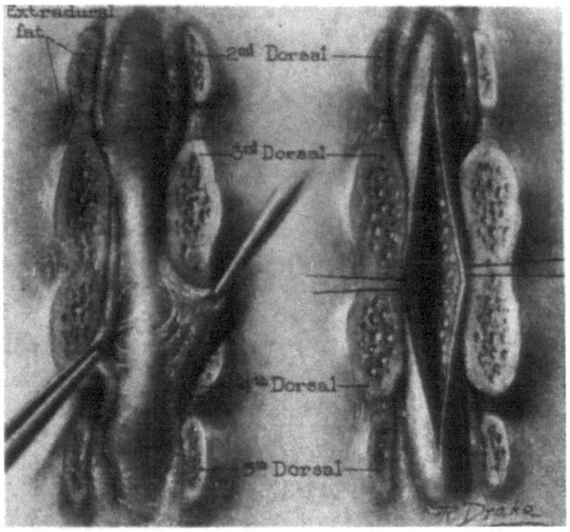

Fig. 1.1 - Hypertrophy of T_3 and T_4 laminae causing spinal cord compression, and inflammatory thickening of the meninges. Drawing of operative findings from Parker and Adson's paper.

marked degenerative changes improved following surgery.

In 1925 Parker and Adson reported on a series of cases, some of whom had marked hypertrophy of the laminae and the spinous processes and narrowing of the spinal canal (Fig. 1.1). These changes, observed in the thoracic as well as in the lumbar spine, were associated with signs of compression of the spinal cord and cauda equina.

Over the same period Putti (1927) emphasized the importance of degenerative changes of the zygoapophyseal joints and to their anomaly of orientation (asintropism) as a possible cause of narrowing of the intervertebral foramina and subsequent compression of the spinal nerve roots. In the 1930's Towne and Reichert (1931) and Spurling *et al.* (1937) drew attention to the thickening of the ligamenta flava as the cause for compression of the caudal nerve roots observed in two, and seven cases, respectively. In the series of Spurling, however, thickening of the laminae of the fourth lumbar vertebra was constantly noticed, which leads to the belief that the bony spinal canal was abnormally narrow.

Some years later, Sarpyener (1945, 1947) described a number of children and adolescents with congenital narrowing of the spinal canal, often associated with spina bifida or other vertebral anomalies. Most of these patients had presented with leg pain, bladder incontinence and spastic paraparesis or paraplegia. The author interpreted these symptoms as the consequence of a congenital narrowing of the spinal cord itself (and not of the spinal canal), which during growth would tend to become larger, with consequent clinical improvement. These observations, however, have never been confirmed subsequently by other authors. It is likely

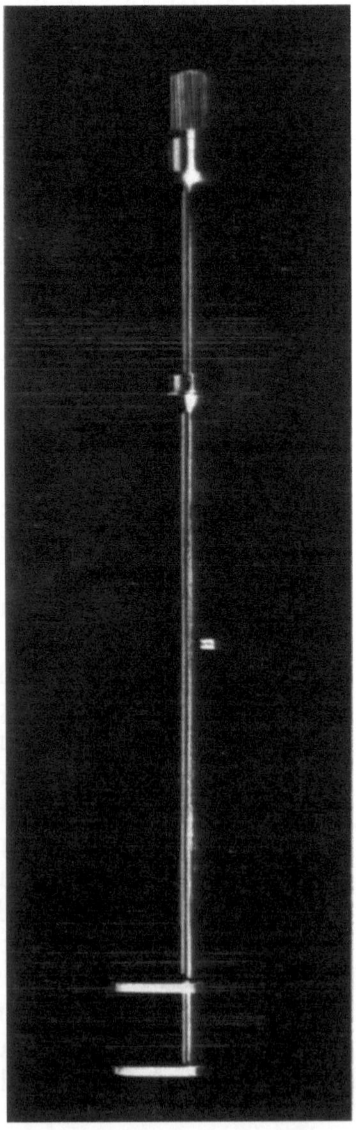

Fig. 1.2 - Stenosimeter used by Verbiest to measure the midsagittal dimensions of the spinal canal during surgery.

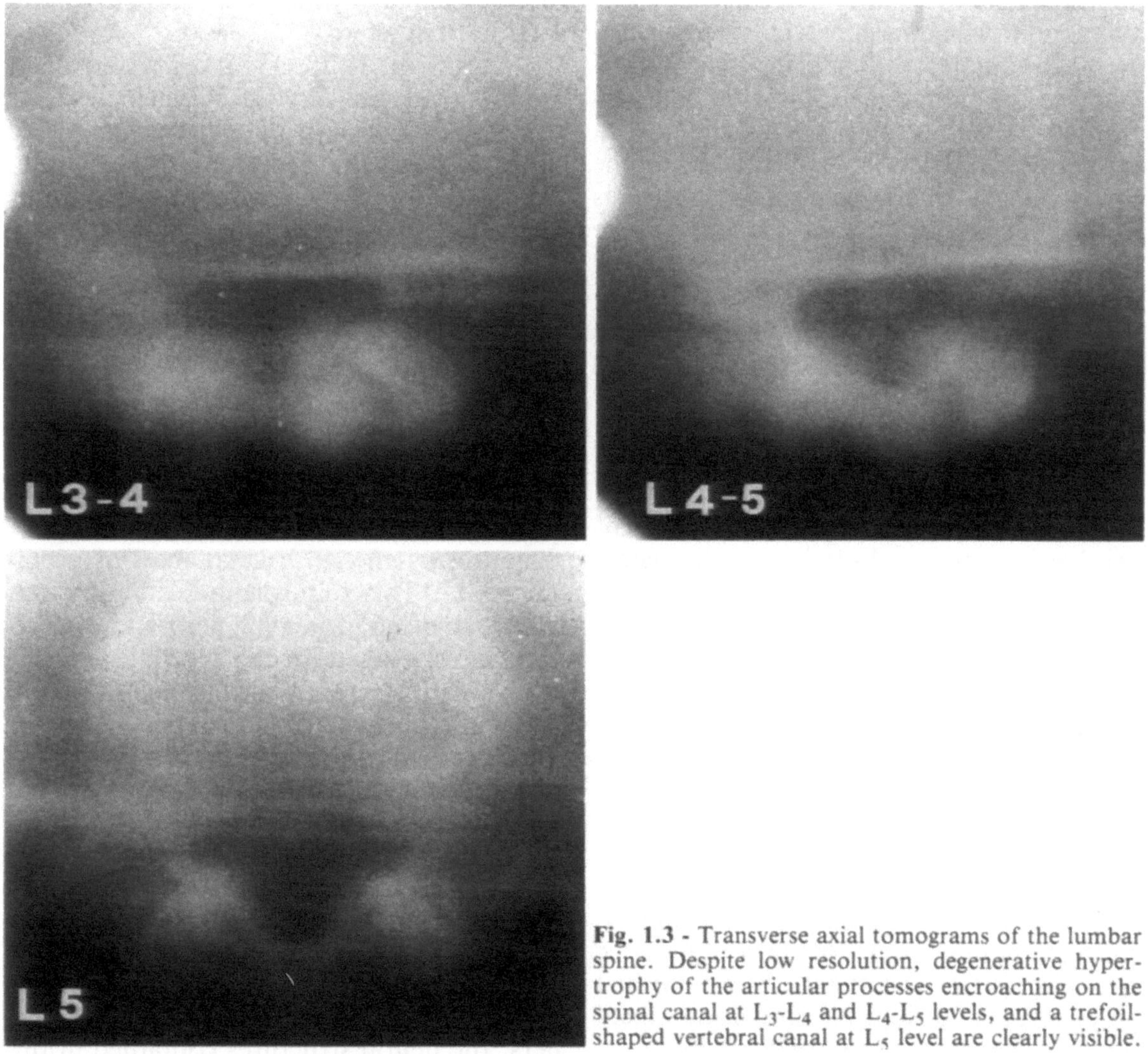

Fig. 1.3 - Transverse axial tomograms of the lumbar spine. Despite low resolution, degenerative hypertrophy of the articular processes encroaching on the spinal canal at L_3-L_4 and L_4-L_5 levels, and a trefoil-shaped vertebral canal at L_5 level are clearly visible.

that at least some of Sarpyener's patients were suffering from disorders not classifiable as forms of spinal stenosis.

During the same period Van Gelderen (1948) reported the cases of two elderly patients who had presented with paraesthesiae and weakness in the lower limbs after standing or walking for a few minutes and in whom the symptoms rapidly improved with sitting.

Both cases had normal peripheral pulses in the lower limbs, whilst the knee and ankle reflexes were absent. One of the two could ride a bicycle for a long distance with his hands holding the handle bars, but was unable to extend his lumbar spine without feeling immediate weakness and paraesthesiae in both legs. At operation the author found a marked thickening of the ligamenta flava at L_3-L_4 level and interpreted this «standing syndrome» of the cauda equina as a consequence of compression of the neural elements exerted, in the standing position, by hypertrophic ligamenta flava or a bulging disc. With this first precise description of the typical stenotic syndrome, the history of spinal stenosis moved forward into the present area.

In 1950 MacNab reported on a series of 22 patients showing spondylolisthesis with an intact neural arch, a condition — already described by Junghanns (1930) in cadavers and called «pseudospondylolisthesis» —

which is presently referred to as degenerative spondylolisthesis. Reports of single cases of this condition had been previously published by other authors, the first being Lane in 1893 who, in the preradiographic era, had performed a laminectomy on a patient with progressive weakness and paraesthesiae of the lower limbs; at operation a spondylolisthesis of the fifth lumbar vertebra was found in the presence of an intact neural arch. MacNab, on the basis of his large series of cases, described the various types of clinical presentation of degenerative spondylolisthesis, focusing attention on the importance of the osteoarthritic changes of the facet joints in the genesis of olisthesis as well as compression of the caudal nerve roots.

With Verbiest (1954, 1955), lumbar stenosis has become a well-defined pathological entity. He introduced the concept of developmental stenosis, caused by an abnormally short midsagittal diameter of the spinal canal, resulting from a disturbance of vertebral growth of unknown aetiology. To measure the size of the spinal canal, Verbiest designed a special instrument, the stenosimeter, with which he could record the sagittal dimensions of the spinal canal at each vertebral level explored during surgery (Fig. 1.2). On the basis of these measurements, collected in many years of surgical practice on a large series of patients, he established his concepts of absolute, relative and mixed stenosis (Verbiest, 1973; 1975; 1976).

In 1962 Epstein *et al.* reported on a large series of patients with lumbar spinal stenosis, drawing attention to the narrowing of the lateral recess as a cause of nerve root compression. Ten years later the same authors (Epstein *et al.*, 1972) defined the concept of narrowing of the nerve root canal, emphasizing that it can represent an isolated feature in a spinal canal with a normally sized midsagittal diameter.

During the 1970's a marked difference in opinion emerged between Verbiest, with his concept of developmental pathogenesis of stenosis, and the vast majority of other authors, mostly American, who identified the most frequent cause of narrowing of the lumbar spinal canal in degenerative changes of the vertebrae and intervertebral discs (Ehni 1965; Kirkaldy-Willis *et al.*, 1974; Arnoldi *et al.*, 1976).

Transverse axial tomography, allowing the vertebral canal to be visualized in transverse section, contributed significantly to the knowledge of these «degenerative» forms of lumbar spinal stenosis (Gargano *et al.*, 1974, Jacobson *et al.*, 1975; Urso and Postacchini, 1978). This tomographic examination, although often producing poor and distorted images, offered for the first time a means of evaluating directly the size of the spinal canal and particularly of assessing its alterations caused by the degenerative changes of the facet joints (Fig. 1.3). Transverse axial tomography, however, was rapidly made obsolete by computerized tomography (Sheldon *et al.*, 1977, Glenn *et al.*, 1979; Postacchini *et al.*, 1980). The latter, in fact, not only proved able to give more precise and detailed transaxial images of the vertebral canal, but also to visualize, with high resolution scanners, the neural structures contained in the canal. With the advent of computerized tomography, a decisive step forward was made in the morphological definition of vertebral structures, leading to a more precise identification of the pathological characteristics of the various forms of lumbar stenosis.

REFERENCES

ARNOLDI C.C., BRODSKY A.E., CAUCHOIX J., CROCK H.V., DOMMISSE G.A. et al.: Lumbar spinal stenosis and nerve root entrapment syndromes. Definition and classification. *Clin. Orthop.* **115**: 4, 1976.

BAILEY P., CASAMAJOR L.: Osteo-arthritis of the spine as a cause of compression of the spinal cord and its roots. With a report of five cases. *J. Nerve Ment. Dis.* **38**: 588, 1911.

CRAMER F.: A note concerning the syndrome of cauda equina radiculitis. *Bull. Neurol. Inst. N.Y.* **3**: 501, 1943.

EHNI G.: Spondylotic cauda equina radiculopathy. *Texas Med. J.* **61**: 746, 1965.

EPSTEIN J.A., EPSTEIN B.S., LEVINE L.: Nerve root compression associated with narrowing of the lumbar spinal canal. *J. Neurol. Neurosurg. Psych.* **25**: 165, 1962.

EPSTEIN J.A., EPSTEIN B.S., ROSENTHAL R.C., LEVINE S.L.: Sciatica caused by nerve root entrapment in the lateral recess: the superior facet syndrome. *J. Neurosurg.* **36**: 584, 1972.

GARGANO F.P., JACOBSON R.E., ROSOMOFF H.L.: Transverse axial tomography of the spine. *Neuroradiology* **6**: 254, 1974.

GLENN W.V. Jr., RHODES M.L., ALTSCHULER E.M., WILTSE L.L., KOSTANEK C., MING KUO Y.: Multiplanar display computerized body tomography applications in the lumbar spine. *Spine* **4**: 282, 1979.

JACOBSON R.E., GARGANO F.P., ROSOMOFF H.L.: Transverse axial tomography of the spine. Part 2: The stenotic spinal canal. *J. Neurosurg.* **42**: 412, 1975.

JUNGHANNS H.: Spondylolisthesis ohne Spalt im Zwischengelenkstück. *Arch. Orthop. Unfallchir.* München **29**: 118, 1930.

KIRKALDY-WILLIS W.H., PAINE K.W.E., CAUCHOIX J., MCIVOR G.: Lumbar spinal stenosis. *Clin. Orthop.* **99**: 30, 1974.

LANE W.A.: Spondylolisthesis associated with progressive paraplegia: laminectomy. *Lancet* **1**: 991, 1893.

MCNAB I.: Spondylolisthesis with an intact neural arch - The so-called pseudo-spondylolisthesis. *J. Bone and Joint Surg.* **32-B**: 325,1950.

OLLIVIER C.P.: De la moelle épinière et de ses maladies. *Arch. Gén. Méd* (Paris) **4**: 153, 1824.

PARKER J.L. and ADSON A.W.: Compression of the spinal cord and its roots and hypertrophic osteoarthritis. *Surg. Gynecol. Obstet.* **41**: 1, 1925.

PORTAL A.: *Cours d'Anatomie Médicale ou Eléments de l'Anatomie de l'homme*, vol. 1, Paris, Baudovin, 299, 1983.

POSTACCHINI F., PEZZERI G., MONTANARO A., NATALI G.: Computerized tomography in lumbar stenosis. A preliminary report. *J. Bone and Joint Surg.* **62-B**: 78, 1980.

PUTTI V.: New conceptions in the pathogenesis of sciatic pain. *Lancet* **2**: 53, 1927.

SACHS B., FRAENKEL J.: Progressive ankylotic rigidity of the spine (spondylose rhizomelique). *J. Nerve Ment. Dis.* **27**: 1, 1900.

SARPYENER M.A.: Congenital stricture of the spinal canal. *J. Bone and Joint Surg.* **27**: 70, 1945.

SARPYENER M.A.: Spina bifida aperta and congenital stricture of the spinal canal. *J. Bone and Joint Surg.* **29**: 817, 1947.

SHELDON J.J., SERSLAND J., LEBORGNE J.: Computed tomography of the lower lumbar vertebral column: normal anatomy and the stenotic canal. *Radiology* **124**: 113, 1977.

SPURLING R.G., MAYFIELD F.H., ROGERS J.B.: Hypertrophy of the ligamenta flava as a cause of low-back pain. *J. Am. Med. Ass.* **109**: 928, 1937.

SUMITA M.: Beiträge zur Lehre von der Chondrodystrophia foetalis (Kaufmann) und Osteogenesis imperfecta (Vrolik) mit besonderer Berücksichtigung der anatomischen und klinischen Differential Diagnoses. *Dtsch. Z. Chir.* **107**: 1, 1910.

TOWNE E.B., REICHTER F.C.: Compression of the lumbosacral roots of the spinal cord by thickened ligamenta flava. *Ann. Surg.* **94**: 527, 1931.

URSO S., POSTACCHINI F.: The value of transverse axial stratigraphy in the diagnosis of lumbar stenosis. *Italian Journal* of *Orthopaedics and Traumatology* **4**: 213, 1978.

VAN GELDEREN CHR.: Ein Orthotisches (lordotisches) Kondasyndrom. *Acta Psychiat.* (Kbh) **23**: 57, 1948.

VERBIEST H.: A radicular syndrome from developmental narrowing of the lumbar vertebral canal. *J. Bone and Joint Surg.* **36-A**: 230, 1954.

VERBIEST H.: Further experiences on the pathological influence of a developmental narrowness of the bony lumbar vertebral canal. *J. Bone and Joint Surg.* **37-B**: 576, 1955.

VERBIEST H.: Neurogenic intermittent claudication in cases with absolute and relative stenosis of the lumbar vertebral canal (ASLC and RSLC), in cases with narrow lumbar intervertebral foramina, and in cases with both entities. *Clin. Neurosurg.* **20**: 204, 1973.

VERBIEST H.: Pathomorphologic aspects of developmental lumbar stenosis. *Orthop. Clin. North Am.* **6**: 177, 1975.

VERBIEST H.: *Neurogenic intermittent claudication.* Amsterdam, North Holland Publishing Co., New York, American Elsevier, 1976.

Chapter II

Anatomy of the vertebral canal and the neural structures in the lumbar spine

F. Postacchini, W. Rauschning

VERTEBRAL FORAMEN

MORPHOLOGY

The vertebral foramen is the hole, in the isolated vertebra, bounded by the vertebral body and the posterior arch. The walls of the foramen are formed anteriorly by the posterior aspect of the vertebral body, laterally by the pedicles, and posteriorly by the apophyseal joints, the partes interarticulares, the laminae and the base of the spinous process.

The posterior aspect of the vertebral body is concave in the sagittal plane. The concavity is less marked in the midsagittal plane than in the lateral sagittal planes, i.e. near the pedicular attachments. The concavity in the sagittal plane increases progressively from L_1 to L_4 and then decreases at L_5, whereas that in the lateral sagittal planes shows a progressive increment from L_1 to L_5 (Larsen, 1985a). Evaluated in the axial plane, the posterior aspect of the vertebral body is concave at L_1 to L_3, approximately flat at L_4 and generally convex at L_5 (Larsen, 1985b).

The pedicles originate from the vertebral body adjacent to the superior end-plate. The superior vertebral notch, therefore, is significantly less deep than the inferior (Fig. 2.1). The height (vertical diameter) and the length (sagittal diameter) of the pedicles vary considerably from individual to individual. Usually the length decreases in a craniocaudal direction and is shortest at L_5.

The articular processes are obliquely orientated in relation to the sagittal axis of the vertebra. The angle formed by their anteroposterior axis with the midsagittal axis of the vertebral body varies considerably in different subjects, at different levels in the same subject and, occasionally, on the two sides of the same vertebra (Fig. 2.2). The angle formed by a tangent line to the anterior and posterior margins of the superior articular process on one side, with the same line on the opposite side, is on average 74° at L_3, 96° at L_4, and 106° at L_5 (Van Schaik *et al.*, 1985). The superior articular process contributes to delimit, with its anteromedial

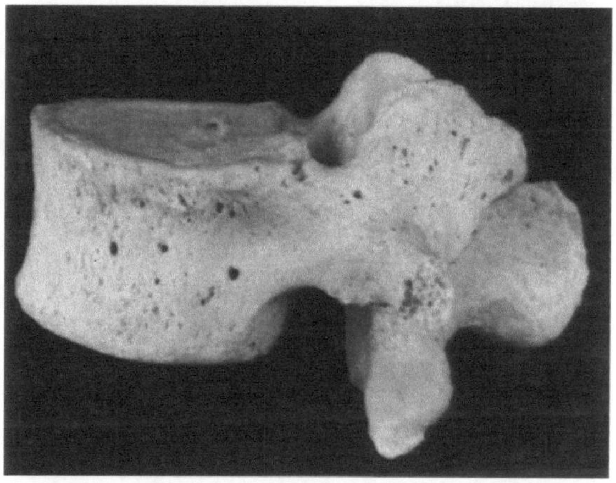

Fig. 2.1 - The superior and inferior border of the pedicle form the two vertebral notches, the inferior of which is considerably deeper than the superior.

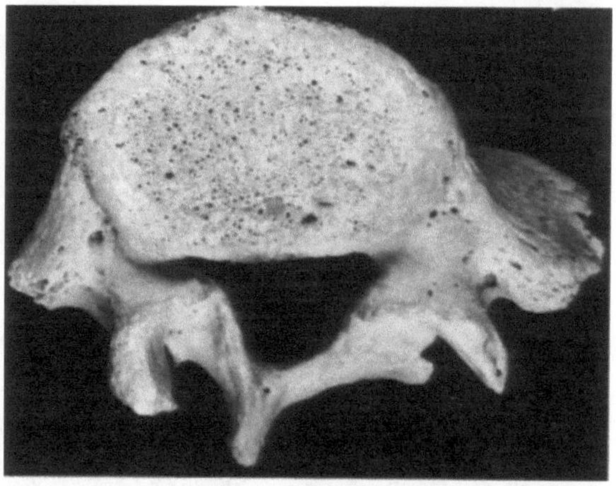

Fig. 2.2 - Asymmetric orientation of the articular processes on the two sides and different orientation and length of the laminae.

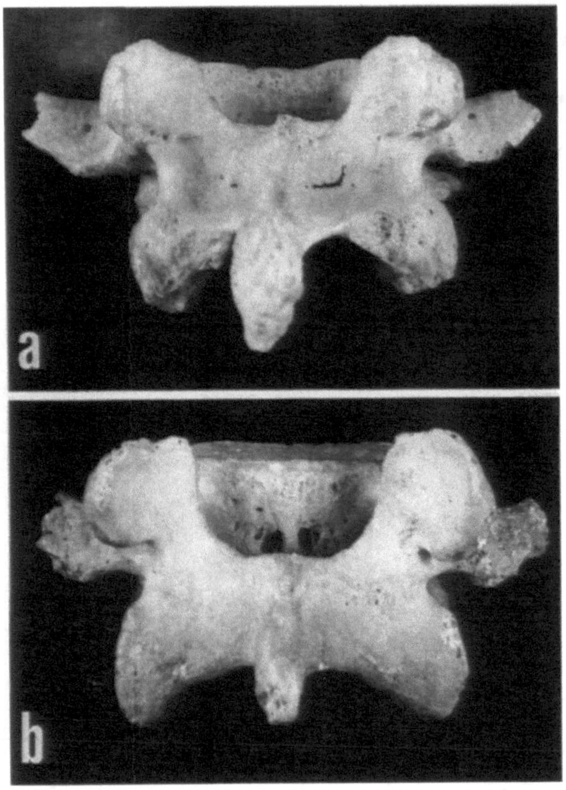

Fig. 2.3 - Different location of the laminae with respect to the vertebral body in two L_4 vertebrae. **a.** The laminae are entirely comprised within the limits of the body. **b.** The upper border of the laminae is located at the level of the middle portion of the vertebral body. In these cases, the inferior margin of the laminar arch is located caudally to the inferior vertebral end-plate.

border, the lateral portion of the vertebral foramen, and the inferior articular process, the inferolateral part of the foramen.

The laminae can be contained for the whole of their height within the limits of the posterior aspect of the vertebral body, or can extend distally to the inferior end-plate (Fig. 2.3). The anteroposterior axis of the laminae shows, with respect to the coronal plane, a highly variable degree of obliquity in both different lumbar vertebrae and omologous vertebrae of different individuals (Fig. 2.4). Sometimes the laminae of the same vertebra can have different orientations (Fig. 2.2). The angle formed by the anteroposterior axis of the two laminae is, on average, 91° at L_3, 99° at L_4 and 106° at L_5 (Van Schaik *et al.*, 1985). The vertical axis may lie on the coronal plane or, more often, particularly in the two lower lumbar vertebrae, can be directed obliquely downwards and backwards. In the latter case the distal half of the vertebral foramen is usually wider, in the sagittal plane, than the proximal half. On the

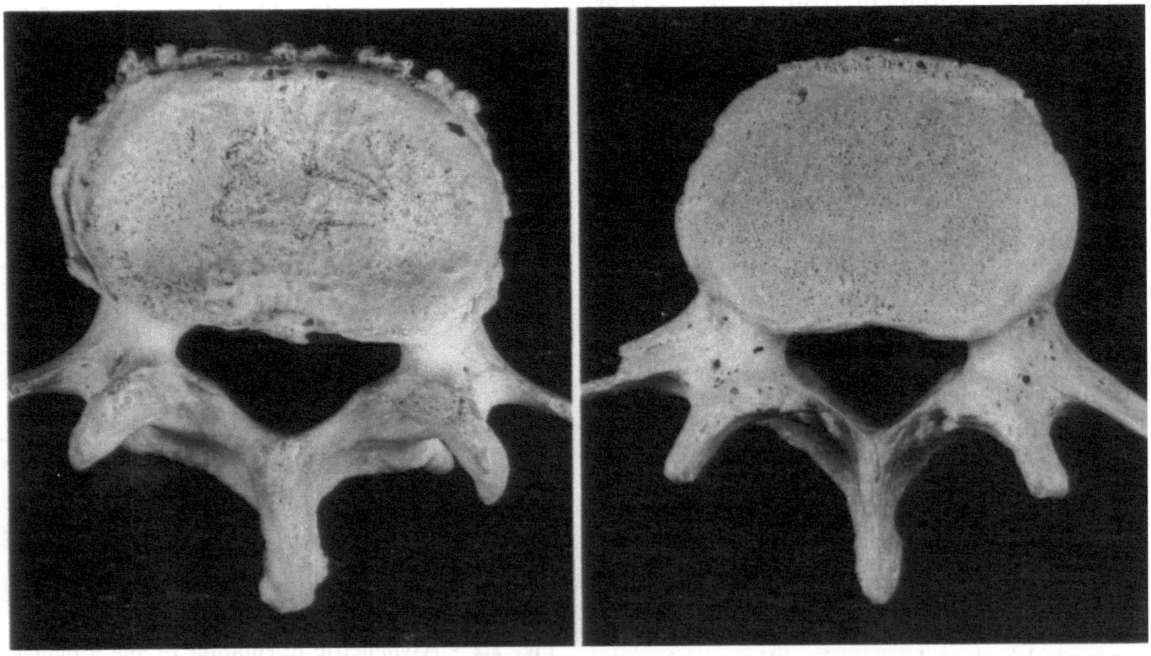

Fig. 2.4 - Different orientation of the laminae in two L_4 vertebrae.

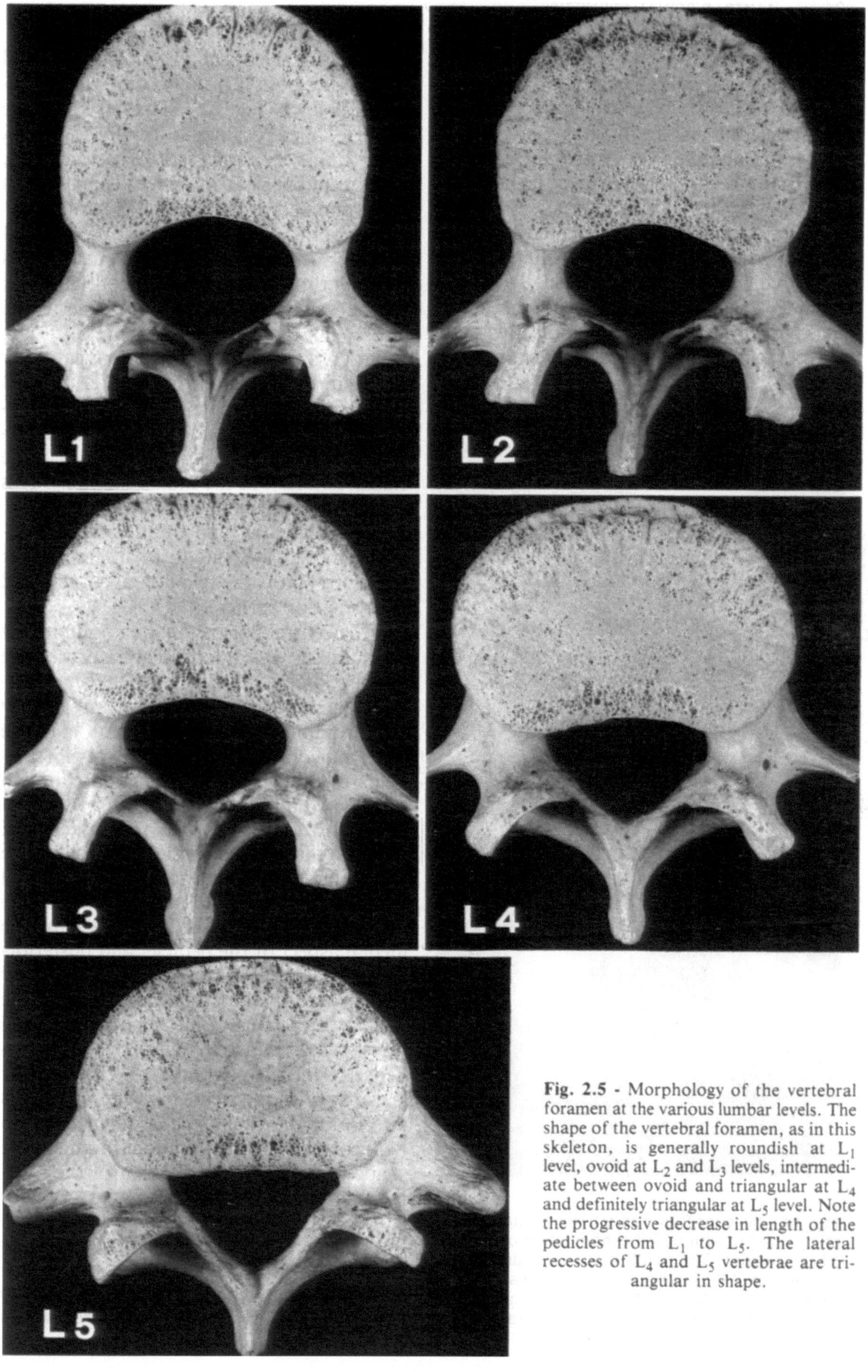

Fig. 2.5 - Morphology of the vertebral foramen at the various lumbar levels. The shape of the vertebral foramen, as in this skeleton, is generally roundish at L_1 level, ovoid at L_2 and L_3 levels, intermediate between ovoid and triangular at L_4 and definitely triangular at L_5 level. Note the progressive decrease in length of the pedicles from L_1 to L_5. The lateral recesses of L_4 and L_5 vertebrae are triangular in shape.

anterior surface of the lamina a crest is present, dividing this surface into a superior smooth portion, which is in contact with the dural sac, and an inferior rough part, generally more oblique in a ventro-dorsal direction than the former, on which the ligamentum flavum has its insertion.

The vertebral foramen can be round, ovoidal, triangular or trefoil-shaped. The first two lumbar vertebrae usually have a round or ovoidal foramen with the major axis lying transversally, whilst the lower two vertebrae more often have a triangular foramen. The shape of the foramen of the third lumbar vertebra is usually somewhat in between the two (Fig. 2.5). The relatively rare trefoil-shaped foramen is usually seen at L_5 (Fig. 2.6); very rarely is it observed at L_4, and exceptionally at L_3. Eisenstein (1980), in a morphometric study on 2,373 lumbar vertebrae of 485 South African skeletons (113 white Caucasian, 204 black Zulu, and 168 black Sotho), found a trefoil configuration of the vertebral foramen in 74 vertebrae (7.1%). Of these vertebrae, 68 were L_5, five L_4 and only one L_3. In an anatomical study of the lumbar vertebrae of 121 skeletons (63 Italians, and 58 Indians from India) Postacchini *et al.* (1983) found a trefoil configuration of the vertebral foramen in 16% of the Italian and 12% of the Indian skeletons. This shape was noticed almost always at L_5.

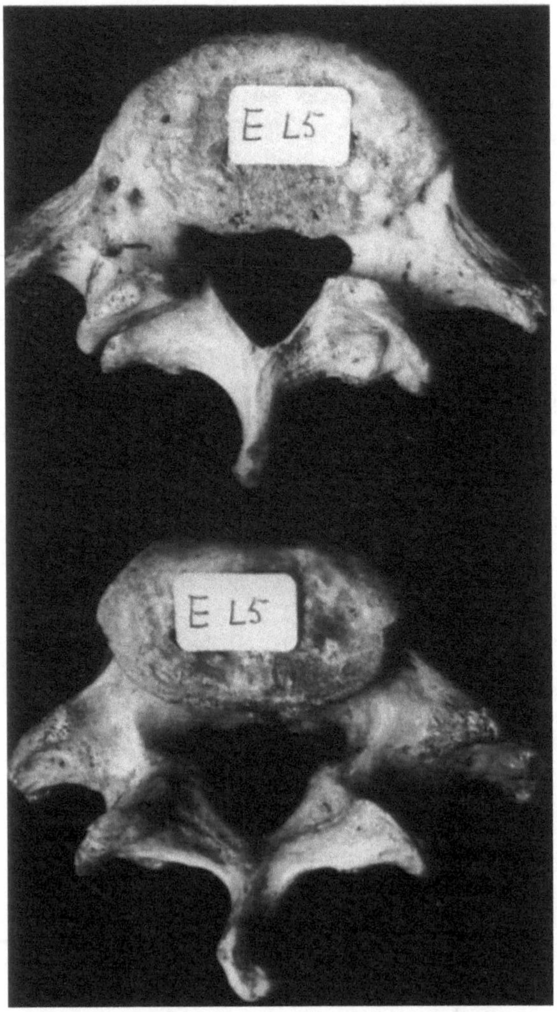

Fig. 2.6 - Superior (top) and inferior (bottom) views of L_5 vertebra with trefoil configuration of the vertebral foramen. The trefoil shape is produced by a prominence of the superior articular processes and the partes interarticulares in the vertebral foramen. The dome-like lateral corners represent the lateral recesses.

The triangular and trefoil-shaped foramen can be divided into three different parts: the central part, the two lateral corners and the posterior corner.

The central part is the area occupied by the dural sac. It is bounded anteriorly by the vertebral body, laterally by the medial margin of the superior articular processes (if they are prominent in the foramen) and the posteromedial aspect of the partes interarticulares, and posteriorly by the anterior two thirds of the laminae.

The two lateral corners form the lateral recesses, through which the nerve roots have their course before entering the intervertebral foramen. These corners are bounded anteriorly by the vertebral body, laterally by the medial aspect of the pedicle, and posteriorly by the base of the superior articular process and the anterolateral aspect of the pars interarticularis. The shape of the lateral recess is determined by the degree of prominence of the medial border of the superior articular process and the pars interarticularis into the spinal canal. If these structures do not protrude into the vertebral foramen, the shape of the recesses, like that of the foramen, is approximately triangular, while a marked protrusion of these structures into the foramen creates a dome-like configuration of the recesses and a trefoil-shaped vertebral foramen (Figs. 2.5 and 2.6). The posterior corner (or posterior recess) is

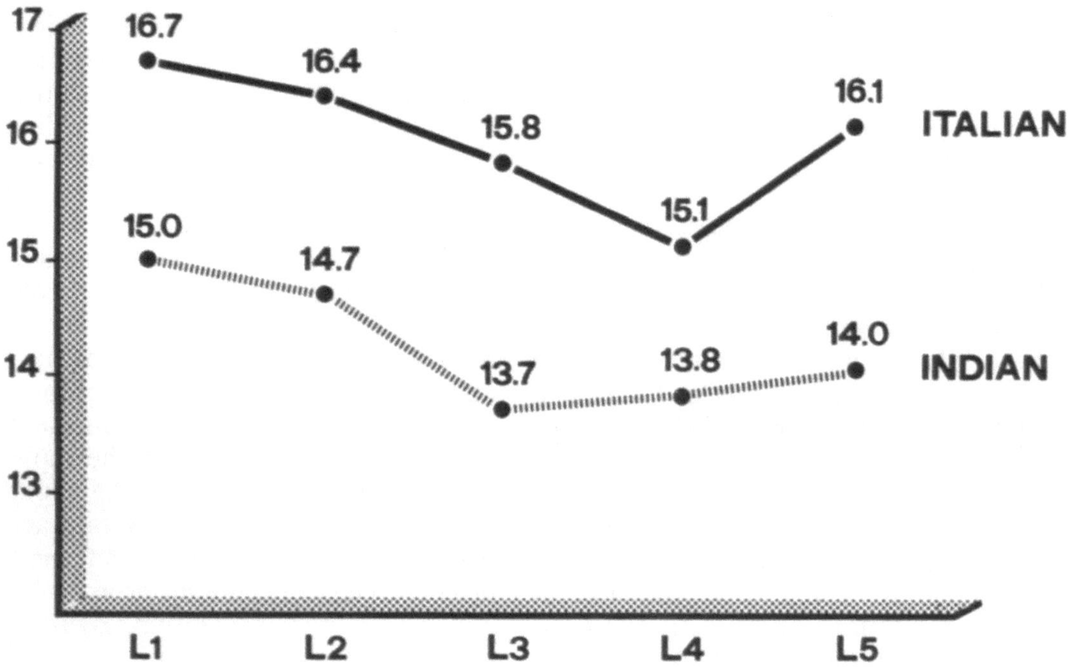

Fig. 2.7 - Mean values of the cranial midsagittal diameter of the vertebral foramen at the various lumbar levels in 63 Italian, and 58 Indian, skeletons.

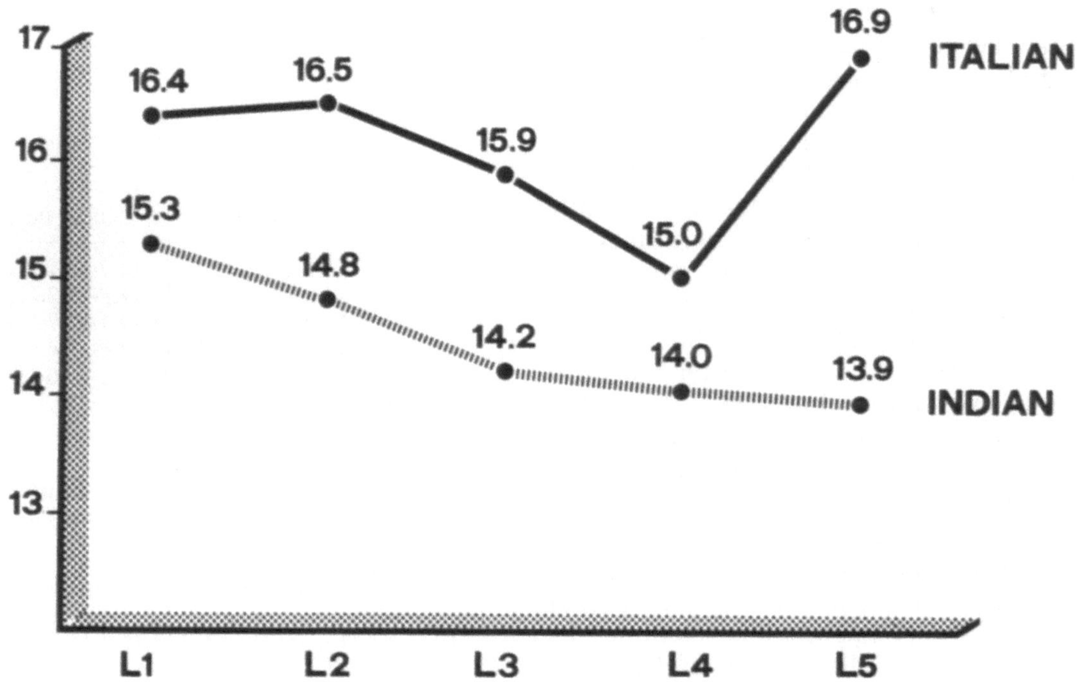

Fig. 2.8 - Mean values of the caudal midsagittal diameter of the vertebral foramen at the various lumbar levels in 63 Italian, and 58 Indian, skeletons.

bounded by the posterior aspect of the laminae and the base of the spinous process, and is occupied *in vivo* by epidural fat.

DIMENSIONS

Huizinga *et al.*, in 1952, measured the midsagittal diameter of the vertebral foramen in 47 Dutch skeletons and obtained the following minimum and maximum values: 14 and 22 mm at L_1, 13 and 20 mm at L_2, 12 and 27 mm at L_3, 11 and 22 mm at L_4, 12 and 22 mm at L_5. In this series of skeletons the shortest interpedicular diameter was 19 mm at L_1 and L_4, and 20 mm at L_1, L_3 and L_5.

Epstein *et al.* (1962), in measurements carried out on the lumbar vertebrae of fifty adult skeletons, found that the anteroposterior dimensions of the vertebral foramen varied within a range of 15 to 23 mm.

More recently Eisenstein (1977) measured the anteroposterior and transverse dimensions of the vertebral foramen and the vertebral body in 443 adult skeletons of both sexes. Amongst these skeletons, 113 belonged to Caucasian subjects and 330 to black South Africans, half of whom were from Zulu and half from Sotho ethnic group. In the Caucasian skeletons the average value of the midsagittal diameter, measured near the superior margin of the posterior arch, was 17 mm, and the limits of normal (mean value ∓ standard deviation) were 13 and 21 mm in females and 14 to 20 mm in males. In the Zulu and Sotho skeletons the limits of normal, depending on sex, were 12 or 13 mm and 19 or 20 mm, respectively. The mean value of the midsagittal diameter of the vertebral foramen in the total population examined was 16 mm and the lower limit of normal (mean value minus standard deviation) was 13 mm. The lowest mean values were generally found at L_3 and L_4, and the highest at L_1 and L_5. Of the vertebrae examined, 1.3% had a midsagittal diameter below the lower limit of normal. However, none of these vertebrae, classified as «stenotic» by the author, had dimensions of less than 11 mm. The mean interpedicular distance in the whole population was 23 mm and the lower limit of normal was 18 mm. Based on the interpedicular distance, 0.8% of vertebrae were «stenotic», but none had a value of less than 16 mm. In total, 6.3% of the skeletons examined had at least one vertebra with the midsagittal and/or interpedicular diameter shorter than the lower limit of normal and approximately half of them had two or more «stenotic» vertebrae.

Postacchini *et al.* (1983) examined the lumbar vertebrae of 121 adult skeletons, (63 Italians and 58 Indians). In each vertebra both the cranial and caudal midsagittal diameter of the vertebral foramen was measured. The cranial diameter was measured between the vertebral body and the upper border of the posterior arch. The caudal diameter was taken as the shortest distance between the vertebral body and the bony prominence in the anterior aspect of the laminae where the ligamentum flavum has its insertion. When this prominence was located at a lower level than the vertebral body, the caudal diameter was measured opposite the lower end-plate of the vertebral body. For both ethnic groups the highest mean values of the cranial midsagittal diameter of the vertebral foramen were at L_1 and L_2 and the lowest at L_3 and L_4 (Fig. 2.7). The highest mean value of the caudal midsagittal di-

Table 2.I

LOWEST AND HIGHEST VALUES, AND STANDARD DEVIATIONS (IN BRACKETS) OF THE SPINAL MIDSAGITTAL DIAMETER IN ITALIAN SKELETONS

	Cranial (mm)	Caudal (mm)
L1	15.2-18.2 (1.5)	14.7-18.1 (1.7)
L2	14.7-18.1 (1.7)	14.8-18.2 (1.7)
L3	14.0-17.6 (1.8)	14.1-17.7 (1.8)
L4	12.6-17.6 (2.5)	12.6-17.4 (2.4)
L5	13.6-18.6 (2.5)	13.8-20.0 (3.1)

Table 2.II

LOWEST AND HIGHEST VALUES, AND STANDARD DEVIATIONS (IN BRACKETS) OF THE SPINAL MIDSAGITTAL DIAMETER IN INDIAN SKELETONS

	Cranial (mm)	Caudal (mm)
L1	13.7-16.3 (1.3)	13.8-16.8 (1.5)
L2	13.3-16.1 (1.4)	13.1-16.5 (1.7)
L3	12.5-14.9 (1.2)	12.4-15.8 (1.7)
L4	12.2-15.4 (1.6)	12.2-15.8 (1.8)
L5	11.9-16.1 (2.1)	11.5-16.3 (2.4)

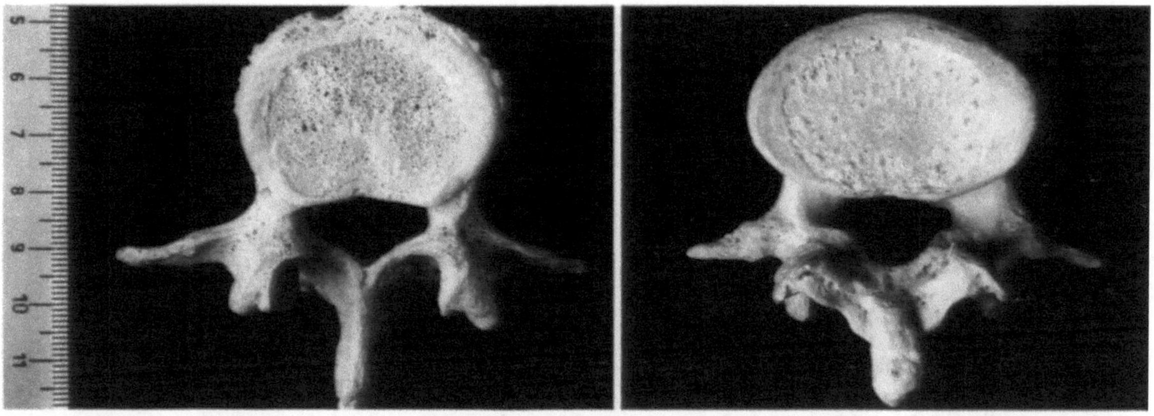

Fig. 2.9 - Superior (left) and inferior (right) views of L_4 vertebra of an Italian skeleton. The cranial midsagittal diameter of the vertebral foramen measured 10.8 mm and the caudal 11.2 mm.

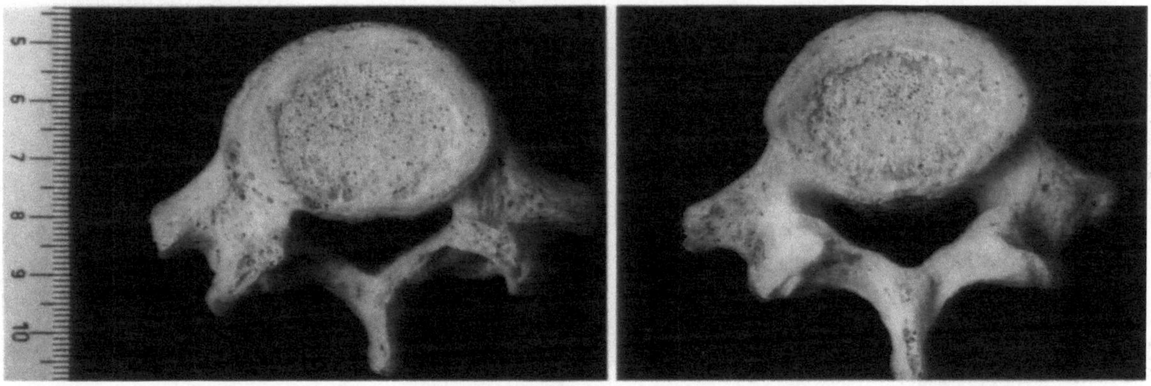

Fig. 2.10 - Superior (left) and inferior (right) views of L_5 vertebra of an Italian skeleton. The cranial and caudal midsagittal diameters of the vertebral foramen measured, 10.1 mm and 10.6 mm, respectively.

ameter was at L_1 in both ethnic groups, while the lowest mean value was at L_4 in the Italian population and at L_5 in the Indian (Fig. 2.8). The mean values of both sagittal diameters (cranial and caudal) were significantly higher in the Italian spines (Figs. 2.7 and 2.8). In both groups the highest standard deviations were found at L_4 and L_5 (Tables 2.I and 2.II), and, as a whole, the standard deviations were higher in the Italian series (Tables 2.I and 2.II). The lower limit of normal (mean value minus standard deviation) was 12.6 mm at L_4 in the Italian skeletons and 11.5 mm at L_5 in the Indian (Tables 2.I and 2.II). In the Italian series three spines (5%) had one or more vertebrae with cranial and/or caudal midsagittal diameters of less than 11 mm (from 10.1 to 10.8 mm) (Figs. 2.9 and 2.10). In the Indian series six spines (10%) had one or more vertebrae with anteroposterior dimensions of the vertebral foramen between 9 mm and 10.5 mm (Figs. 2.11, 2.12 and 2.13). Furthermore, in another spine from the Indian series the foramen of L_4 had a cranial sagittal diameter of 10.8 mm. Of the 10 skeletons (in the two ethnic groups) with dimensions of less than 11 mm at one or more levels, seven had at least one other vertebra with anteroposterior dimensions below the lower limit of normal. All vertebrae with sagittal dimensions of less than 11 mm were L_4 or L_5.

In the vertebrae with midsagittal dimensions below the lower limit of normal, the small size of the vertebral foramen was due to one or more of the following factors: short

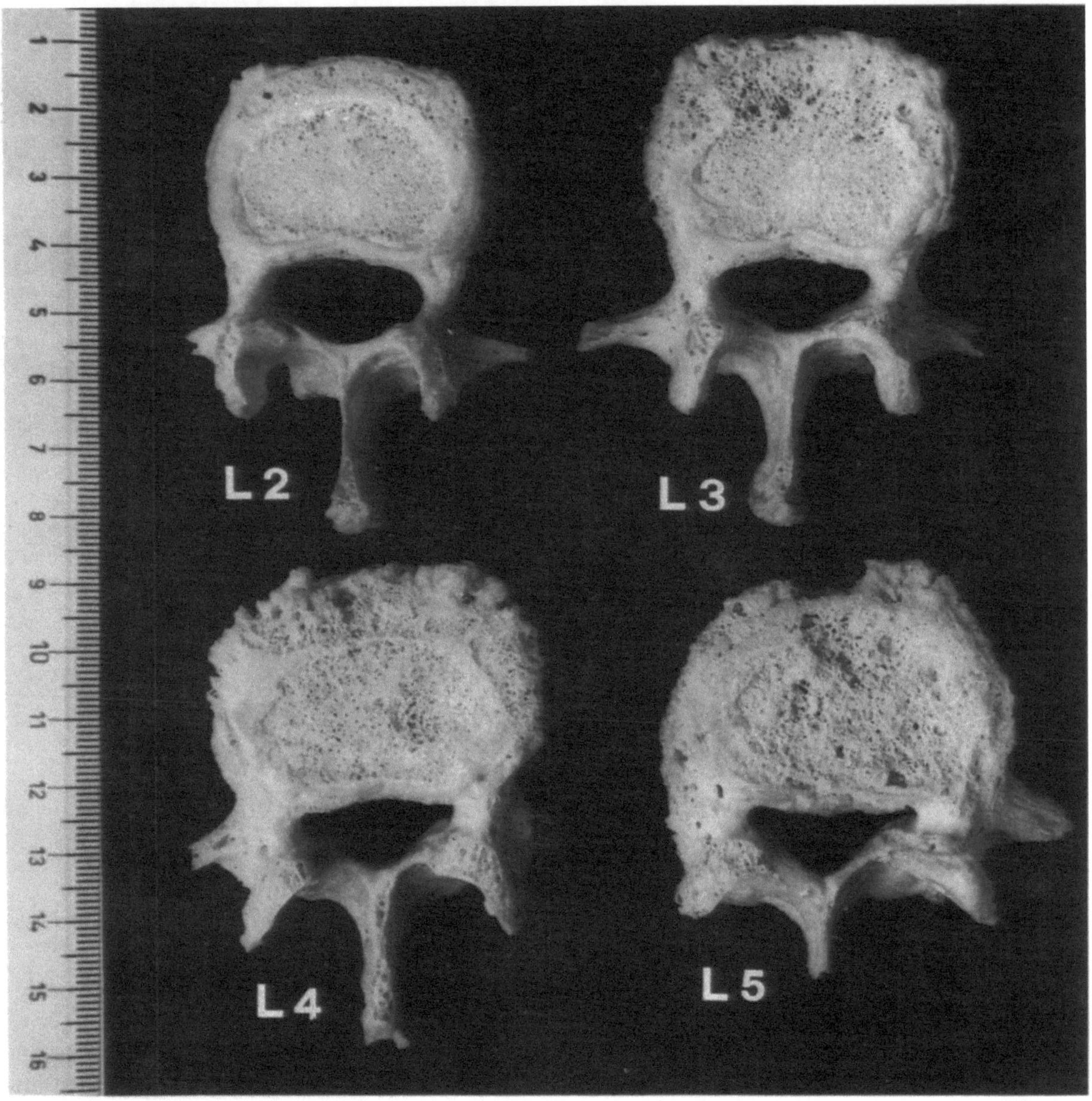

Fig. 2.11 - Lower four lumbar vertebrae of an Indian skeleton. The midsagittal diameter of the vertebral canal ranged from 10.5 mm at L_2 to 9.5 mm at L_5.

Table 2.III
VALUES OF THE INTERPEDICULAR DIAMETER OF THE VERTEBRAL CANAL

	Italian skeletons (mm)*	Indian skeletons (mm)*
L1	21.7±1.5	19.1±1.7
L2	22.2±2.1	19.5±1.8
L3	22.7±2.0	19.9±2.1
L4	25.9±2.4	21.2±2.6
L5	24.8±2.7	22.8±2.6

* mean value ± standard deviation.

pedicles, short laminae, more frontal orientation of the laminae. In some of the vertebrae with «narrow» vertebral foramen, the vertebral body showed marginal posterior osteophytes but in no cases did the osteophytes contribute to significantly reduce the size of the vertebral foramen.

The lowest mean values of the interpedicular diameter were at L_1 and highest at L_4 (Italian spines) or at L_5 (Indian spines) (Table 2.III). The average values of the interpedi-

Table 2.IV
DIMENSIONS OF THE VERTEBRAL BODY

	Italian skeletons			Indian skeletons		
	SD	TD	H	SD	TD	H
L1	29±3	41±4	26±2	25±2	36±3	21±2
L2	31±3	43±5	27±5	27±2	37±3	22±2
L3	30±3	44±4	28±3	28±2	40±3	23±1
L4	32±3	47±4	28±3	29±2	41±4	23±2
L5	33±3	49±4	30±4	29±2	43±4	24±1

* mean value ± standard deviation.
SD = Sagittal Diameter; TD = Transverse Diameter; H = Height.

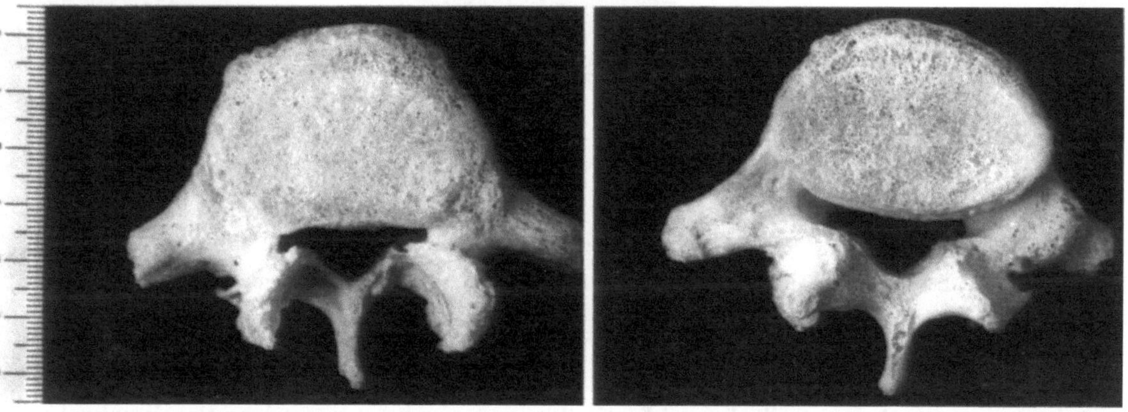

Fig. 2.12 - Superior (left) and inferior (right) views of L_5 vertebra of an Indian skeleton. The cranial and caudal midsagittal diameters of the vertebral foramen were 9 mm and 9.5 mm, respectively.

cular diameter, as for the midsagittal diameter, were significantly higher in the Italian, as compared with the Indian, spines at all lumbar levels. In the Italian series the interpedicular distance was never below 19 mm, whilst in 35% of the Indian vertebrae the interpedicular distance was 17 mm or less. The thickness of the laminae varied from 4.7 to 6.6 mm in the vast majority of the vertebrae examined, including those in which the sagittal diameter was below 11 mm.

The dimensions of the vertebral body increased regularly from L_1 to L_5 in the Indian spines and irregularly in the Italian spines (Table 2.IV). In the latter, the mean values and standard deviations were greater than in the Indian spines at all lumbar levels.

WIDTH OF THE LATERAL RECESSES

The width of the lateral recesses, measured as the sagittal distance between the edge of the superior end-plate (or the vertebral body) and the medial tip of the superior articular process, varies significantly between different individuals of similar ethnic groups as well as between individuals of different races. Normally it ranges from 5 mm to 9 mm at L_4 level and 4.5 mm to 8 mm at L_5 level.

The dimensions of the lateral recesses are mainly related to two factors: the length of the pedicles and the shape of the vertebral foramen. A marked shortening of the pedicles or a trefoil configuration of the vertebral foramen, as isolated conditions, have little or no influence on the dimensions of the lateral recesses. Their association, however, may cause a marked narrowing of the recesses, which may be further narrowed by osteophytes from the superior articular process or the posterior border of the vertebral body (Figs. 2.14 and 2.15). The two lateral recesses

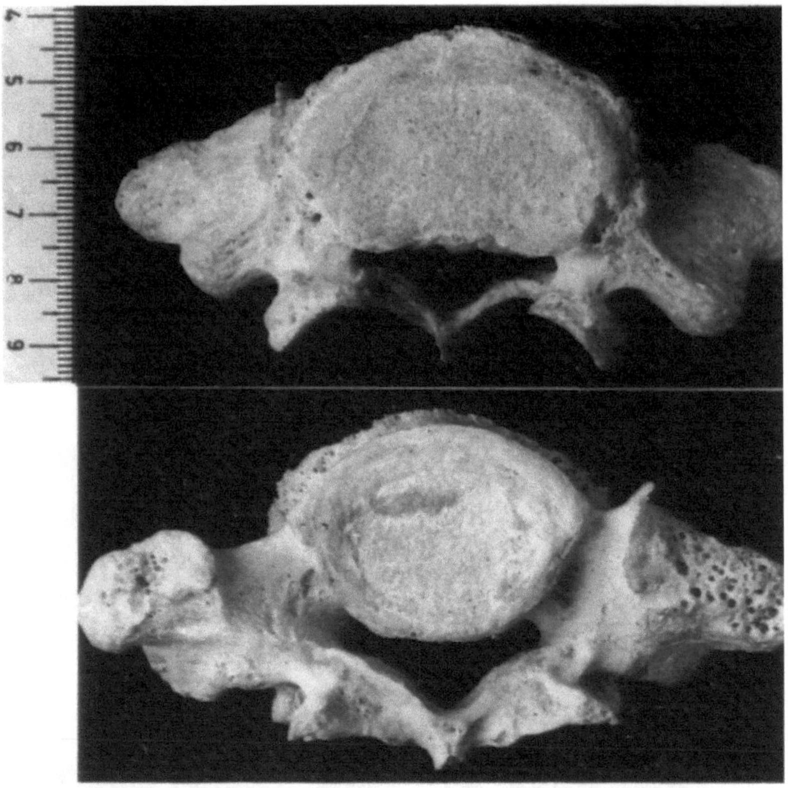

Fig. 2.13 - Superior (top) and inferior (bottom) views of L_5 vertebra of an Indian skeleton. The caudal midsagittal diameter of this vertebra, showing bilateral sacro-transverse articulation, was 9.1 mm. The cranial diameter measured 10.6 mm.

of the same vertebra usually have identical shapes and dimensions. Asymmetry can be due to different lengths of the pedicles or a different degree of prominence of the superior articular process into the vertebral canal. Lateral recess asymmetry can also be due to different size or location of osteophytes on the two sides.

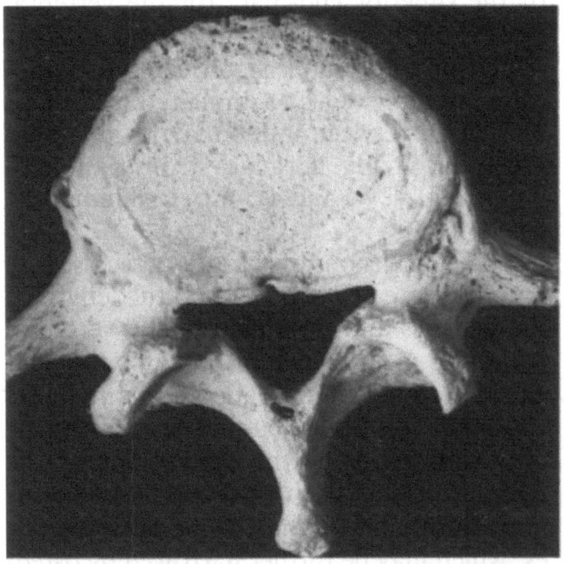

Fig. 2.14 - L_5 vertebra of an Indian skeleton with a trefoil shaped vertebral foramen and narrow lateral recesses in the absence of spondylotic changes.

The width of the recesses is related, although not strictly, to the sagittal dimensions of the vertebral foramen. In the Italian and Indian spines examined by Postacchini *et al.* (1983), the width of the lateral recesses was at, or below, the lower limit of normal in 68% of the L_4 and L_5 lumbar vertebrae with a midsagittal diameter of the vertebral foramen of less than 11.5 mm. However, extremely narrow lateral recesses (3-3.5 mm) were also found in three vertebrae with normal sagittal dimensions of the vertebral foramen (one L_4 and two L_5).

These findings indicate that marked narrowing of the lateral recesses may well be an isolated feature in an otherwise normal vertebra but the likelihood of lateral recess narrowing is significantly higher in those vertebrae with an abnormally short midsagittal diameter of the vertebral foramen.

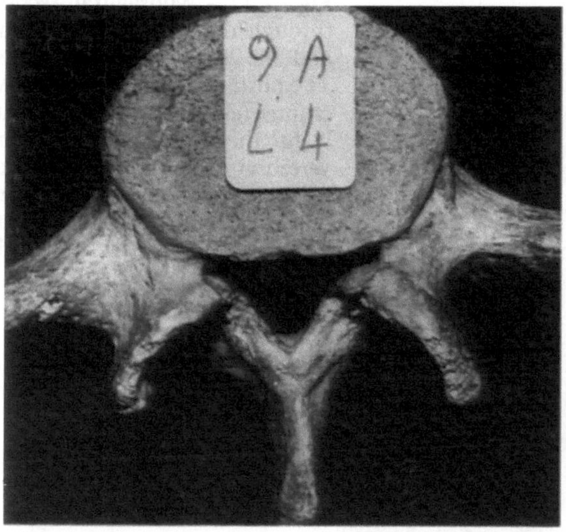

Fig. 2.15 - L_4 vertebra of an Italian skeleton. The marked narrowing of the lateral recesses is due to the trefoil configuration of the vertebral foramen and degenerative changes of the superior articular processes.

VERTEBRAL CANAL

The vertebral canal is constituted by the sequence of the single vertebral foramina and the interposed non-osseous structures, such as the intervertebral discs and ligamenta flava. In normal conditions the dimensions and shape of the spinal canal are similar to those of the vertebral foramina, as the intervertebral discs do not protrude, or protrude only slightly, into the canal, and the ligamenta flava are disposed in the same plane as the proximal and distal lamina, into which they have their insertion (Figs. 2.16 and 2.17).

Examined in a transverse section, the spinal canal can be divided into three different portions: pedicular, subpedicular, and intervertebral. In the pedicular portion the canal is bounded entirely by bony structures, represented anteriorly by the posterior aspect of the vertebral body, laterally by the pedicles, and posteriorly by the superior articular processes and/or the partes interarticulares, the laminae and the base of the spinous process (Fig. 2.18). In the subpedicular portion, which corresponds approximately to the caudal half of the vertebral body, the posterior aspect of the body of the vertebra is separated from the posterior arch by two symmetrical spaces corresponding to the intervertebral foramina (Fig. 2.19). The dimensions of these spaces vary according to the level of the transverse section, reaching a maximum in proximity to the inferior endplate of the vertebral body. The posterior wall of the canal is formed by the base of the inferior articular process or both articular processes (according to the level of the transverse section), by the laminae, and the

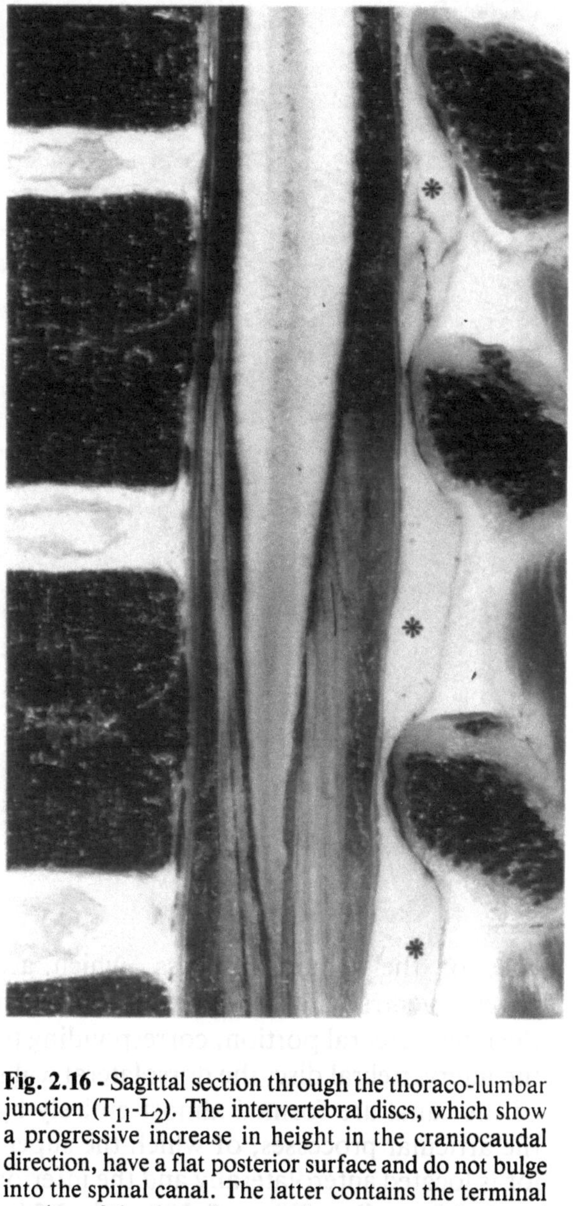

Fig. 2.16 - Sagittal section through the thoraco-lumbar junction (T_{11}-L_2). The intervertebral discs, which show a progressive increase in height in the craniocaudal direction, have a flat posterior surface and do not bulge into the spinal canal. The latter contains the terminal portion of the thoracic cord, the conus medullaris and the nerve roots of the cauda equina. The asterisks indicate the fat pad filling, at each intervertebral level, the space between the ligamenta flava.

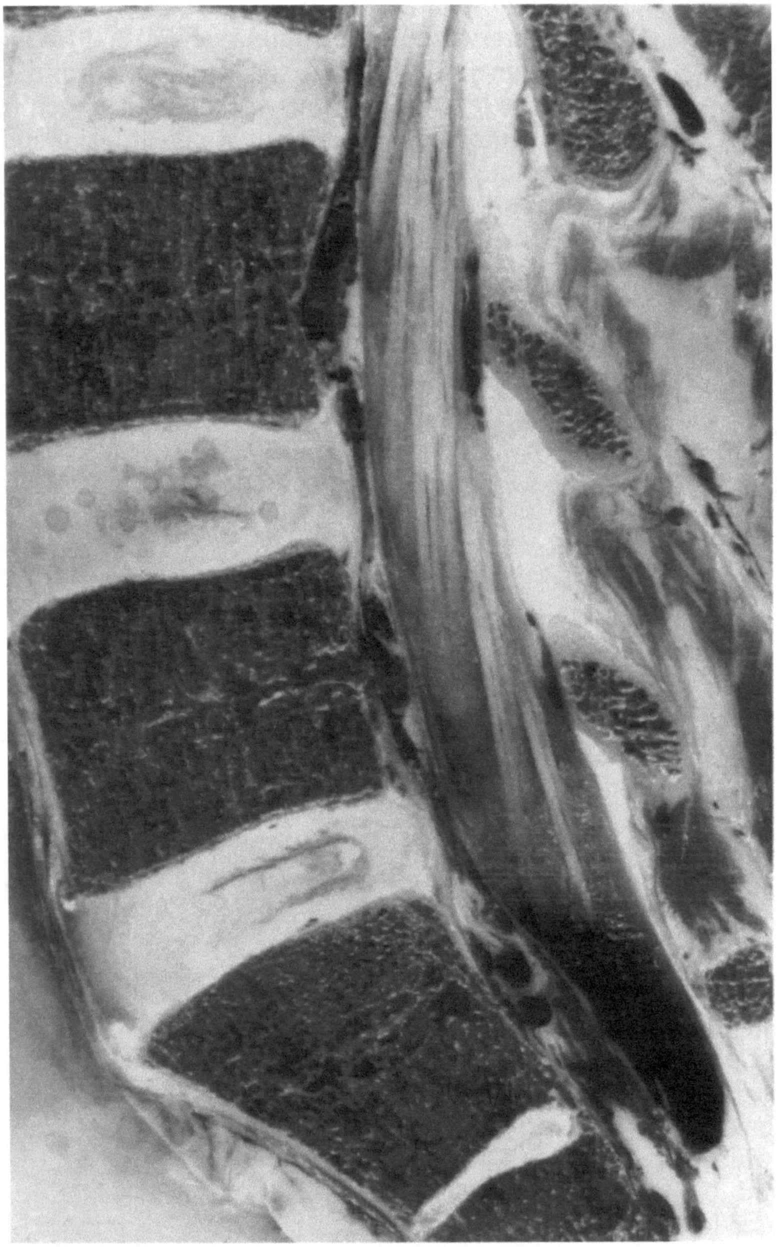

Fig. 2.17 - Midsagittal section through the lower lumbar spine and the upper sacral segments. The posterior surface of the lower three lumbar discs bulges slightly into the spinal canal. The intervertebral discs and the vertebral bodies are covered by a thick posterior longitudinal ligament. Large epidural vessels are visible behind the vertebral bodies.

base of the spinous process, which are covered ventrally by the ligamenta flava. In the intervertebral portion, corresponding to the intervertebral disc, the dorsolateral walls of the canal are formed almost entirely by the articular processes, of which the superior is located anterolaterally and the inferior posterolaterally (Figs. 2.20 and 2.21). Posteriorly, according to the level of the transverse section, the canal may be bounded by the ligamenta flava covering the laminae and the base of the spinous process (Fig. 2.20) or by the ligamenta flava alone (Fig. 2.21).

NERVE ROOT CANAL

As with the vertebral foramen, the lumbar spinal canal can be divided into a cen-

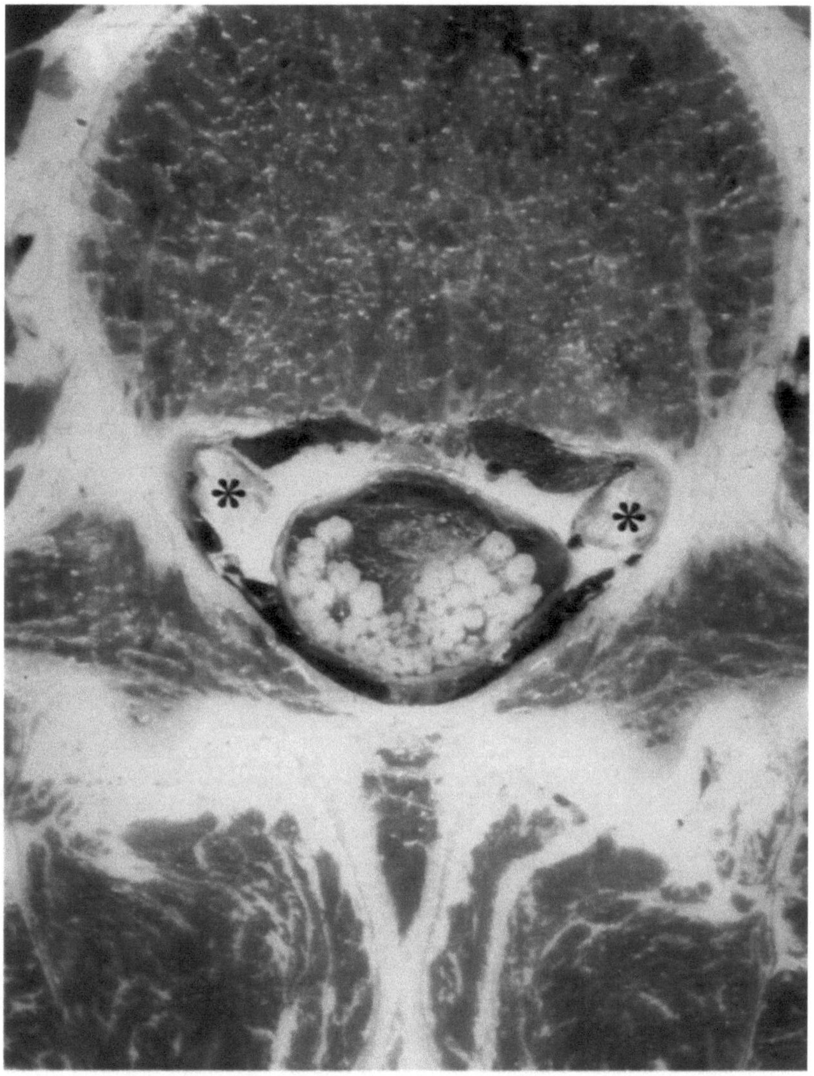

Fig. 2.18 - Axial section immediately below the lower margin of the pedicles of L_4 vertebra. The spinal canal is entirely delimited by bony structures. The L_4 nerve roots (asterisks), which have already emerged from the sac and are about to enter into the L_4-L_5 intervertebral foramen, are visible alongside the thecal sac. The latter is separated from the vertebral body by fat tissue and epidural vessels.

tral portion, two lateral portions, and a posterior portion corresponding to the interlaminar corner.

The central portion represents the *central spinal canal*, whereas each lateral portion constitutes the so-called *nerve root canal.* This canal, more an anatomical concept than a real canal, is the tubular structure in which the nerve root has its course from the lateral aspect of the dural sac to the intervertebral foramen. The distinction between the central spinal canal and the nerve root canal is based on physiopathological and clinical considerations rather than anatomical principles, as these two portions can become stenotic independently from each other and produce different clinical syndromes.

The nerve root canal consists of two parts: the proximal, subarticular or intervertebral, and the distal, constituted by the lateral recess.

The proximal part is bounded anteriorly by the intervertebral disc and posterolaterally by the anterior border of the superior articular process, covered by the ligamentum flavum, which at this level merges with the articular capsule of the zygoapophyseal joint. The distal part begins at the level of the superior end-plate and ends at the entrance of the intervertebral foramen. In this second part the nerve root canal is bounded posteriorly by the base of the superior articular

Fig. 2.19 - Axial section 7 mm below the pedicles. **a.** Laterally to the spinal canal are the intervertebral foramina containing the spinal nerve roots. The posterior wall of the vertebral canal is formed by the ligamenta flava, a short portion of the laminae and the base of the spinous process. **b.** Spinal canal at higher magnification. Anteriorly, the thecal sac is in close contact with the vertebral body, whereas posteriorly the sac is separated from the spinous process by fat tissue. The asterisks indicate the spinal nerve roots in the intervertebral foramina.

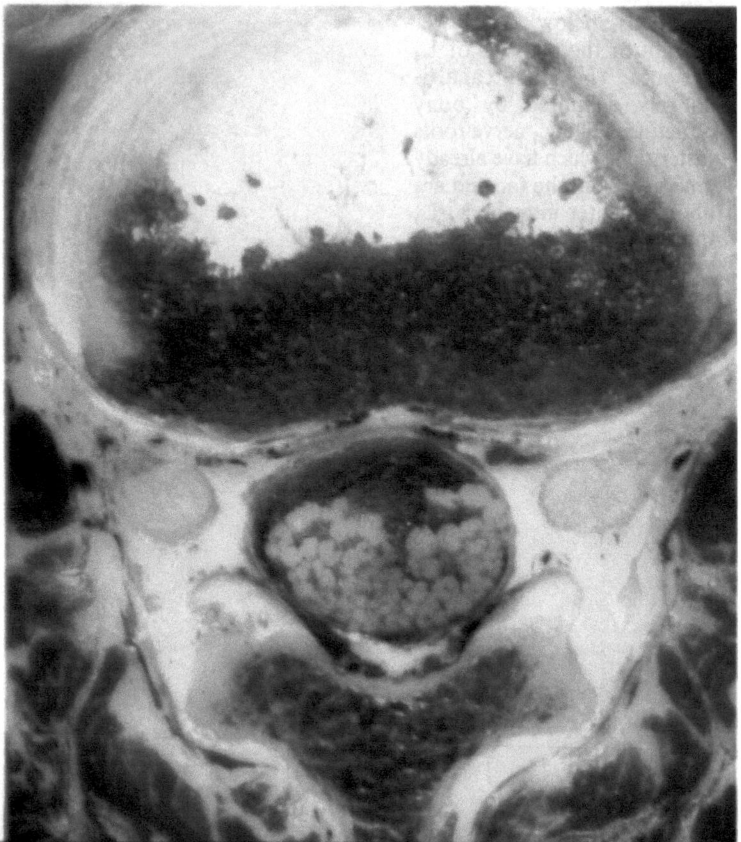

a

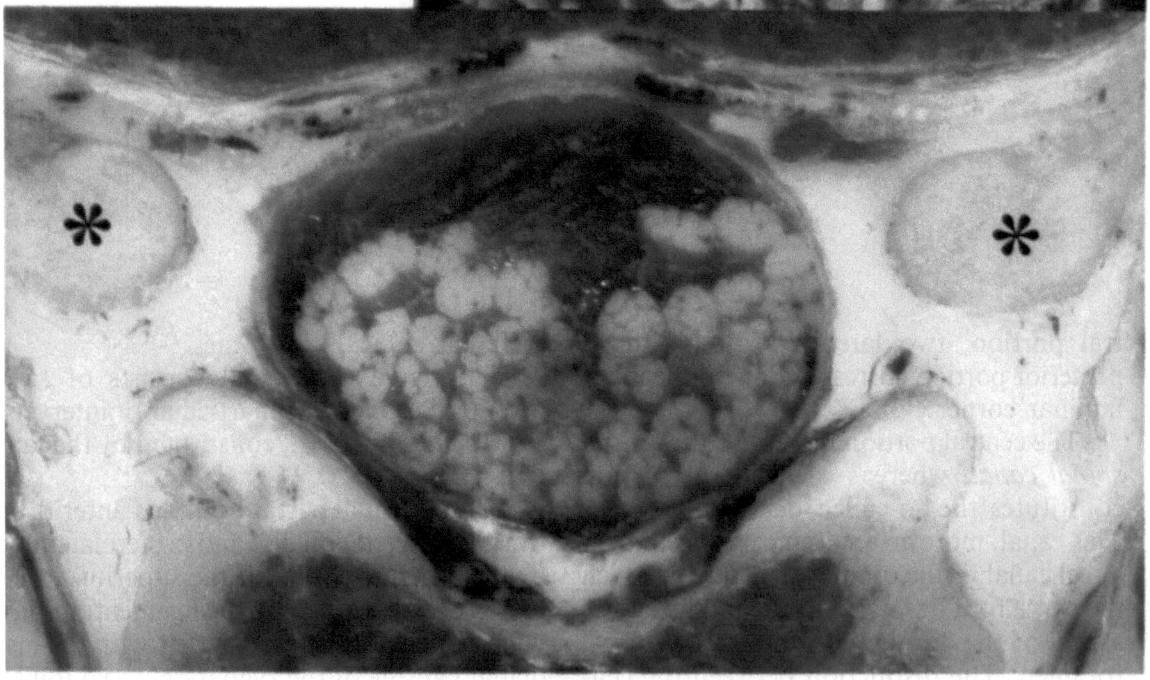

b

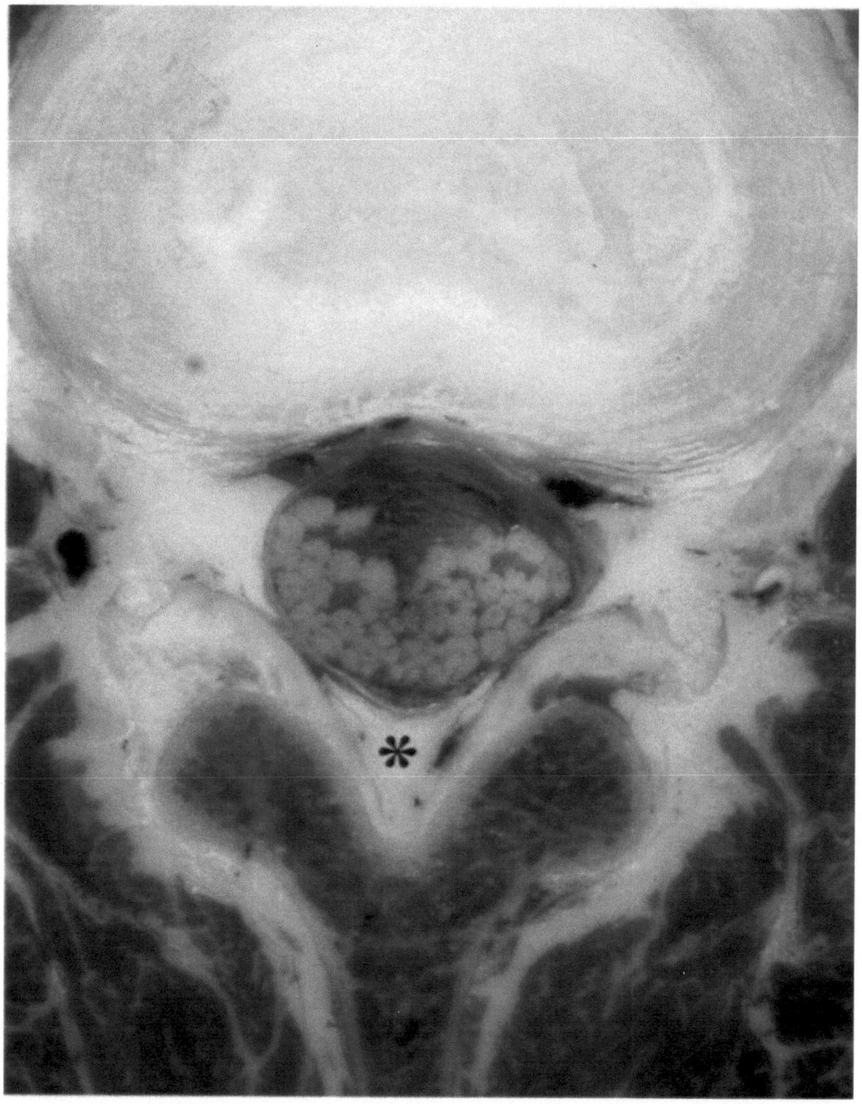

Fig. 2.20 - Axial section through the proximal portion of the L_4-L_5 disc. The spinal canal is delimited posterolaterally by the base of the inferior articular processes of L_4 and the laminae; these bony structures are covered ventrally by the ligamenta flava, which run anteriorly to the proximal portion of the facet joints. The posterior corner of the spinal canal is occupied by fat tissue (asterisk).

process and the pars interarticularis and laterally by the pedicles (Figs. 2.21 and 2.22). The nerve root canal does not have a real medial wall; this may be identified, for both the proximal and distal portion, with the lateral aspect of the dural sac (Fig. 2.22). The lateral recess exists as an identifiable anatomical structure only for the lower two lumbar nerve roots, especially for the fifth, and for the first sacral root. The first three lumbar roots, in fact, go almost immediately, after their emergence, through the intervertebral foramen, the entrance of which is almost in contact with the dural sac.

INTERVERTEBRAL FORAMEN

The intervertebral foramen, which is in reality more an osteofibrous canal than a real foramen, is formed by two adjacent vertebrae and the intervertebral disc in between.

The anterior wall of the foramen is formed by the subpedicular portion of the body of the proximal vertebra, the intervertebral disc, and the short suprapedicular portion of the body of the distal vertebra. The superior wall is constituted by the inferior border of the pedicle of the proximal vertebra, and the inferior wall by the superior

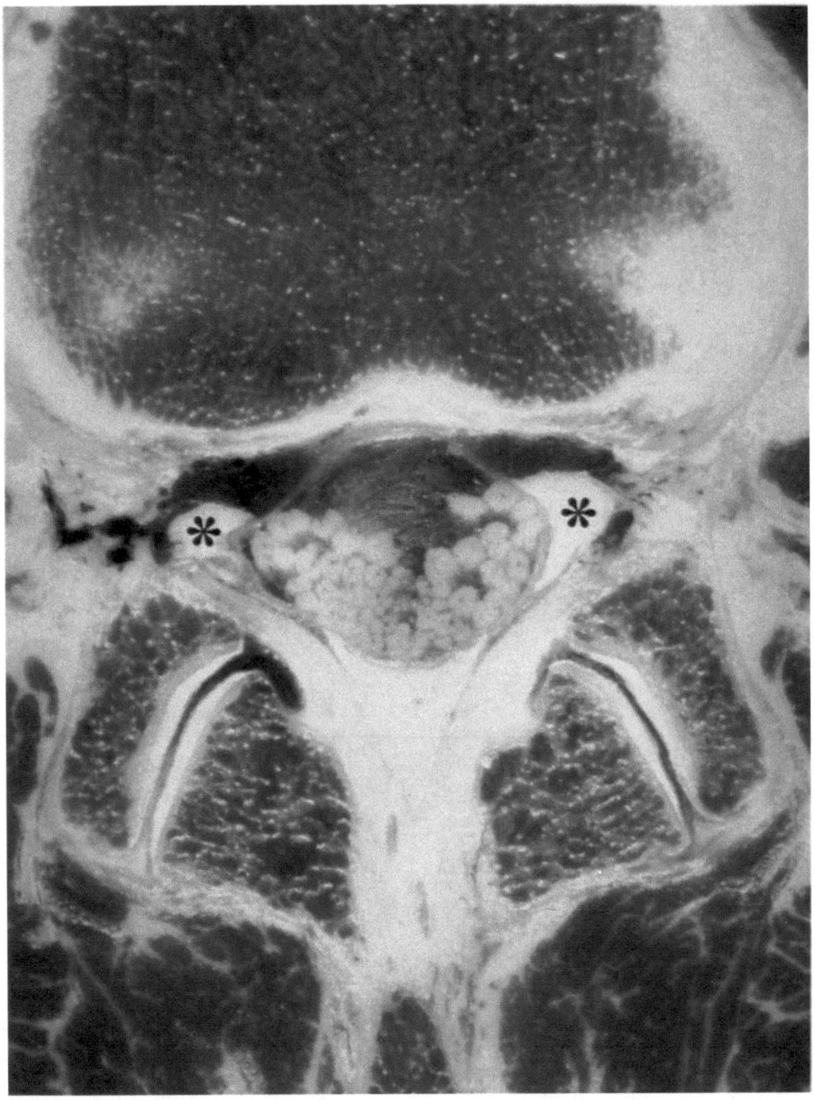

Fig. 2.21 - Axial section through the upper end-plate of L_5. The facet joints are covered anteriorly by the ligamenta flava, which form the posterior wall of the spinal canal. The L_5 nerve roots are visible (asterisks) in the intervertebral portion of the radicular canal alongside the thecal sac.

margin of the pedicle of the distal vertebra. The posterior wall is formed by the lateral end of the ligamentum flavum, behind which is the pars interarticularis, by the base of the inferior articular process, the capsule of the apophyseal joint and the superior articular process. The entrance and exit of the foramen correspond respectively to the medial and lateral aspect of the pedicle.

The lumbar intervertebral foramina have an inverted tear-drop shape, the proximal part being larger than the distal (Fig. 2.23). The sacral foramina are rounder. The vertical dimensions of the foramina are essentially related to the height of the intervertebral disc. The sagittal dimensions depend on the length of the pedicle, the thickness of the ligamentum flavum, the volume of the superior articular process and orientation of the latter in the sagittal plane. This first four lumbar foramina have similar dimensions and their anteroposterior axis is almost parallel to the sagittal axis of the vertebra. The fifth intervertebral foramen generally has a smaller vertical diameter than the others, because of the tall fifth lumbar pedicle, and its sagittal axis

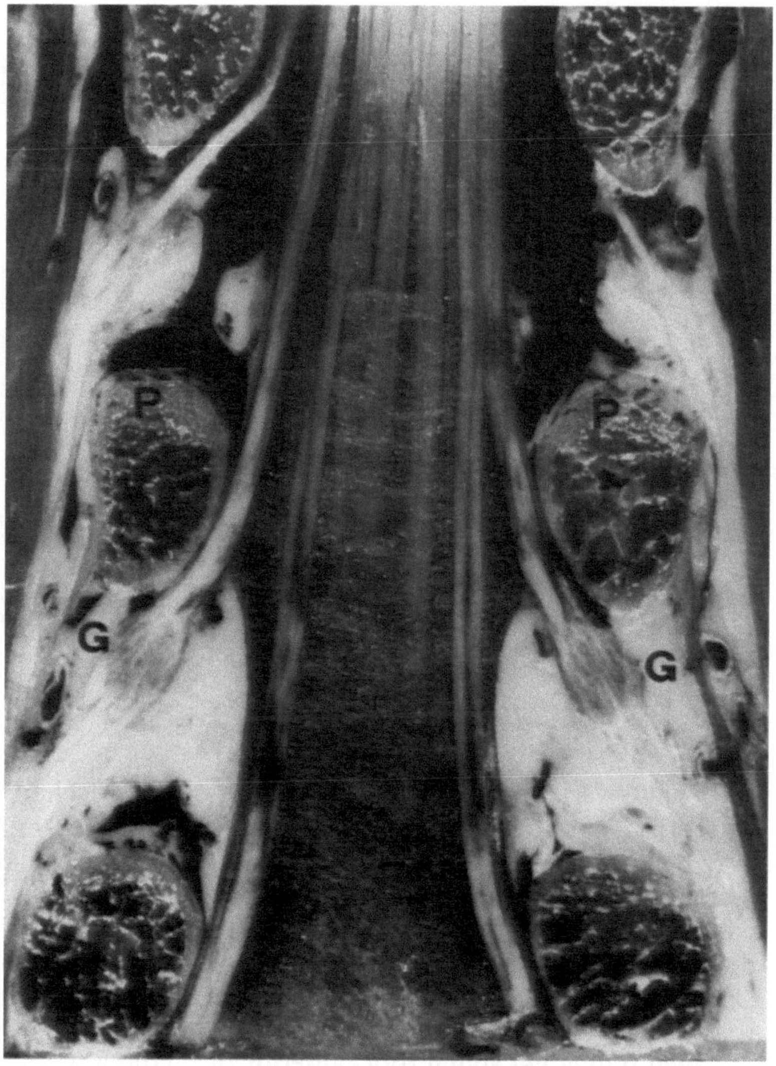

Fig. 2.22 - Coronal section through the pedicles (P) of L_3, L_4 and L_5 vertebrae. The nerve roots of the cauda equina are clearly visible in the intrathecal course. The roots emerging from the sac at each vertebral level run along the radicular canal in direct contact with the medial surface of the pedicle and the lateral wall of the thecal sac. The nerve root encounters the dorsal ganglion (G) within, or immediately outside, the intervertebral foramen.

is orientated on a slightly oblique plane in the dorso-ventral and inward-outward direction.

In the lumbar spine the nerve roots occupy only the proximal third or half of the foramen (Bose and Balasubramaniam, 1982; Rauschning, 1985) (Fig. 2.24). The remaining space is occupied by the spinal branch of the lumbar artery and the radicular veins, and is also used by the apophyseal joints for their reciprocal movements in spinal flexion and extension. In the sacrum, due to the absence of movement of the single vertebral segments, the relatively small intervertebral foramina are occupied almost entirely by the nerve roots surrounded by the radicular vessels.

NEURAL STRUCTURES IN THE VERTEBRAL CANAL

SPINAL CORD AND CAUDA EQUINA

In the vast majority of individuals the proximal portion of the lumbar spinal canal contains the terminal part of the lumbar widening of the cord and the conus medullaris, which is the short terminal segment of cord from which the last three sacral nerve roots and the coccygeal nerve originate. Normally, the conus medullaris is located at the level of the L_1 vertebral body and the L_1-L_2 intervertebral disc or, less frequently, at the

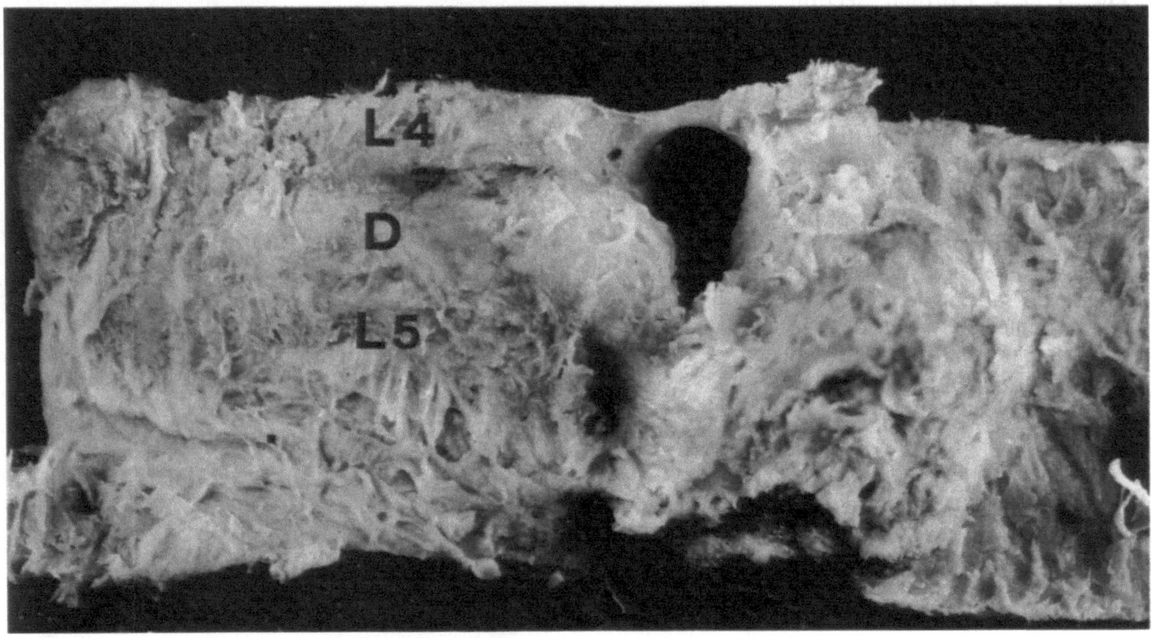

Fig. 2.23 - Typical inverted tear-drop shape of the intervertebral foramen. The L_4 vertebra was sectioned near the inferior border of the pedicle. D: intervertebral disc.

level of L_2 vertebral body and L_2-L_3 intervertebral disc (Louis, 1983). Very rarely it may be at T_{12}-L_1 level and the lumbar vertebral canal would not therefore contain spinal cord. Distally to the conus medullaris the dural sac contains the filum terminale, which extends as far as the base of the coccyx, and the nerve roots of the cauda equina.

Each individual spinal root, anterior or posterior, originates from the cord as thin rootlets. These, after a short distance, unite to form the nerve root common bundle (anterior and posterior). Each rootlet is surrounded by an extension of the pial covering of the spinal cord, which follows the rootlets throughout their course as root fascicles, taking the name of fascicular pial sheath (Parke and Watanabe, 1985). As the rootlets converge to form the nerve root, they are encircled by a common pial sheath — radicular pial sheath — which merges with the fascicular pial sheath at the periphery of the root fascicles (Fig. 2.31). These pial sheaths, however, do not constitute a closed membrane. They are formed by a thin openmeshed structure with openings of variable size — larger in the radicular sheath and smaller in the fascicular — which allow metabolic exchange between the nerve fibers and the cerebrospinal fluid.

The spinal roots, constituted by densely packed nerve fibers, do not have a precise location within the theca, with the exception of the emerging roots, which occupy the anterolateral portion of the dural sac (Figs. 2.25, 2.26). The latter is formed by parallel columns of fibroblast-like cells and by bundles of collagen fibres orientated vertically, which occupy the space between the cell rows. Amongst the collagen fibres, numerous elastic fibres, with both a horizontal and vertical course, are present, which give high elasticity to the dural tissue. The inner surface of the dural sac is covered by the arachnoid membrane, separating the dura mater from the cerebrospinal fluid.

The length of the dural sac, i.e. the vertebral level at which its bottom arrives, is highly variable. In the majority of individuals the sac ends between the first and the second sacral vertebra or at the level of the second sacral vertebra. Less frequently it terminates at the level of the L_5-S_1 intervertebral disc or the proximal half of the first sacral vertebra, or continues as far as the body of the third sacral vertebra.

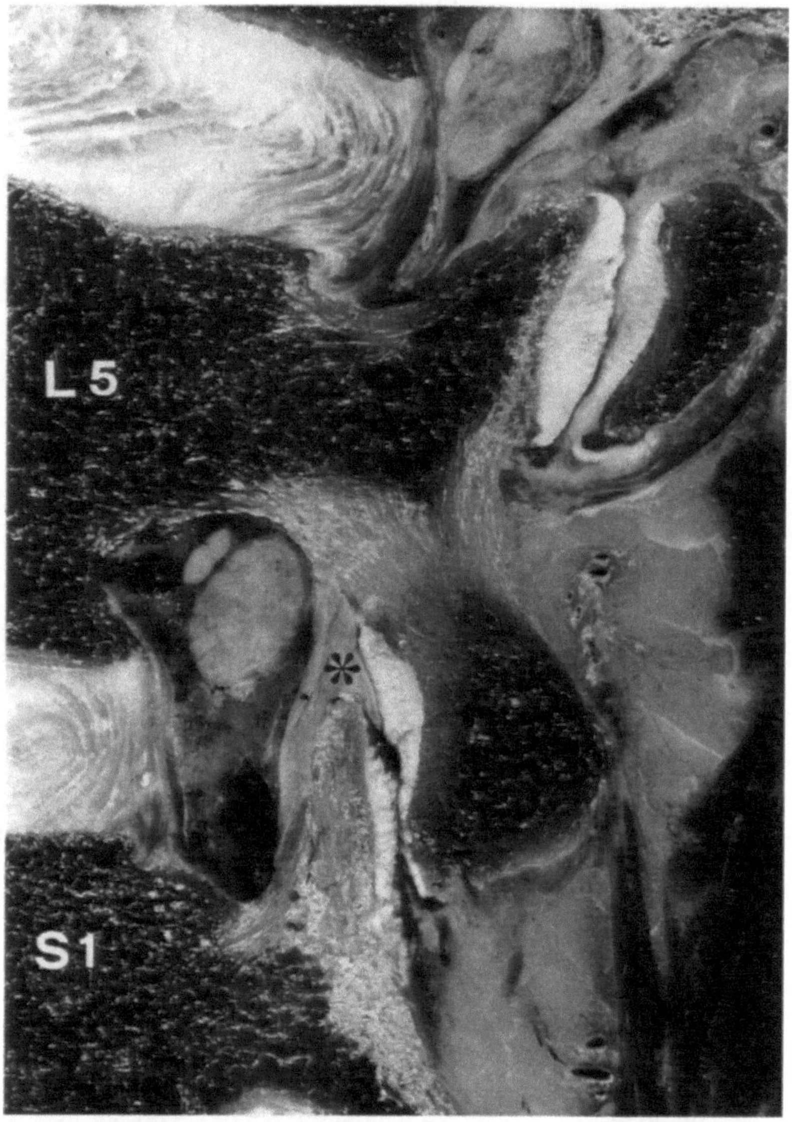

Fig. 2.24 - Sagittal section through the central portion of the L_5-S_1 intervertebral foramen (center) and the outer portion of the L_4-L_5 foramen (top). Normally, the nerve root occupies, as in the L_5-S_1 foramen, the cranial portion of the neuroforamen. The caudal portion is filled by fat tissue and vessels. The ligamentum flavum (asterisk), forming the anterior portion of the facet joint capsule, is seen behind the L_5 nerve root.

EXTRADURAL COURSE OF THE SPINAL NERVE ROOTS

The anterior and posterior spinal nerve roots emerging from the dural sac penetrate the dura through two separate openings: the ventral opening, which is occupied by the motor root, and the dorsal, through which the sensory root passes. Once out of the dural sac, the two radicular branches (which more correctly should be called radicular nerves rather than, as is usually the case, spinal nerve roots) are encircled by a common fibrous sheath, representing an extension of the dura mater, inside which the two roots are separated by a fibrous septum. This dural covering, as for the spinal dura mater, is internally lined by an extension of the arachnoid membrane. Distally to the spinal ganglion the two roots merge to form the spinal nerve and whilst the dural sheath extends into the epineurium, the arachnoid continues into the neurilemma.

The first three lumbar nerve roots emerge from the dural sac at the level of the proximal half of the homologous vertebral body. In particular, the L_1 root emerges at the level of the centre of the L_1 vertebral body,

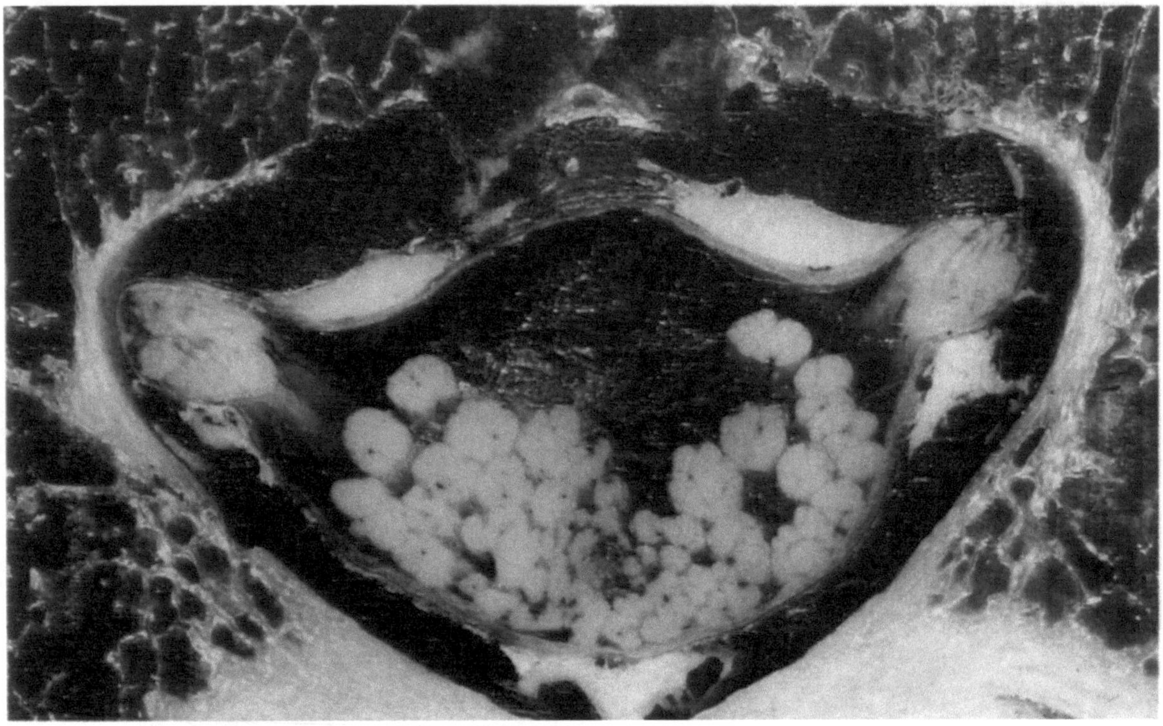

Fig. 2.25 - Axial section of the spinal canal through the lower portion of the pedicle of the L_4 vertebra. The anterior and posterior roots of the cauda equina do not appear to have any precise arrangement. The L_5 nerve roots, already formed by anterior and posterior rootlets, are located in the lateral portions of the thecal sac, which they are about to leave.

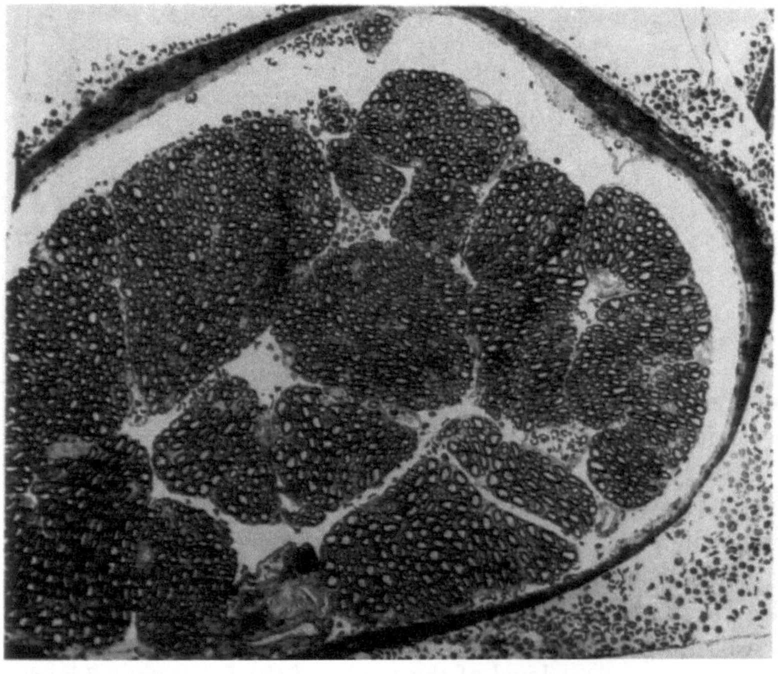

Fig. 2.26 - Histologic axial section of the terminal portion of the dural sac and cauda equina. Nerve rootlets, formed by nerve fibres grouped in fascicles, are in close contact with one another without any precise topographic arrangement.

whilst the L_2 and L_3 roots emerge opposite the pedicle of the second and third lumbar vertebra, respectively. The extradural path in the vertebral canal is therefore very short and essentially transverse, as these roots go almost immediately through the foramen, which faces their emergence from the dural sac.

The L_4 nerve root emerges from the thecal sac opposite to the upper border of the pedicle of L_4 and rapidly reaches the intervertebral foramen, but with a slightly longer and more oblique course than the upper lumbar nerve roots. However, the length of the extradural course of this nerve root, as for the L_5 and S_1 nerve roots, is related to the level at which the thecal sac ends. If the sac terminates more cranially than normal, these three roots will have a longer extradural course, whereas the opposite occurs when the theca ends more distally.

The L_5 nerve root usually emerges at the level of the L_4-L_5 intervertebral disc, heading downwards and laterally with a 45° oblique orientation and a course of approximately 3 cm (Crock, 1981). The anterior wall of the L_5 nerve root canal is formed by the L_4-L_5 intervertebral disc and the posterior aspect of the fifth lumbar vertebral body. The posterior wall is formed, from top to bottom, by the L_4-L_5 ligamentum flavum, the inferior articular process of L_5, if this process is prominent in the spinal canal, and the pars interarticularis. The medial wall is formed by the dural sac and the S_1 nerve root, if this has a very proximal emergence. The lateral wall is formed by the pedicle.

The S_1 nerve root generally emerges at the level of the inferior half of the L_5 vertebral body, the obliquity of this root being approximately 30°. The length of the S_1 nerve root is on average 3.5 cm (Crock, 1982). The anterior wall of the S_1 nerve root canal is formed, from top to bottom, by the posterior aspect of the L_5 vertebral body, the L_5-S_1 intervertebral disc, and the posterior aspect of the body of S_1 in the portion located medially to the pedicle. The relationship of the nerve root with the posterior anatomical structures depends on: the site of emergence of the root; the position of the neural arch in relation to the vertebral body (facing the vertebral body entirely or being partly distal to its lower end-plate); and the orientation of the lamine (oblique rearwards or vertical). Generally, the posterior wall is formed by the bony crest at the site of the proximal insertion of the ligamentum flavum on the anterior aspect of the lamina of L_5, by the L_5-S_1 ligamentum flavum, the anteromedial portion of the superior articular process of S_1 and the lamina of the first sacral vertebra. The medial wall is formed by the dural sac or the S_2 nerve root, if this has a proximal emergence. Laterally to the S_1 nerve root there is the L_5 root first, then

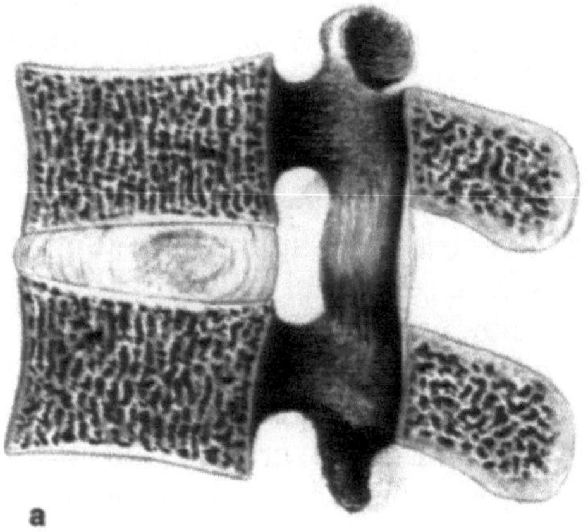

a

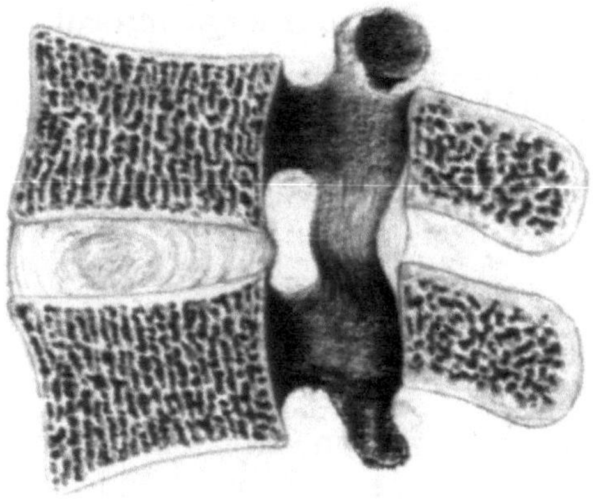

b

Fig. 2.27 - Functional changes of the vertebral canal in spinal flexion and extension. **a.** In flexion, the spinal canal lengthens and increases in width in the sagittal plane due both to separation of the laminae and the consequent decrease in thickness of the ligamenta flava, and the distension of the posterior annulus fibrosus. **b.** Opposite changes occur in extension.

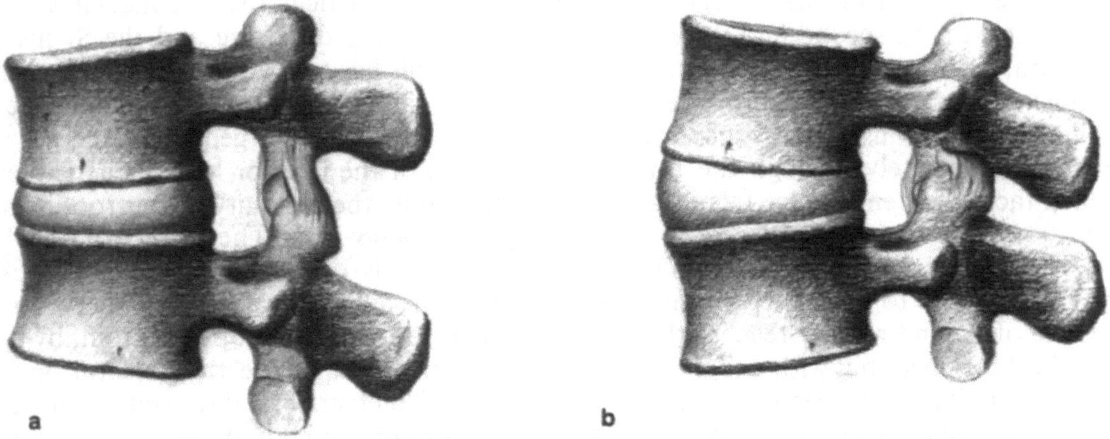

Fig. 2.28 - Changes in size of the intervertebral foramen in spinal flexion and extension. **a.** In flexion, the foramen increases in height. **b.** In extension, it decreases in height and width due to bulging of the annulus fibrosus, increase in thickness of the anterior capsule of the facet joint and nearing of the tip of the superior articular process to the pedicle of the vertebra above.

the L_5-S_1 intervertebral foramen, and finally the medial aspect of the pedicle of S_1.

Through the intervertebral foramen, the lumbar nerve roots have an oblique course from top to bottom, and from inside outwards. The degree of obliquity increases progressively from the first to the fifth lumbar root depending on the different level of emergence from the dural sac with respect to the intervertebral foramen. The root, within the foramen, is bordered initially by the inferior margin of the pedicle and the vertebral body, and subsequently by the posterolateral aspect of the intervertebral disc. The contact with the disc can increase if the root's course is more vertical. In the intervertebral foramen, the dorsal root meets the spinal ganglion and converges on the ventral root to form the spinal nerve at the exit of the foramen.

FUNCTIONAL CHANGES OF THE VERTEBRAL CANAL AND NERVE ROOTS

In spinal flexion, the laminae of two adjacent vertebrae move apart and the interlaminar space widens, thus producing lengthening and thinning of ligamentum flavum. At the same time the two adjacent vertebral bodies move closer anteriorly and further apart posteriorly, stretching the posterior portion of the annulus fibrosus (Fig. 2.27). This increases the length and the sagittal dimensions of the spinal canal. The opposite occurs in extension of the spine. The ligamenta flava shorten, become thicker and buckle in the canal, which becomes shorter and narrower (Fig. 2.27). Tajima and Kawano (1986) in an anatomic study on the functional variations of the thickness of the ligamentum flavum at the L_4-L_5 level, found a range of values between 1.9 mm to 3.3 mm in flexion, and 4.5 mm to 5.9 mm in extension.

The intervertebral foramen increases its vertical dimensions in flexion, whereas it narrows by approximately one fourth in both vertical and sagittal diameters in extension (Tajima and Kawano, 1986). The narrowing is due to buckling in the foramen of the annulus fibrosus and the ligamentum flavum covering ventrally the apophyseal joint, and to the associated cranial sliding of the superior articular process (Fig. 2.28).

Parallel with the modification of the spinal canal, the intradural nerve roots stretch, straighten, and move cranially in flexion, whereas they shorten, become winding, and move caudally in extension (Breig and Marions, 1963). In their extradural course the roots undergo similar functional modifications which, however, are less marked due to their close relationship with the dural structures.

BLOOD SUPPLY

VASCULAR PATTERN OF THE SPINAL CORD AND CAUDA EQUINA

The thoracolumbar spinal cord derives its arterial blood supply from arterial trunks (called radicular or radiculo-medullary) which originate from the parietal intercostal, lumbar and lateral sacral arteries and reach the cord following the course of the spinal nerve roots. At the level of the dorsal root ganglion each spinal arterial trunk divides into two branches (anterior and posterior radicular artery), which follow the anterior and posterior spinal root, respectively. The anterior radicular artery reaches the anterior median fissure of the spinal cord and divides into an ascending and a descending branch, which anastomose with the homologous branches of the adjacent radicular arteries to form the anterior spinal artery. The posterior branch reaches the dorsolateral portion of the cord and divides into an ascending and a descending branch which, through similar anastomoses as for the anterior branches, contribute to form the posterior spinal arteries. The latter consist on each side of two longitudinal trunks — one medial and the other lateral to the posterior nerve roots — linked together by transversal branches. The anterior spinal artery and the posterior spinal arteries are connected by numerous transverse anastomotic branches called vasa corona, which form a perimetral vascular network around the cord. According to the classic description, the radicular arteries in post-embryonic life are less numerous than the spinal roots or, in other words, only some roots are accompanied by an artery. As far as the anterior roots are concerned, a radicular artery is found only every three or four roots on each side (Testut and Latarjet, 1963). The arteries of the posterior roots are more numerous, on average two arteries every three pairs of roots, but thinner than those of the anterior roots. The distal portion of the dorsal spinal cord and the conus medullaris derive most of their blood supply from an anterior artery, the artery of Adamkiewicz or of Lazorthes. This originates at a variable level, generally between T_{10} and L_2, or more rare-

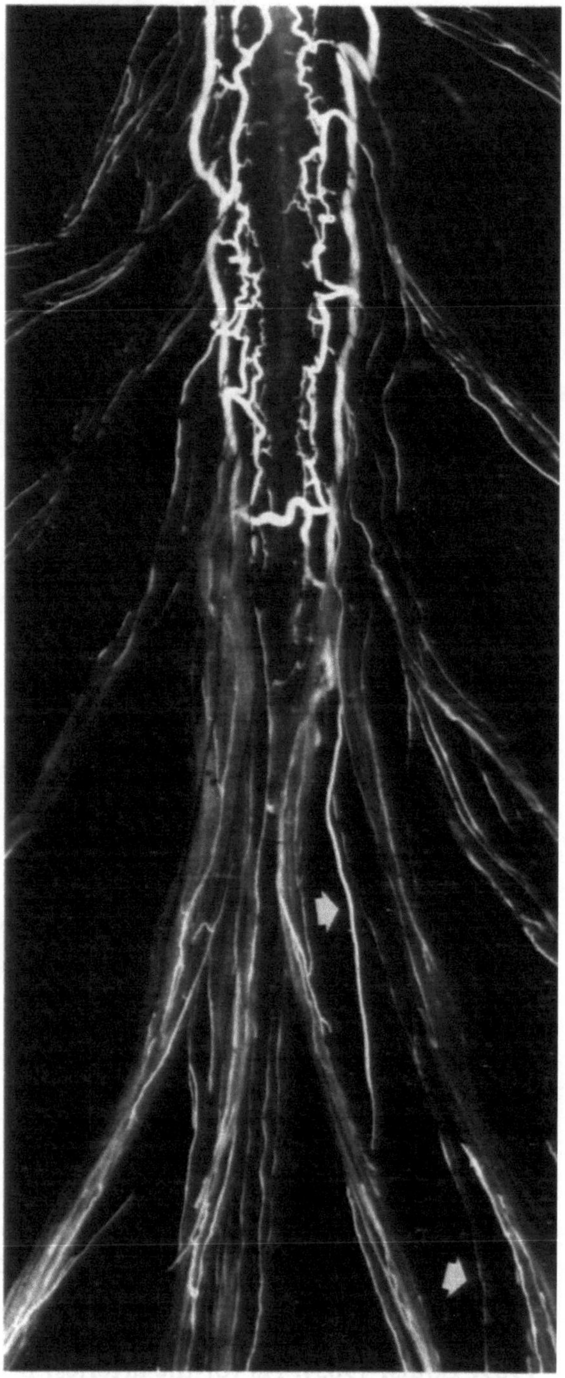

Fig. 2.29 - Dorsal view of the lower thoracic cord, the conus medullaris and cauda equina with their arterial network. Each caudal nerve root is accompanied by a radicular artery and collateral branches of the latter. The radicular arteries are in continuity with the posterior spinal arteries or, in some instances, with the vasa corona. The arrows point to interradicular vessels. (From Crock H.V. *et al.*, *The conus medullaris and cauda equina in man*, 1986).

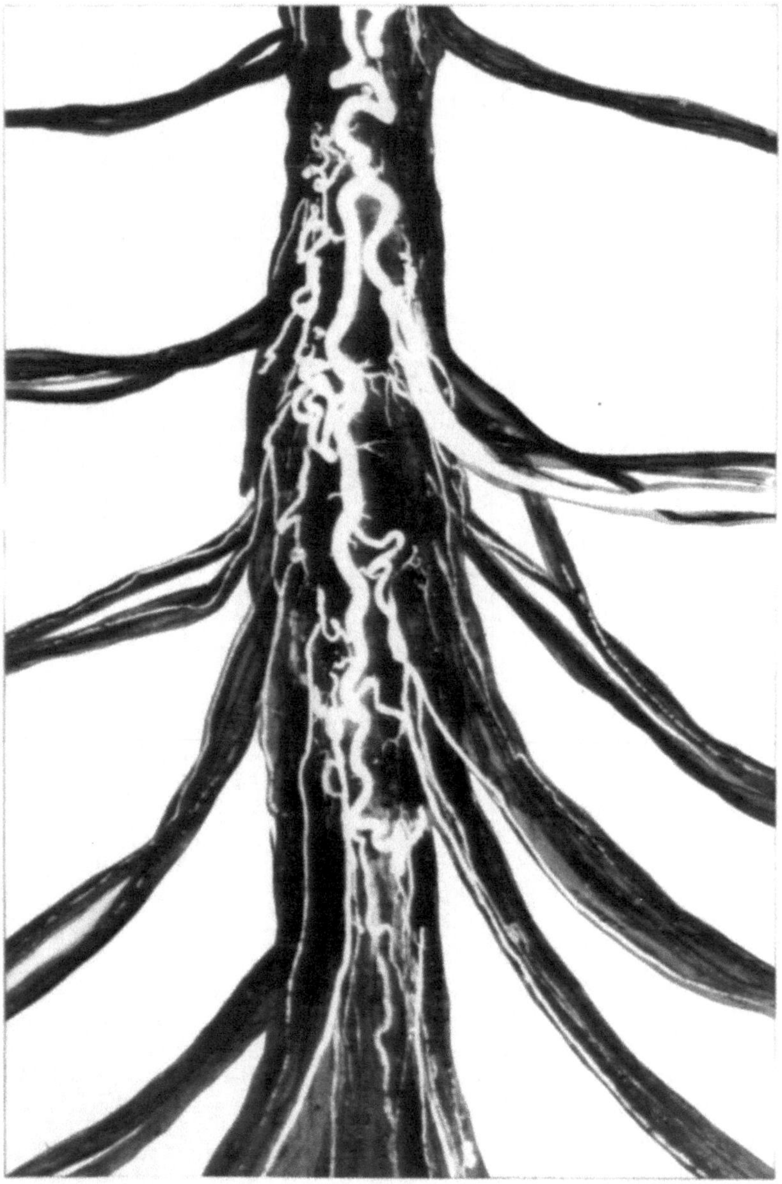

Fig. 2.30 - Venous system of the dorsal aspect of the lower thoracic cord and conus medullaris, and the cauda equina. A radicular vein, which is in continuity with the perimedullary venous network (dorsal median longitudinal venous channel, postero-lateral longitudinal venous channels and vasa corona), runs along each nerve root. One of the roots on the right side is accompanied by a large venous trunk (dorsal vena radiculo-medullaris magna). (From Crock H.V. *et al.*, *The conus medullaris and cauda equina in man*, 1986).

ly at L_4 or S_1 level, and is generally found on the left side (Adamkiewicz, 1882; Lazorthes *et al.*, 1957; Obounou-Akong, 1969; Louis, 1983). As for the arteries, not all spinal nerve roots are accompanied by veins. There is, on average, a radicular vein every two or three roots. The radicular veins drain the blood from the perimedullary venous network. This network, in the conus medullaris, is constituted by the anterior and posterior median veins, which are of large calibre, and by the anterior and posterior lateral veins, which are of smaller calibre. At the level of the intervertebral foramen, the radicular veins drain into the foraminal veins and, through these, into the parietal veins.

More recently Parke *et al.* (1981) have suggested a new terminology and described a more complex vascular architecture than the classic. According to these authors all nerve roots, anterior and posterior, are accompanied by at least one artery. These arteries can be of two types: large calibre arteries (medullary arteries), which supply the anterior spinal artery or the posterior spinal arteries; and smaller arteries (true radicu-

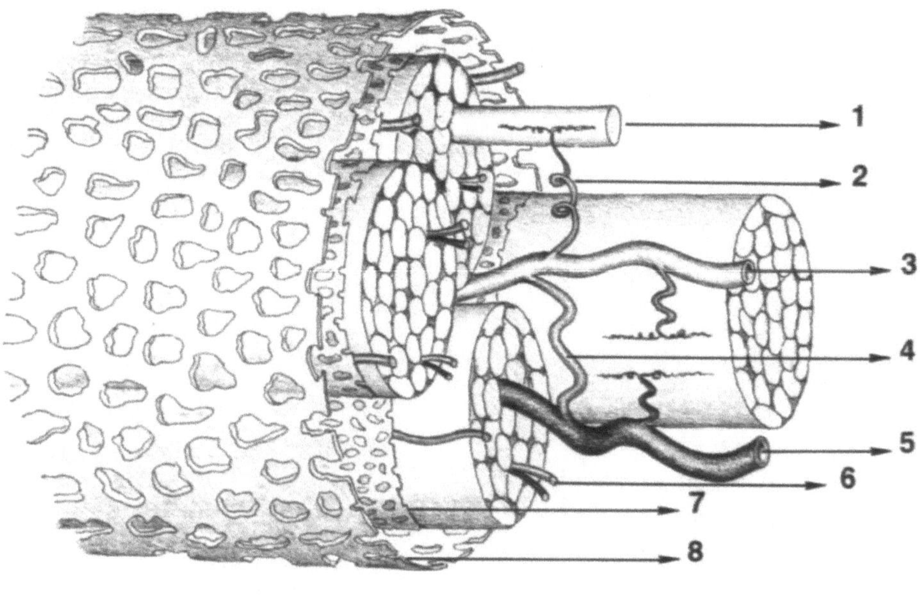

Fig. 2.31 - Intrinsic vasculature of the spinal nerve root. **1.** Portion of a nerve fascicle. **2.** Transverse arterial branch with spiraling coils. **3.** Radicular artery running between the nerve root fascicles. **4.** Artero-venous shunt. **5.** Radicular vein. **6.** Collateral radicular arteries running along the peripheral area or within the nerve fascicles. **7.** Perifascicular pial sheath. **8.** Periradicular pial sheath with large openings (From Parke W.W. and Watanabe R., 1985).

lar arteries) which supply only the nerve root. In the lumbrosacral region, of the anterior roots, only one or two are accompanied by a medullary artery, whilst the posterior roots are more frequently associated with arteries classifiable as medullary, although smaller than the anterior vessels. The radicular arteries are of two types, distal and proximal. The distal arteries are branches of the lumbar and sacral arteries for the roots not accompanied by medullary vessels. For the roots that have medullary arteries, the distal radicular arteries originate from the medullary branch at the level of the dorsal root ganglion. These arteries feed the caudal portion of the root, whereas the cranial portion is fed by the proximal radicular arteries which, in the thoracolumbar cord, are

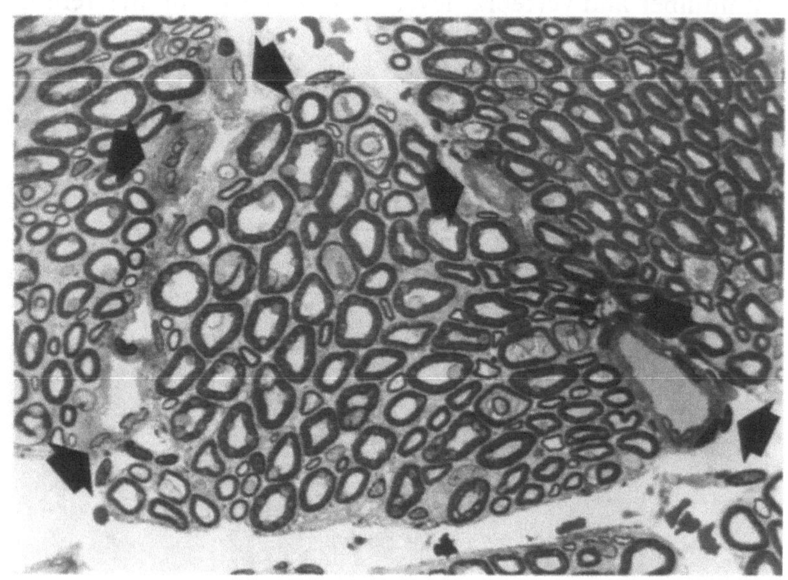

Fig. 2.32 - Histologic axial section of a portion of a nerve root in the intrathecal course. Nerve fascicles, formed by closely packed nerve fibres, are separated by septa, occupied by arterioles arranged in an undulating course (arrows). The vessels are arranged transversely to the longitudinal axis of the fascicles.

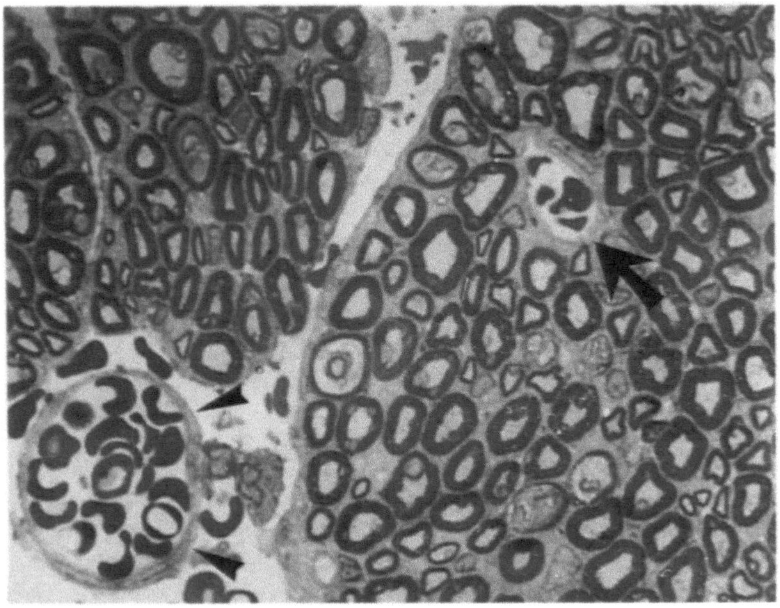

Fig. 2.33 - Histologic pattern of a nerve root in the intrathecal course. A vein (arrowheads) is visible at the periphery of the fascicles; between the nerve fibres of one of the fascicles, a transversely sectioned capillary (arrow) can be seen.

branches of the anterolateral longitudinal arteries, derived from the vasa corona, or branches of the posterior spinal arteries. The spinal roots, therefore, are fed by arterious blood originating from the medullary network in the proximal part, and directly from the parietal circulation in the distal part. The venous system follows inversely the structure of the arterious circulation. The proximal radicular veins end into the veins of the perimedullary network, which join the nerve root medullary veins (which are inconstant in number and vertebral level). These veins drain into the parietal. The distal radicular veins end into the medullary veins of the nerve roots or directly into the parietal.

The theory of duplicity of the radicular arteries (medullary arteries and radicular arteries proper) has been disputed by Crock *et al.* (1986), according to whom all nerve roots are accompanied by a radicular artery, which originates from the parietal vessels and reaches, with an interrupted course, the perimedullary arterial systems (Fig. 2.29). The radicular arteries are of different calibre in different nerve roots. Along their course

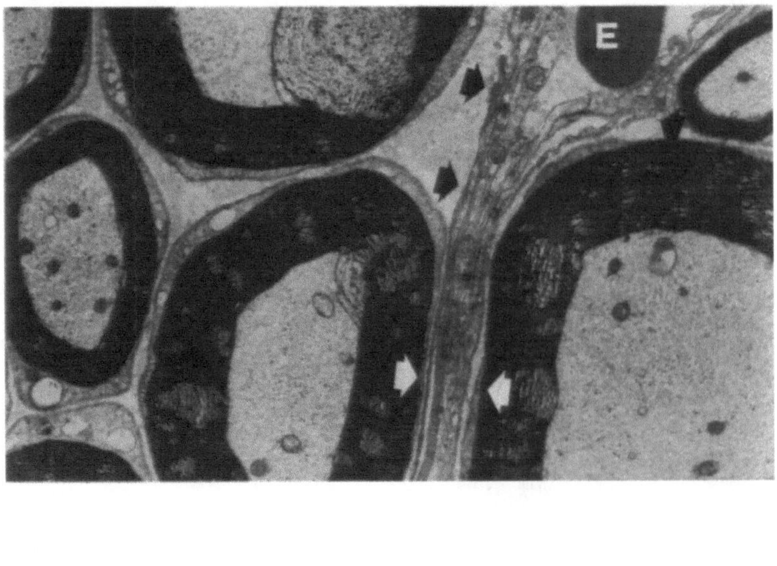

Fig. 2.34 - A capillary (arrows) penetrating, with a transverse course, between the fibres of a nerve fascicle. E: erythrocyte.

they issue, at regular intervals, collateral branches destined to supply the root. Furthermore, they can sometimes give origin to branches which anastomose with radicular arteries of adjacent roots (Fig. 2.29). In contrast to what was previously thought, therefore, the spinal cord would not be fed by few large arteries but by as many arteries as the spinal anterior and posterior nerve roots. The roots, in addition, would be entirely fed by branches of the radicular arteries. According to this vascular architecture the venous system is formed by radicular veins, one for each root, which drain the blood from the perimedullary venous network as well as nerve root (Fig. 2.30). Like the arteries, the lumbosacral radicular veins have a highly variable calibre.

INTRINSIC VASCULATURE OF THE CAUDAL NERVE ROOTS

In each single spinal root there are generally two or three arterious vessels of large calibre that deserve the name of radicular arteries. Their course is generally at the periphery of the larger neural fascicles which form the root (Parke and Watanabe, 1985). In addition to these, there are vessels of minor calibre which can be defined as collateral radicular arteries. These, as the main vessels, have a longitudinal course and are generally located at the periphery of the neural fascicles (Figs. 2.31 and 2.32). From the main radicular arteries, and especially the collateral vessels, numerous transverse branches originate, which are destined to anastomose with radicular arteries of adjacent fascicles and to penetrate into the fascicles to give origin to precapillary branches with longitudinal course (Fig. 2.33). The capillaries originating from these vessels course between the single nerve fibres of the fascicles both longitudinally and transversely (Fig. 2.34). A peculiar characteristic of the collateral radicular arteries and their transverse branches is the presence of coils, which in the longitudinal vessels are located immediately adjacent to the origin of the transverse branches (Parke and Watanabe, 1985) (Fig. 2.31). Such coils probably have the role of allowing reciprocal motion of the neural fascicles during lengthening and shortening of the spinal nerve roots, occurring, respectively, in flexion and extension of the spine. Another characteristic differentiating the radicular circulation from that of peripheral nerves is the presence of numerous arterovenous shunts. These probably represent a protective mechanism in the presence of circulatory obstruction in a portion of the root. The radicular veins do not accompany the associated arteries, as is the case in peripheral nerves, but tend to have a spiraling course within the neural fascicles (Parke and Watanabe, 1985). The smaller-calibre radicular veins end into two or three major branches which drain the blood into the parietal network.

REFERENCES

ADAMKIEWICZ A.: Die Blutgefässe des menschlichen Rückenmarks. II Teil. Die Gefässe der Rückenmarkesoberfläche. *Sitzungs Math. Naturwiss. Classe Akd. Wissensch.* **85:** 101, 1882.

BOSE K., BALASUBRAMANIAM P.: Nerve root canals of the lumbar spine. *Spine* **9:** 16, 1984.

CROCK H.V.: Normal and pathological anatomy of the lumbar spinal nerve root canals. *J. Bone and Joint Surg.* **63-B:** 487, 1981.

CROCK H.V., YAMAGISHI M., CROCK M.C.: *The conus medullaris and cauda equina in man. An atlas of the arteries and veins.* Springer Verlag, Wien, New York, 1986.

EISENSTEIN S.: The morphometry and pathological anatomy of the lumbar spine in South African Negroes and Caucasoids with specific reference to spinal stenosis. *J. Bone and Joint Surg.* **59-B:** 173, 1977.

EISENSTEIN S.: The trefoil configuration of the lumbar vertebral canal. A study of South African skeletal material. *J. Bone and Joint Surg.* **62-B:** 73, 1980.

EPSTEIN J.A., EPSTEIN B.S., LEVINE L.S.: Nerve root compression associated with narrowing of the lumbar spinal canal. *J. Neurol. Neurosurg. Psych.* **25:** 165, 1962.

HUIZINGA J., HEIDEN J.A.D.V., VINKEN P.J.J.G.: The human lumbar vertebral canal. A biometric study. *Proc. Kon. Med. Akad. Wet. C.* 55-22, 1952.

LARSEN J.L.: The posterior surface of the lumbar vertebral bodies. Part 1. *Spine* **10:** 50, 1985.

LARSEN J.L.: The posterior surface of the lumbar vertebral bodies. Part 2. An anatomic investigation concerning the curvatures in the horizontal plane. *Spine* **10:** 901, 1985.

LAZORTHES G., POULHES J., BASTIDE G., ROULLEAU J., CHANCOLLE A.R.: Recherches sur la vascularization artérielle de la moelle. Applications à la pathologie médullaire. *Bull. Acad. Nat. Med.* (Paris) **41:** 464, 1957.

LOUIS R.: *Surgery of the spine.* Springer Verlag, Berlin, Heidelberg, New York, 1983.

OBOUNOU-AKONG D.: *Contribution à l'étude topographique des artères rachidiennes et médullaires.* (110 pièces anatomiques). These, Dakar.

PARKE W.W., GAMMEL K., ROTHMAN R.H.: Arterial vascularization of the cauda equina. *J. Bone and Joint Surg.* **63-A:** 53-62, 1981.

PARKE W.W., WATANABE R.: The intrinsic vasculature of the lumbosacral spinal nerve roots. *Spine* **6:** 508, 1985.

POSTACCHINI F., RIPANI M., CARPANO S.: Morphometry of the lumbar vertebrae. An anatomic study in two Caucasoid ethnic groups. *Clin. Ortoph.* **172:** 296, 1983.

RAUSHNING W.: *Detailed sectional anatomy of the lumbar spine.* In: «*Multiplanar CT of the spine*». Ed. by Rothman S.L.G. and Glenn W.V., University Park Press, Baltimore, 1985.

TESTUT L., LATARJET A.: *Trattato di Anatomia Umana.* Utet, Torino, 1963.

VAN SCHAIK J.P.J., VERBIEST H., VAN SCHAIK F.D.J.: The orientation of laminae and facet joints in the lower lumbar spine. *Spine* **10:** 59, 1985.

Chapter III

Definition and classification

STENOSIS AND PSEUDOSTENOSIS

The possibility, in recent years, of visualizing the spinal canal in transverse section by means of tomographic transaxial studies has considerably contributed to our knowledge of the pathological anatomy of the various forms of lumbar stenosis. However, controversy still exists both on the definition, and thus the concept, of lumbar stenosis and the classification of the different forms of stenosis. The lack of a uniform interpretation of pathology and the frequently inappropriate use of the term stenosis produce confusion in the taxonomy of lumbo-radicular diseases and do not allow reliable comparison of different clinical series.

Attempts to rigorously define the concept of lumbar spinal stenosis arise from the need for this term to be universally employed to indicate a well determined group of pathological conditions. This is necessary not only for the need for precision and uniformity in terminology, but also to prevent an erroneous interpretation of the concept of lumbar stenosis from leading one to diagnose and treat conditions of different nature as stenosis.

PREVIOUS DEFINITIONS OF LUMBAR STENOSIS

Verbiest (1973,1975,1975) has defined lumbar stenosis as an abnormal narrowing of the lumbar vertebral canal, resulting from an exceedingly short midsagittal diameter of the canal.

The spinal canal is considered stenotic when the midsagittal diameter measures 12 millimetres or less. In particular, stenosis is referred to as «absolute» when this diameter is 10 millimetres or less and «relative» when it measures 10 to 12 millimetres. The distinction is based on the assumption that, in the former instance, the bony canal is so narrow as to be able, in itself, to produce compression of the cauda equina, whereas in the latter compression of the nervous structures occurs only in the presence of additional agents, such as spondylotic changes or disc protrusions, further reducing the dimensions of the spinal canal. According to Verbiest, stenosis is due to a genetic disturbance that reveals its pathological effects only when growth is complete and the vertebrae have reached their full size. This form of stenosis, indicated as developmental, is usually characterized by normal interpedicular diameters and, very often, abnormally thickened laminae, short pedicles and hypertrophic articular processes. Since the aetiology of the growth disturbance is unknown, this form of stenosis is also called idiopathic. This term allows distinction from those forms of stenosis in which the defective vertebral growth, as occurs in achondroplasia, is caused by well determined pathological conditions, responsible for a general disturbance of skeletal development. Lumbar stenosis may also be an element of a congenital malformation of the lumbar spine (congenital stenosis) or may be caused by acquired conditions (acquired stenosis) such as spondylotic changes, systemic bone diseases or late vertebral fractures. As far as concerns acquired stenosis, however, Verbiest's opinion has oscillated between denial of its existence and admission that a pure acquired stenosis may occur, but only very rarely, since in the vast majority of cases an acquired condition may cause stenosis of the spinal canal only when the latter is primarily narrow. These forms of developmental-acquired stenosis are called «complicated developmental stenosis» to emphasize the prevalent role played, in the aetiopathogenesis, by the developmental narrowing of the spinal canal.

Kirkaldy-Willis *et al.* (1974) have defined lumbar stenosis as «a condition in which the antero-posterior and lateral diameters of the bony canal are narrower than normal and/or in which the shape of the canal in cross section is often abnormal». According to this definition, in order that the spinal canal be considered stenotic, it is sufficient that it is deformed in transverse section or the antero-posterior diameter is below the limits of normal. The authors do not define these limits; however, based on myelographic findings, they consider sagittal dimensions of the contrast column of less than 14 millimetres as pathological. This value, which probably refers to measurements carried out on the lateral myelogram, corresponds approximately, taking into account the radiographic magnification, to the real value of 11 millimetres (using a correction coefficient of 0.8).

Eisenstein (1976,1977) considers as stenotic the vertebrae with the midsagittal and/or the interpedicular diameter of the spinal canal below the lower limits of normal. According to this author, these limits vary, depending on the race and ethnic group, between 12 and 14 millimetres for the antero-posterior diameter and between 17 and 19 millimetres for the transverse diameter. This implies that a relatively high proportion of individuals would be affected by lumbar spinal stenosis. In fact, of the skeletons examined by Eisenstein, 6.7% presented one or more vertebrae which were stenotic in the midsagittal diameter (4.7%) and/or the interpedicular diameter (2%).

In 1976, a group of 21 authors (Arnoldi *et al.*) defined lumbar spinal stenosis as «any type of narrowing of the spinal canal, nerve root canals or intervertebral foramina. It may be local, segmental or generalized. It may be caused by bone or by soft tissue and the narrowing may involve the bony canal alone or the dural sac or both». This definition, emphasizing the possibility that stenosis of the nerve root canal or the intervertebral foramen may occur as an isolated condition, extends the concept of stenosis to all the pathological conditions causing a narrowing of the spinal canal, including disc herniations, when these «occur together with other types of stenosis».

THE CONCEPT OF STENOSIS

I have defined lumbar spinal stenosis as an *abnormal narrowing of the osteoligamentous vertebral canal and/or the intervertebral foramina, which is responsible for compression of the dural sac and/or the caudal nerve roots. Narrowing of the vertebral canal may involve one or more levels and, at a single level, may affect the whole canal or part of the canal* (Postacchini, 1983).

Based on this definition, abnormal narrowing of the spinal canal may be regarded as stenosis if two criteria are fulfilled: narrowing involves the osteoligamentous spinal canal, and causes a compression of the nervous structures contained in the canal.

The first criterion implies a sharp distinction between disc pathology and stenosis. This distinction may appear to be arbitrary both on account of the fact that the intervertebral disc contributes to delimit the spinal canal and because, in stenosis, compression of the nervous structures is often caused by a co-existing disc disease, in the form of a more or less marked annular bulging or disc protrusion (Fig. 3.1). However, if the concept of stenosis is not limited to the osteo-ligamentous vertebral canal, even a protrusion or herniation of the nucleus pulposus becomes a stenotic condition. In the strictest sense, in fact, a disc prolapse causes stenosis, that is a pathological narrowing of the whole or part of the spinal canal. However, since the two conditions — disc herniation and stenosis — differ considerably in the pathogenesis and anatomo-clinical characteristics, they cannot be considered as a single pathological entity. The alternative would be to specify, in each instance, whether stenosis is of a discal, osteo-ligamentous or other etiology, but hopefully this were not to be the case since, instead of order and clearness, it would give rise to uncertainty in the taxonomy of lumbo-radicular syndromes. Furthermore, it should be pointed

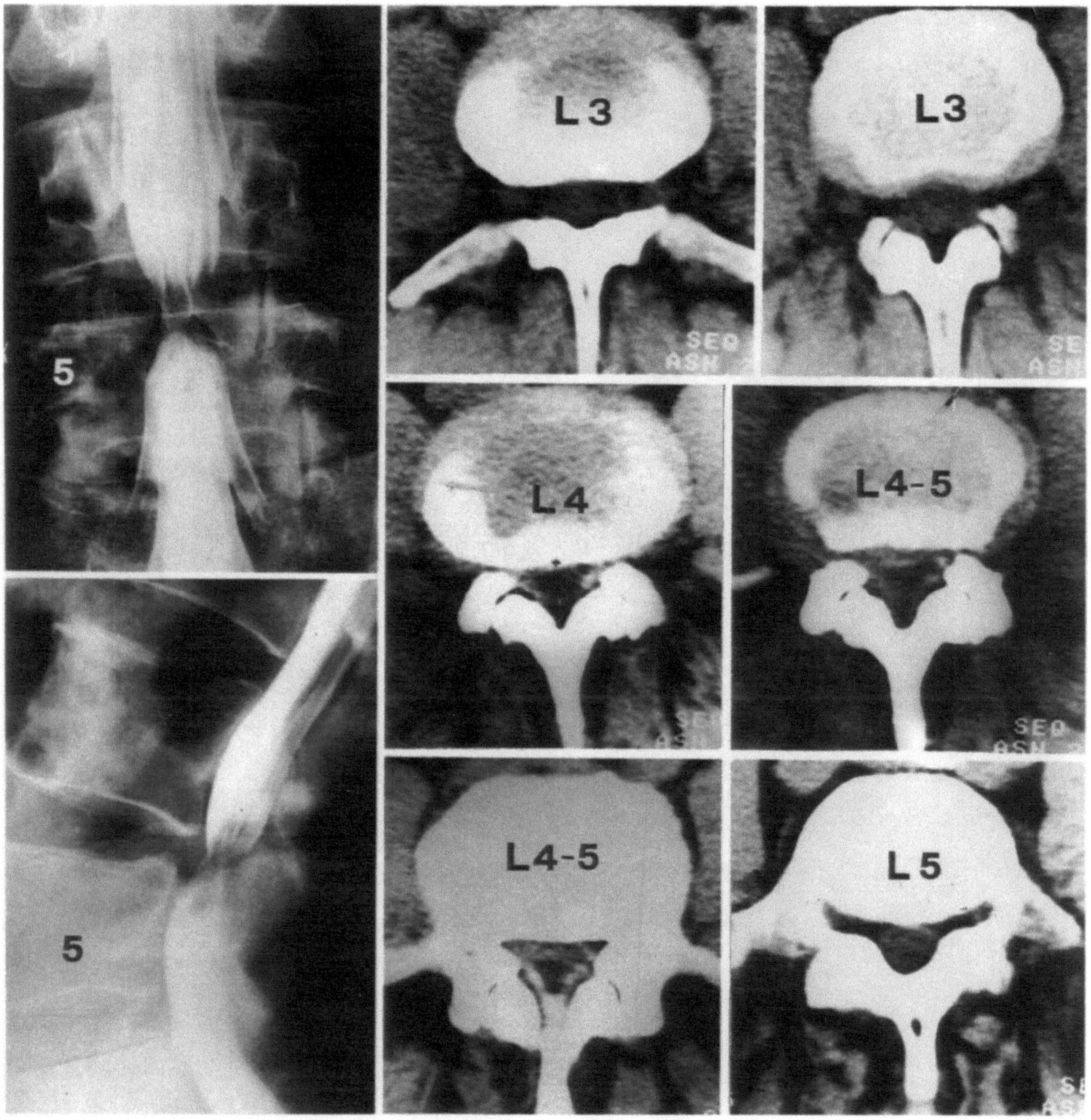

Fig. 3.1 - Single level stenosis of the spinal canal at L_4-L_5. The lateral meylogram shows a marked posterior indentation of the dural sac produced by the osteoligamentous structures of the neural arch and an anterior, relatively mild indentation, caused by a bulging annulus fibrosus. CT scans reveal developmental narrowing of the spinal canal and hypertrophy of the articular processes at L_4-L_5 level. At this level, the posterior bulging of the annulus fibrosus is clearly visible.

out that disc changes represent a marginal element in the pathological anatomy of stenosis. The peculiarity of the latter, in fact, lies in the compression of the dural sac and the spinal nerve roots by the osteoligamentous components of the canal. Anterior compression by the disc, as well as posterior encroachment by thickened ligamenta flava, may increase the narrowing of the spinal canal and contribute to determine clinical symptoms and signs, but do not represent necessary factors in the genesis of stenosis. The distinction between disc herniation and stenosis remains valid even when the two con-

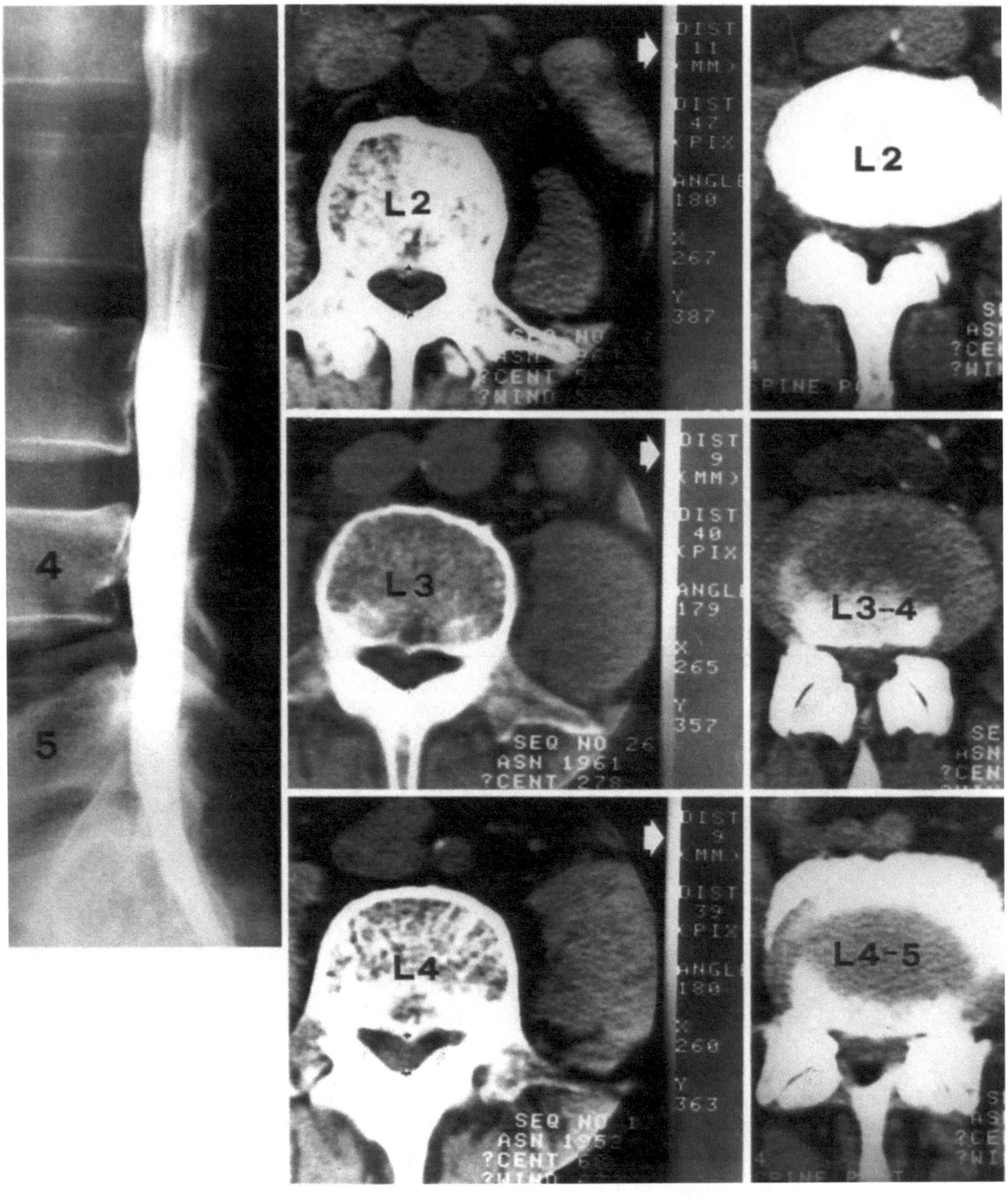

Fig. 3.2 - Narrow spinal canal. The lateral myelogram reveals narrowing of the contrast column in the sagittal direction at all lumbar levels, but shows no compression of the dural sac. Sagittal narrowing of the vertebral canal is confirmed by CT scans. The arrows indicate the midsagittal dimensions of the spinal canal at L_2 (11 mm), L_3 (9 mm) and L_4 (9 mm). At L_3-L_4 and L_4-L_5 levels, no constriction of the dural sac is visible, despite hypertrophy of the articular processes.

ditions are associated at the same level or at different levels, that is when the combined condition of disc herniation in a narrow spinal canal occurs. On the other hand, bulging of the annulus fibrosus at multiple levels cannot be regarded as a stenotic condition, in the absence of an abnormal narrowing of the osteoligamentous spinal canal.

The second criterion emphasizes the concept of compression of the dural sac and nerve roots, which is implicit in the term stenosis. This term, in fact, indicates a dimensional disproportion between the calibre of the container and the volume of the content. If the content is a fluid, as in blood vessels, there is a reduced flow throughout the stenotic area. Conversely, if the content is a solid or semifluid, as in the vertebral canal, the dimensional disproportion results in compression of the content by the walls of the container. The disproportion, however, is not strictly related to the anteroposterior dimensions of the vertebral canal. Severe compression of the nervous structures may occur even if the midsagittal dimensions of the canal are within normal limits. On the other hand, a midsagittal diameter of 10 millimeters or less does not necessarily lead to compression of the cauda equina (Fig. 3. 2).

This is probably due to the fact that, in normal conditions, the nervous structures contained in the spinal canal develop in harmony with the dimensions of the canal. When this does not occur, the reserve space available for the dural sac and/or the nerve roots of the cauda equina is variably reduced and, therefore, acquired constrictive agents of even minor entity will be sufficient to cause stenosis. If narrowing is not severe enough to cause compression of the nervous structures, the spinal canal is to be considered *narrow* but not stenotic. This interpretation is supported by two series of observations: a) of the two skeletal populations — Italian and Asiatic Indian — in which Postacchini *et al.* (1983) measured the midsagittal diameter of the vertebral foramen, the Indian showed a lower limit of normal of 11.5 mm, a value generally considered as pathological; b) the midsagittal diameters of the foramen measured, at one or more vertebral levels, 10.1 to 10.8 mm in 5% of the Italian skeletons and 9 to 10.5 mm in 10% of the Indian skeletons — such high percentages, compared to the incidence of lumbar stenosis syndromes, as to exclude that during life these narrow canals, or at least the majority of them, might have been responsible for cauda equina compression.

The clinical importance of these findings is that diagnosis of stenosis cannot be made on the basis of measurements of the vertebral canal, such as those obtained by computerized tomography, or the finding, on the lateral myelogram, of a uniform narrowing of the dye column throughout the whole, or almost whole, length of the lumbar spinal canal. Diagnosis of stenosis should only be based on the demonstration of compression of the vertebral nervous structures — which may be clinically symptomatic or asymptomatic — by an abnormally narrow osteoligamentous spinal canal.

The nerve root canal, like the spinal canal, should be considered stenotic when compression of the nerve root is only or mainly due to changes in the osteoligamentous components of the canal. The term stenosis, therefore, is appropriate when compression of the nerve root is related, as frequently occurs, to bulging of the annulus fibrosus, unable in itself to produce a radicular syndrome in a normally sized nerve root canal; it is not appropriate when the radicular syndrome is caused by a disc herniation protruding in a more or less narrow nerve root canal.

PSEUDOSTENOSIS

This term should be reserved for a few pathologic conditions — isthmic spondylolisthesis, vertebral tumors and so-called fibrous stenosis — which, though showing several anatomo-clinical similarities with typically stenotic conditions, cannot be considered as true forms of stenosis.

Many classifications of lumbar spinal stenosis include isthmic spondylolisthesis, when this causes compression of the lumbar nervous structures and a clinical pattern of the stenotic type (Schatzker and Pennal, 1968; Kirkaldy-Willis *et al.*, 1974; Arnoldi

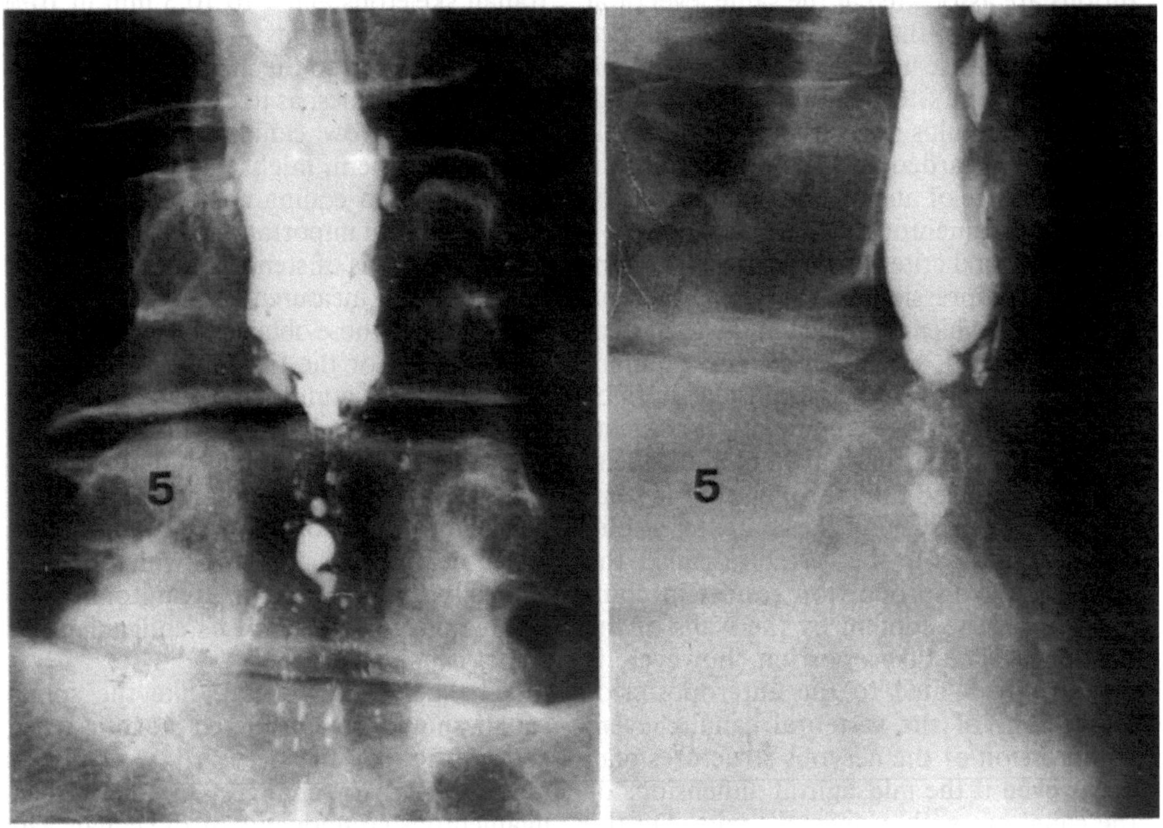

Fig. 3.3 - Complete myelographic block in a patient previously submitted to bilateral laminectomy at L_4-L_5 level. Compression of the nervous structures is caused by peridural scar tissue.

Table 3.I - CLASSIFICATION OF THE VARIOUS FORMS OF LUMBAR STENOSIS

Spinal canal stenosis

Primary
- congenital
- developmental: in achondroplasia or other forms of dwarfism
  idiopathic

Secondary
- degenerative (with or without spondylolisthesis)
- late sequelae of fractures
- late sequelae of infections
- in systemic bone diseases

Combined
- association of primary and secondary stenosis at the same vertebral level

Mixed
- primary and secondary (and/or combined) stenosis at different vertebral levels

Isolated nerve root canal stenosis

Primary
Secondary
Combined

Stenosis of intervertebral foramen

Primary
Secondary
Combined

et al., 1976; Hasue *et al.*, 1977). Indeed, only degenerative spondylolisthesis may be considered as a form of stenosis. In this type of spondylolisthesis, in fact, compression of the nervous structures of the spinal canal is caused not only by vertebral slipping, which is often of mild degree, but rather by osteoarthrotic changes of the articular processes (Perugia and Postacchini, 1980). In isthmic spondylolisthesis, compression of the nervous structures is due to kinking of the dural sac on the vertebra below that presenting olisthesis and the fibrocartilagineous tissue filling the isthmic defect. In this form of spondylolisthesis, in other words, the osteoligamentous spinal canal is deformed, but not narrowed. Indeed, at the level of the olisthetic vertebra, the spinal canal is wider than normal in the sagittal plane, since the dorsal portion of the vertebral arch does not follow the vertebral body in the anterior slipping.

Vertebral tumours may produce narrowing of the spinal canal due to invasion of the canal by neoplastic tissue and/or increase in volume and deformation of the affected vertebral components. In the latter instance, narrowing of the canal caused by a tumour could be included among the true stenotic conditions. Tumours, however, have such peculiar biological, pathological and clinical characteristics that they cannot be associated with the conditions responsible for the true forms of stenosis. The use of the term pseudostenosis to indicate narrowing of the spinal canal caused by tumours underlines the very close affinity that such narrowing may have with stenosis, allowing at the same time the two entities to be kept separate from the taxonomic point of view.

So-called fibrous stenosis is produced by the fibrous or osteofibrous membrane replacing the vertebral arch at the site of a previous laminectomy (Fig. 3.3). In some instances, this membrane may be responsible for compression of the nervous structures, thus causing clinical symptoms and signs of a stenotic type. This particular pathological condition, however, is to be considered at the most a pseudostenotic condition, but not a true stenosis. The most appropriate term to indicate this condition, as indeed any form of compression of the nervous structures by epidural scar tissue, is constrictive epidural fibrosis.

CLASSIFICATION

Lumbar spinal stenosis may be distinguished, on the grounds of anatomopathological features, as: stenosis of the spinal canal, isolated stenosis of the nerve root canal, and stenosis of the intervertebral foramen (Table 3.I).

In stenosis of the spinal canal only the central portion of the canal may be constricted or, as very often occurs, both the latter and the nerve root canal, either on one side or both sides.

In isolated stenosis of the nerve root canal, only this canal is narrowed, whereas the central spinal canal is normal in width or is of such shape and size as not to deter-

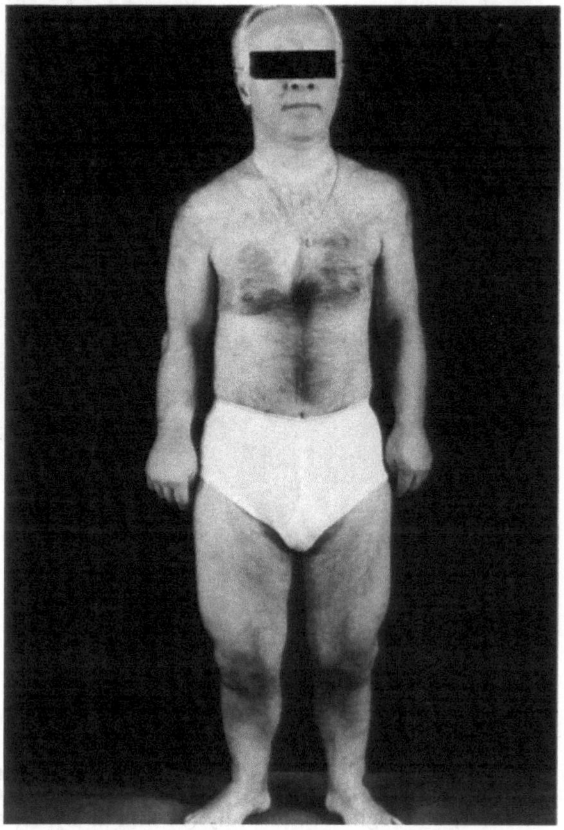

Fig. 3.4 - Achondroplastic dwarf with multilevel lumbar spinal stenosis as shown in Fig. 3.5.

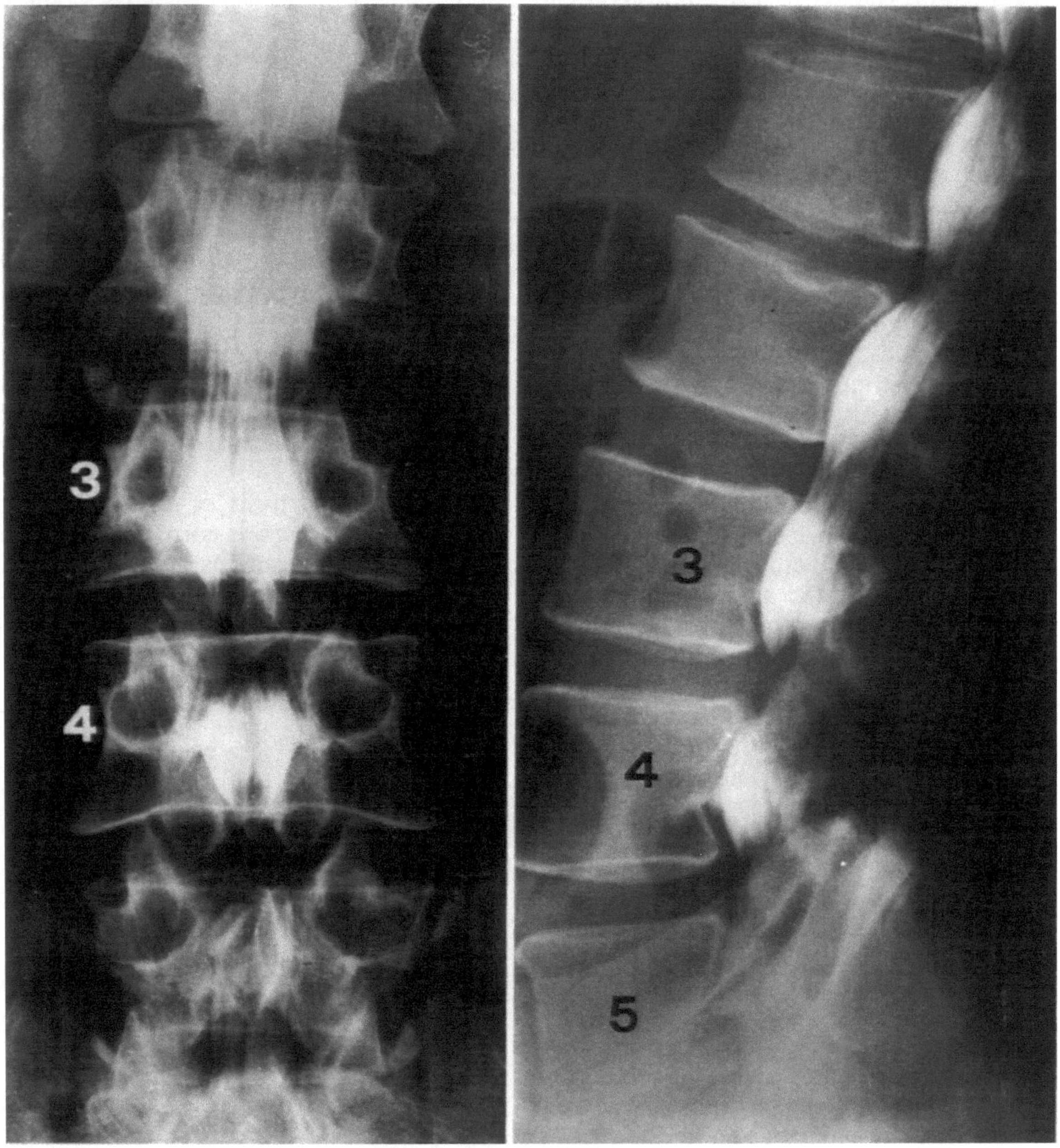

▲

Fig. 3.5 - Lumbar myelograms and CT scans of the achondroplastic dwarf in figure 3.4. Myelograms show ▶ a complete block of the dye column at L_3-L_4 and L_4-L_5. At the supradjacent intervertebral levels, compression of the dural sac is less severe. On CT scans, the midsagittal diameters of the vertebral canal appear to be short, although not markedly (12 mm at L_2, L_3 and L_4). Conversely, the interpedicular diameter is very small at all lumbar levels, and the pedicles are abnormally short. The articular processes make the central spinal canal more narrow, particularly at L_4-L_5 level. Note the narrowing of the nerve root canals at L_3-L_4 and L_4-L_5 levels.

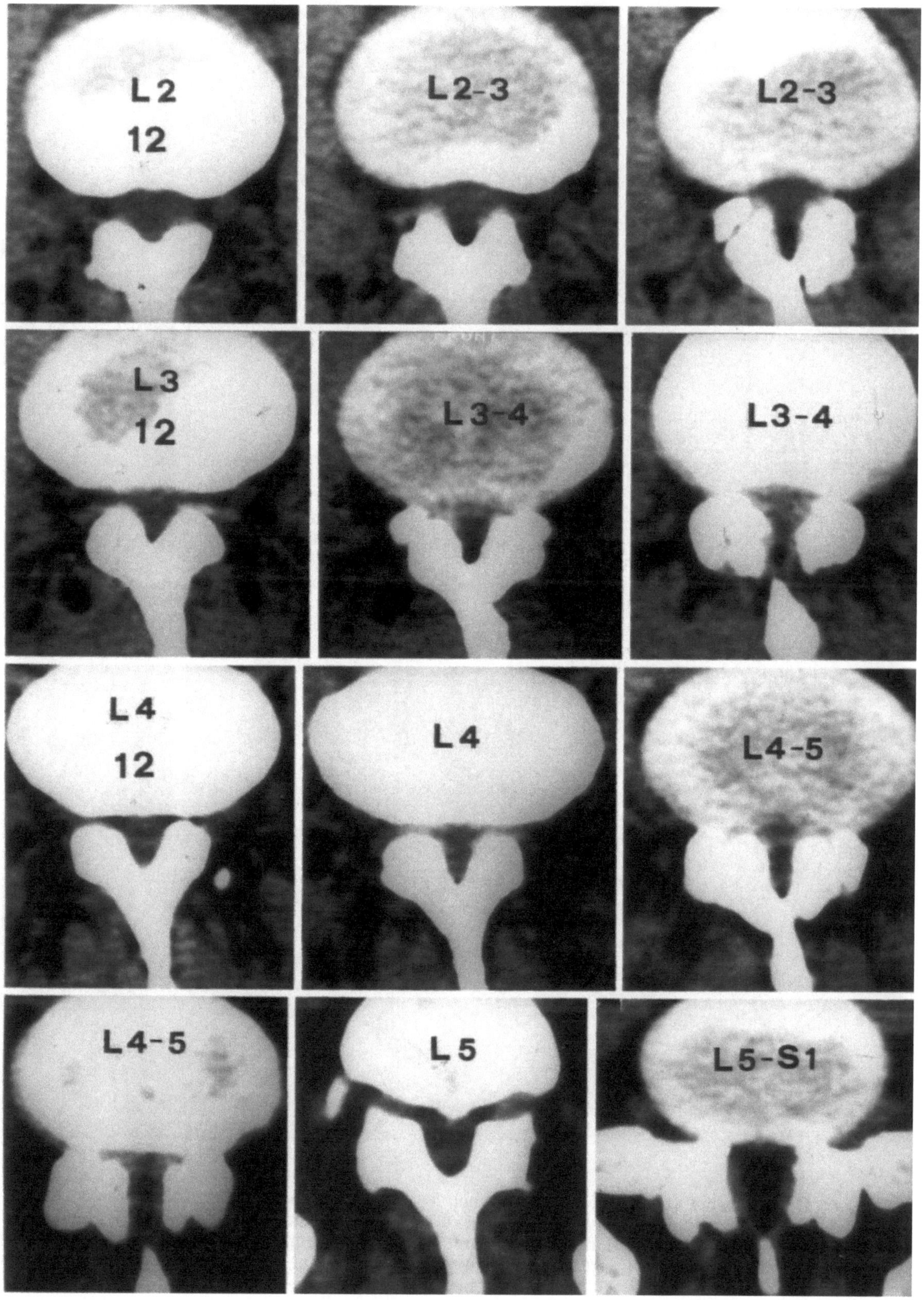

Fig. 3.5

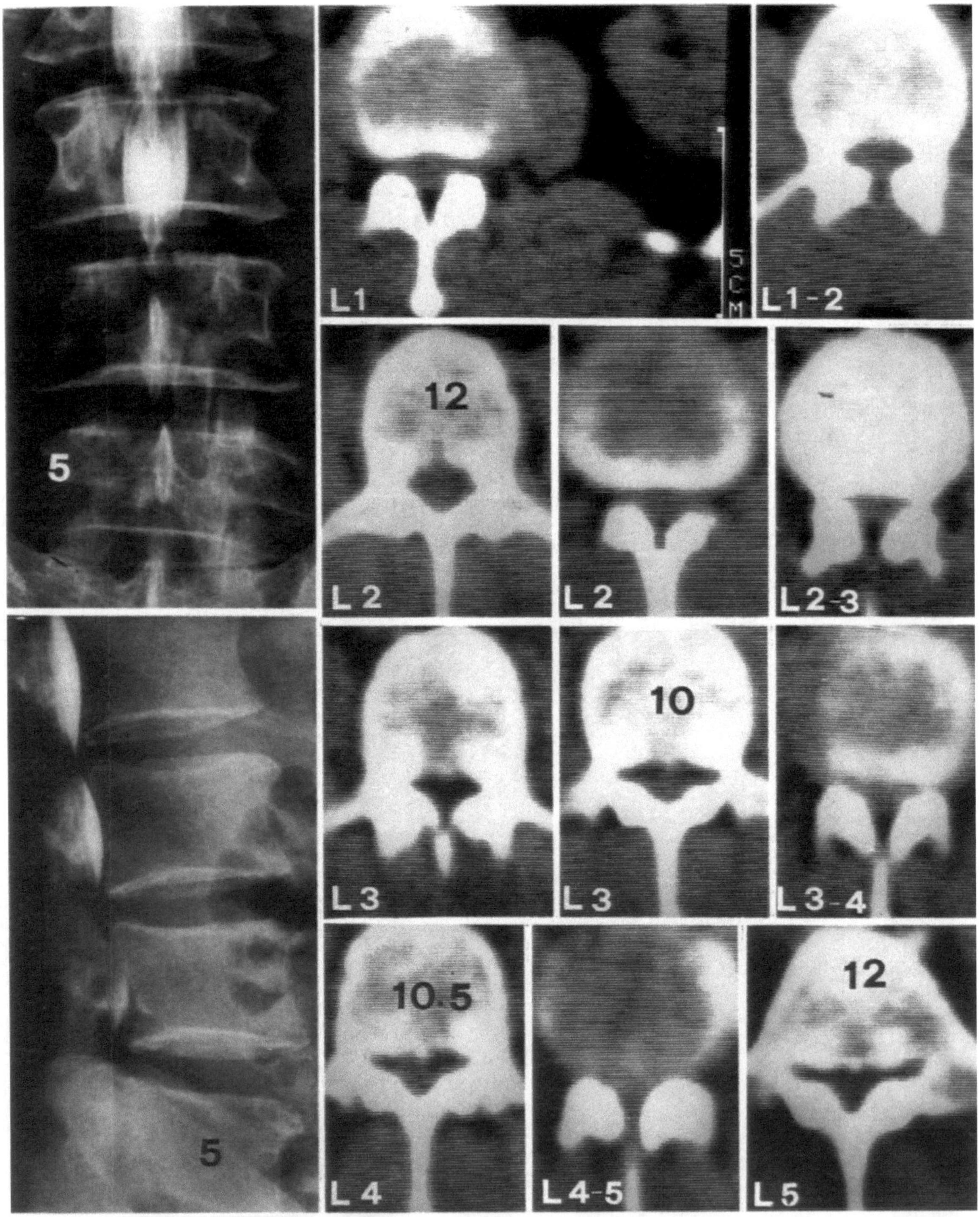

Fig. 3.6 - Developmental stenosis of the spinal canal. Myelograms show multiple blocks of the contrast medium at the four lower lumbar intervertebral spaces. CT scans reveal abnormally short midsagittal diameters of the spinal canal at L_3 (10 mm) and L_4 (10.5 mm) levels, short laminae, and sagittally oriented articular processes. The latter show mild degenerative changes. (The midsagittal diameter of the spinal canal, which is marked on a few vertebral bodies, may be calculated from the scale at L_1 level).

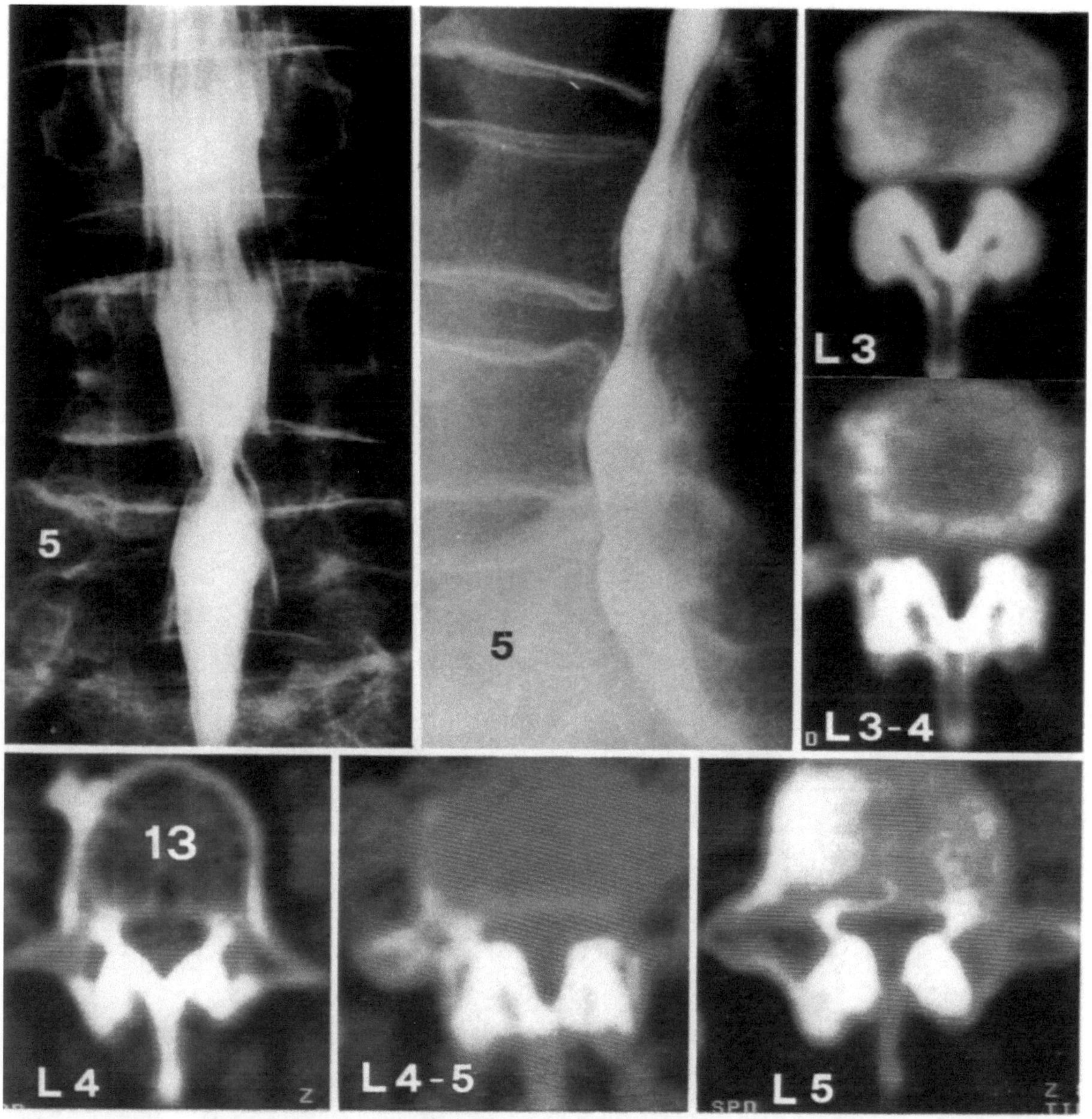

Fig. 3.7 - Degenerative spinal canal stenosis. Myelograms show lateral and posterior constrictions of the nervous structures at L_4-L_5 level and posterior compression of the dye column at L_3-L_4 and L_2-L_3. On CT scans, the vertebral canal displays normal midsagittal dimensions (13 mm at L_4). The articular processes, which appear to be hypertrophic, encroach on the nerve root canals and/or the central portion of the spinal canal at L_4-L_5 and L_3-L_4 levels.

mine any compression of the nervous structures. In these cases, stenosis may be classified as spinal canal stenosis or isolated stenosis of the nerve root canal, depending on the severity of the narrowing of the central spinal canal.

Stenosis of the intervertebral foramen may be isolated or associated with one of the other two forms of lumbar stenosis.

SPINAL CANAL STENOSIS

This includes primary, secondary, combined and mixed forms.

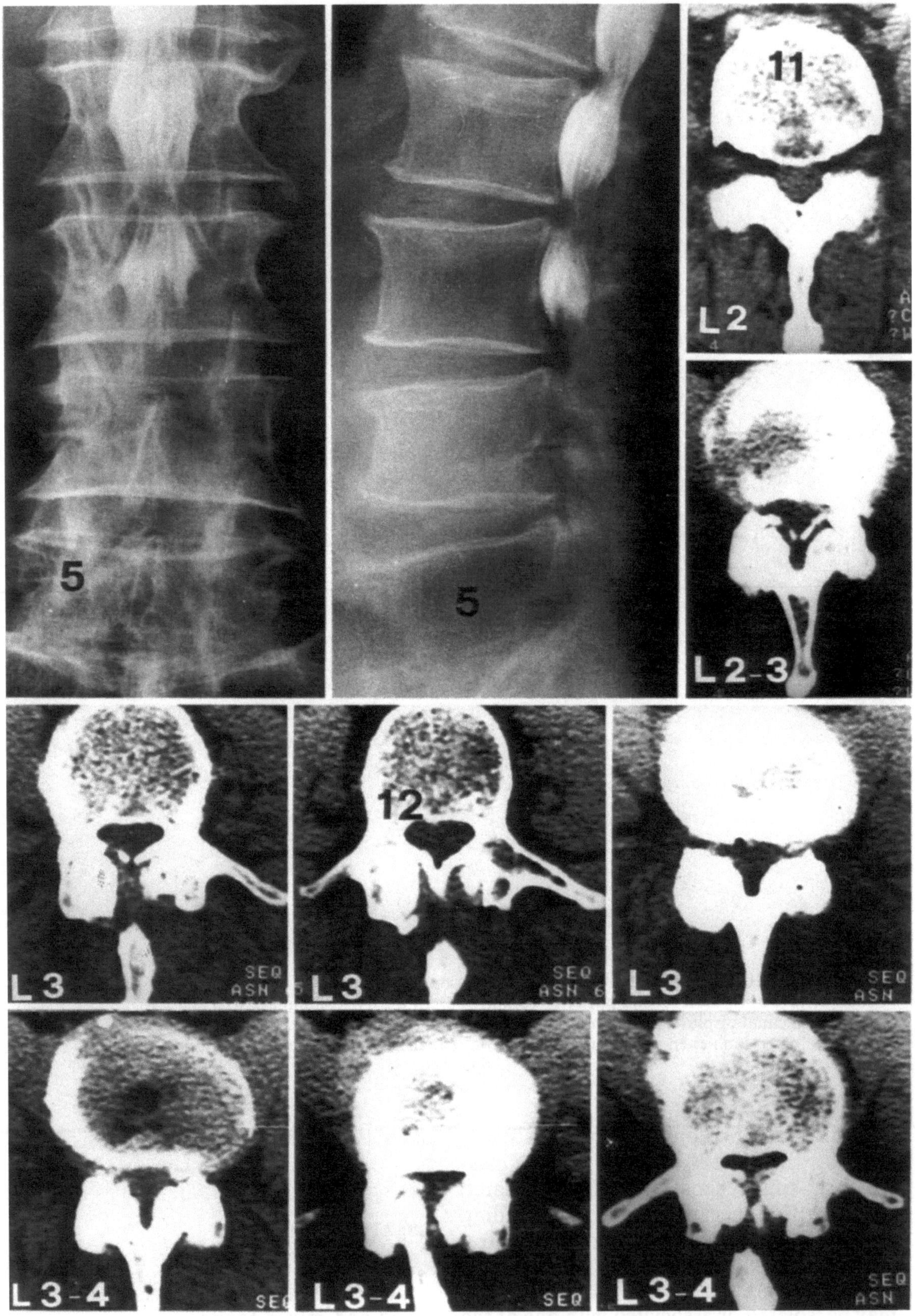
5
5
11
L2
L2-3
L3
SEQ
ASN
12
L3
SEQ
ASN
L3
SEQ
ASN
L3-4
L3-4
SEQ
L3-4
SEQ
ASN

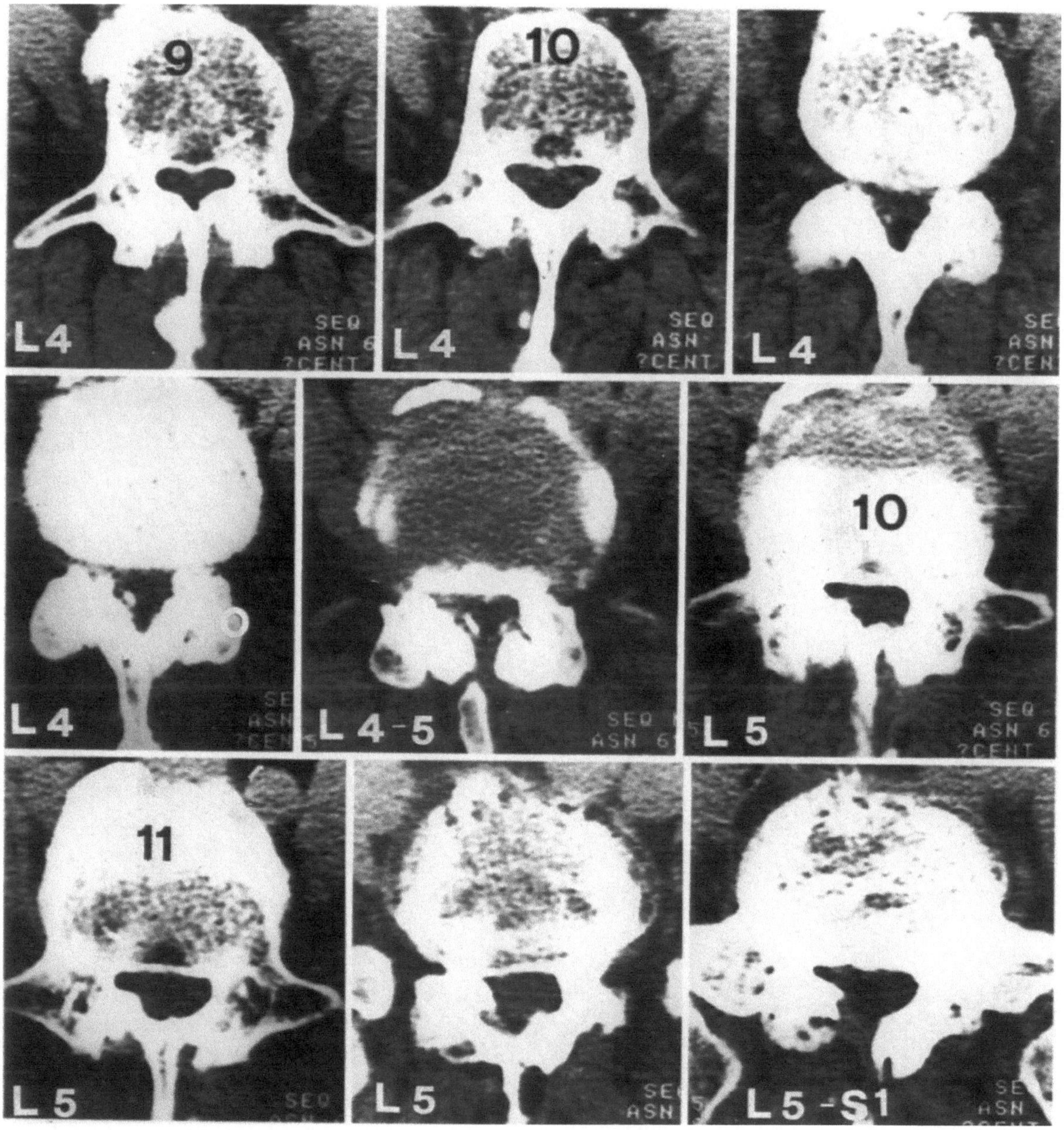

▲

◀ **Fig. 3.8** - Combined spinal canal stenosis, responsible for a complete myelographic block at L_3-L_4 and a subtotal block at L_2-L_3. CT scan: the midsagittal dimensions of the vertebral canal in the transpedicular sections are below the limits of normal; the articular processes show marked arthrotic changes, which further narrow and distort the spinal canal; in many scans the ligamenta flava appear to be calcified. (The midsagittal dimensions, in millimetres, of the spinal canal are marked, in a few scans, on the vertebral bodies).

Primary stenosis

In primary stenosis lumbar spinal canal may be constricted due to congenital malformations or to a disorder in postnatal development of the lumbar vertebrae, compression of the nerve roots of the cauda equina being exclusively or essentially due to the abnormal primary narrowing. Two types of primary stenosis may be identified, congenital and developmental.

Congenital stenosis, which is very rare,

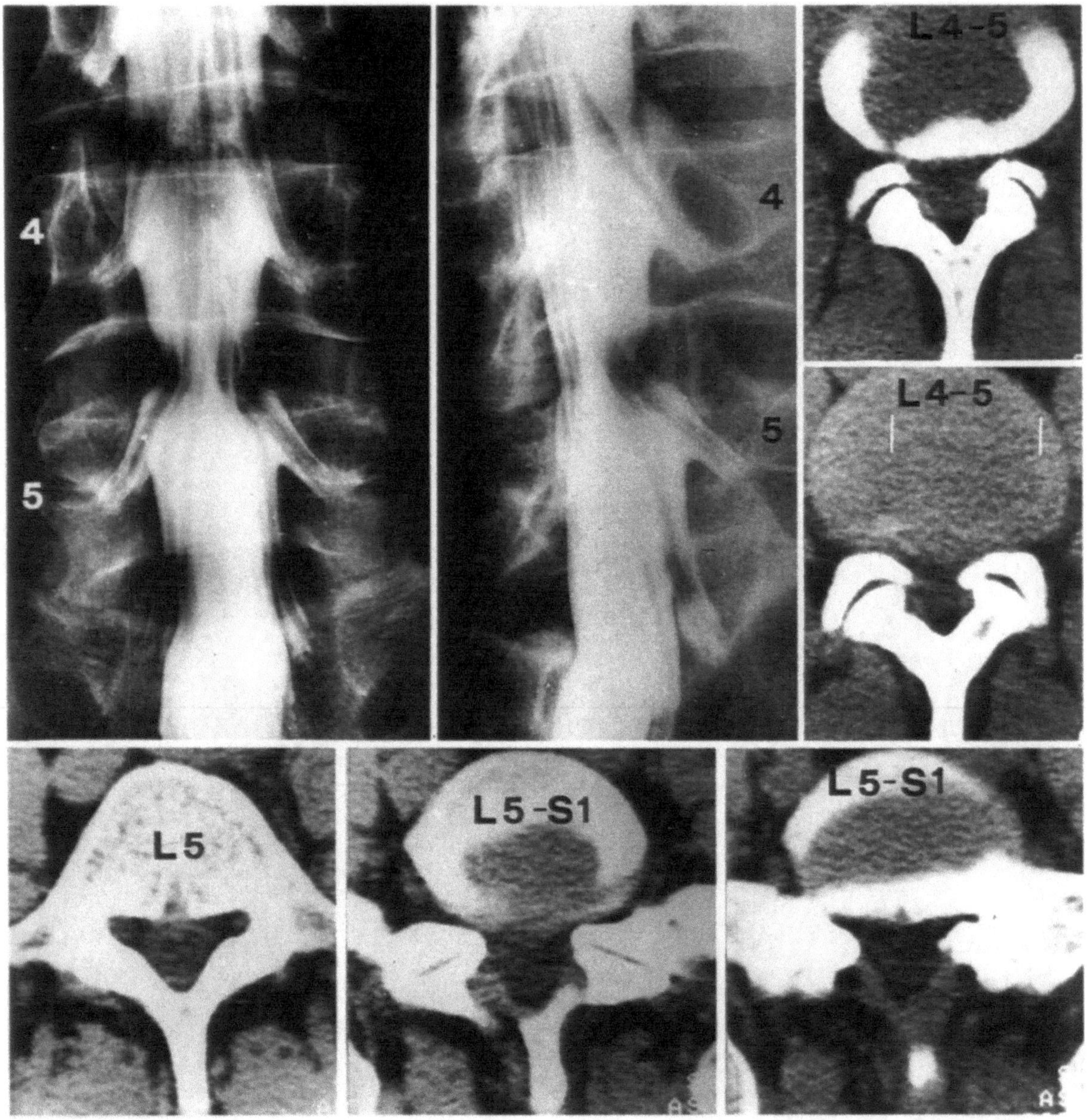

Fig. 3.9 - Isolated stenosis of the nerve root canal at L_4-L_5 and L_5-S_1, bilaterally. Myelograms show filling defects of L_5 and S_1 nerve root sheaths on both sides. On CT scans, the L_5 nerve root canals appear constricted at intervertebral level due not only to hypertrophy of the superior articular processes, the medial border of which encroaches on the vertebral canal, but also to a mild central protrusion of the L_4-L_5 disc. Similar, although less marked, changes can be seen at L_5-S_1 level.

is due to congenital malformations of the vertebral body and/or the posterior arch. The term congenital does not indicate that stenosis is present at birth, but that it is caused exclusively or essentially by a malformative condition. A stenotic condition present at birth has, in fact, never been reported. Compression of the nervous structures usually becomes apparent in adult age, when primary narrowing of the spinal canal is critically accentuated by osteoligamentous or disk changes, which in a normally sized spinal canal would not produce, on account of their mild entity, any pathological effect.

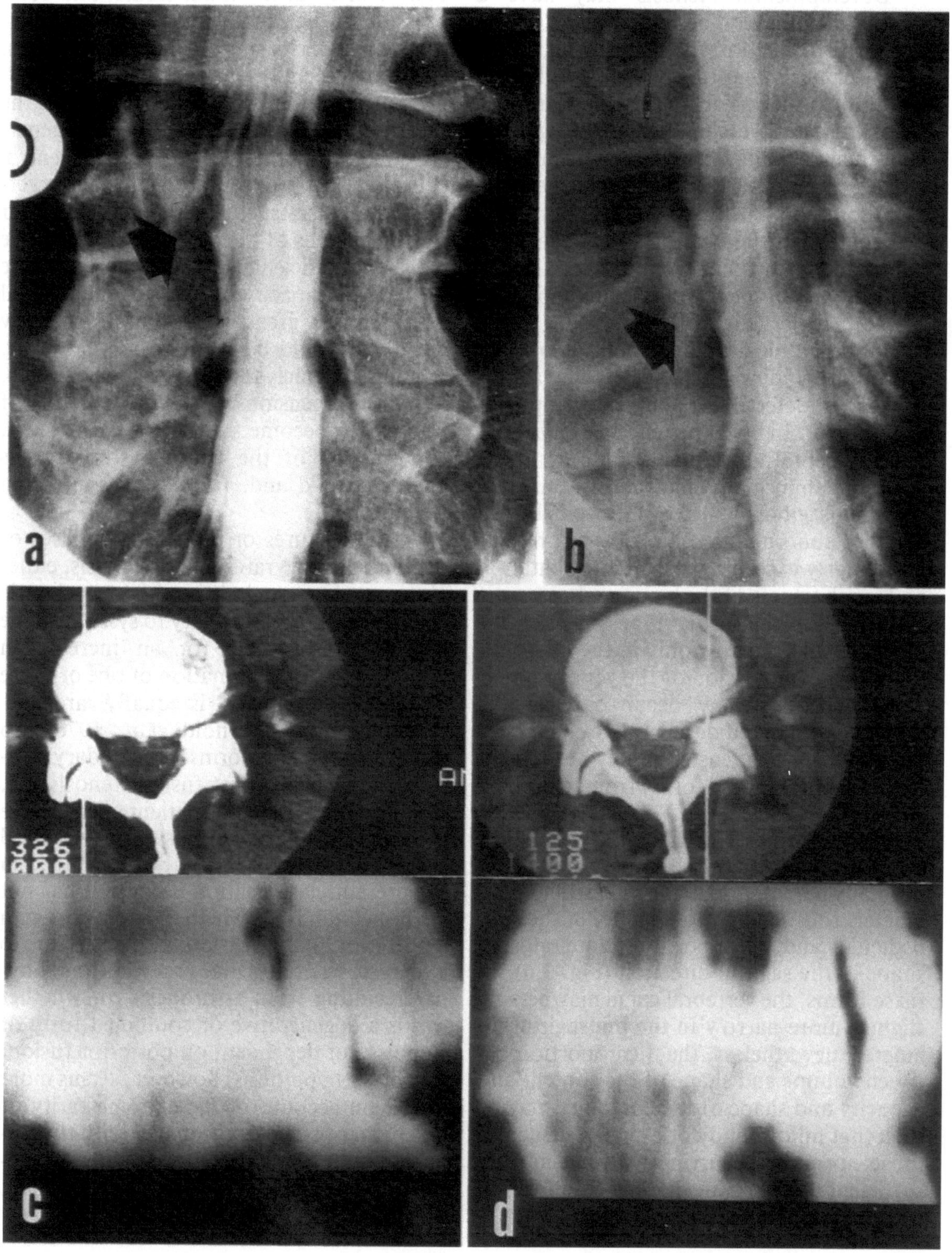

Fig. 3.10 - Isolated stenosis of the right L_4-L_5 intervertebral foramen. **a.** and **b.** Myelograms show non-filling of the L_4 nerve root sheath, which appears to be dilated above the site of compression. **c.** and **d.** On CT scans, the right L_4-L_5 intervertebral foramen (**c**) appears severely narrowed, whereas the left foramen (**d**) appears to be normal.

Developmental stenosis may have a known aetiology or be idiopathic.

In the former instance, narrowing of the spinal canal is due to known pathological conditions, such as achondroplasia or Morquio's disease, which are related to genetic abnormalities with a hereditary transmission. In the achondroplastic forms, which are the most common, the midsagittal and/or interpedicular diameters of the spinal canal are abnormally short and the nerve root canals show a marked narrowing due to shortness of the pedicles (Figs. 3.4 and 3.5).

In idiopathic developmental stenosis, or more simply idiopathic stenosis, the aetiology of the defective vertebral development is unknown. In my experience, two types of developmental abnormality may be identified: the abnormality may consist only in a short midsagittal diameter of the spinal canal or other abnormalities may also be present, particularly exceedingly sagittal orientation and/or shortness of the laminae. In stenotic conditions of the former type, in which the spinal canal is narrow only in the midsagittal plane, compression of the vertebral nervous structures may occur only in the presence of marked degenerative changes of the spine; for this reason, it may be difficult to differentiate these forms from combined stenoses.

In the forms of the second type, which are the most typical, the spinal canal is abnormally narrow also in the interarticular diameter, thus tending to assume, in the subpedicular and discal portions, an elongated shape in the sagittal direction (Fig. 3.6). In these forms, the vertebral canal may be only slightly more narrow in the midsagittal diameter; nevertheless, the disproportion between volume and shape of the content and capacity and shape of the container may be such that mild spondylotic changes (such as those normally occurring with ageing) are sufficient to determine marked compression of the vertebral nervous structures.

Secondary stenosis

In secondary stenosis the midsagittal dimensions of the spinal canal are normal, even if often at the lower limits, and compression of the caudal nerve roots is due exclusively to one or more acquired conditions. These are generally represented by spondylotic changes of the vertebral body and/or the facet joints, associated or not with degenerative spondylolisthesis (Fig. 3.7). As a general rule, in order for compression of the vertebral nervous structures to occur, the wider the dimensions of the canal the more severe the spondylotic changes have to be, because the reserve capacity of a large spinal canal is tendentially greater than that of a narrow canal. It should be pointed out, however, that it is extremely rare for a very wide canal, i.e. with dimensions at the upper limits of normal, to become stenotic; if this occurs, compression of the nervous structures is generally mild and, for this reason, often asymptomatic.

Late fractures or infectious diseases of the lumbar spine rarely cause stenosis, either alone or in association with spondylotic changes. Stenosis secondary to systemic bone diseases, responsible for an increase in volume and/or deformation of one or more vertebral components, is equally rare.

Some authors (Arnoldi *et al.*, 1976) also include, among the forms of secondary stenosis, the so-called post-fusion stenosis, i.e. stenosis presenting in patients who have previously undergone posterior vertebral fusion. This form has not been included in the present classification because it has not yet been established whether, in patients with a posterior lumbar fusion, stenosis is due to hyperostosis of articular processes and laminae resulting from arthrodesis, or whether this is a degenerative or combined form of stenosis not dependent on posterior fusion. The latter hypothesis, however, seems more likely, on account of the extreme rarity of this form of stenosis compared with the frequency with which posterior fusions are performed, particularly in the surgical treatment of scoliosis.

Combined stenosis

Primary narrowing of the spinal canal is associated, at the same vertebral level, with a secondary narrowing, generally spondylotic in nature (Fig. 3.8). Combined stenosis can be differentiated from primary stenosis by the fact that, in the former, developmental narrowing is usually relatively mild and the degenerative changes are more marked than in the primary forms. The distinction between the various forms of secondary stenosis and combined stenoses is very clear-cut for the degenerative forms, but not for the other secondary forms. In degenerative stenosis, in fact, the finding of a normal midsagittal diameter of the vertebral canal in the axial tomograms excludes the possibility that stenosis is combined in nature. In contrast, in the other secondary forms, in which also the midsagittal diameter is generally short, it may be difficult to exclude a primary narrowing.

Mixed stenosis

Mixed stenosis is characterized by primary stenosis at one or more vertebral levels and secondary or combined stenosis at other levels. This form of stenosis is, however, identified for taxonomic rather than anatomo-clinical reasons, because it may be difficult or even impossible to differentiate between mixed stenosis and primary or combined stenosis *in vivo*.

ISOLATED STENOSIS OF THE NERVE ROOT CANAL

Stenosis of the nerve root canal may be due to: a) disturbances of vertebral development, particularly abnormal shortness of the pedicles, even more so if associated with a trefoil configuration of the spinal canal, or anomalous orientation and/or shape of the superior articular process; b) acquired factors, such as hypertrophy and/or osteophytosis of the superior articular process, osteophytosis of the posterolateral portion of the vertebral end-plates, retrolisthesis of the upper adjacent vertebra, late post-traumatic changes; c) association — this being the most frequent occurrence — of primary and secondary pathological conditions. Therefore, even in stenosis of the nerve root canal, primary, secondary and combined forms may be identified. Distinction between the various forms, however, is often difficult in the individual patient, and is, in any event, much less clear-cut than in stenosis of the spinal canal.

The nerve root canal may be stenotic at the level of the proximal portion, corresponding to the intervertebral disc, or the caudal portion, represented by the lateral recess.

The most frequent site of stenosis, or at least of symptomatic stenosis, is the portion corresponding to the intervertebral disc, because at this level the narrowing caused by the bony component of the canal may easily be increased, in a critical measure for the root, by a bulge of varying entity of the annulus fibrosus (Fig. 3.9).

The second portion, corresponding to the lateral recess, is more rarely stenotic, because the walls of the nerve root canal, in this portion, are entirely formed by bony structures. Nerve root compression at this level is usually caused by posterior osteophytes of the superior vertebral end-plate and/or degenerative changes of the superior articular process at the level of its basal portion, facing the vertebral body. Stenosis of this second portion of the canal, however, is generally associated with stenosis of the first portion, at least when narrowing is caused by abnormalities of the superior articular process, which usually involve the entire height of the latter.

STENOSIS OF THE INTERVERTEBRAL FORAMEN

Stenosis of the neuroforamen, at one level or more levels, is not rarely associated with stenosis of the spinal canal, particularly in degenerative forms. On the contrary, it is fairly rare to observe isolated stenosis of the intervertebral foramen (Fig. 3.10). In fact, while it is not infrequent to observe abnormal narrowing of the neuroforamen due to excessive shortness of the pedicles, a decrease in height of the intervertebral disc or osteoarthritic changes of the vertebral body and/or the articular processes, compression of the spinal nerve root is rarely caused by such narrowing. This is due to the fact that the intervertebral foramen has a fairly large reserve capacity. Therefore, the association of two or more pathological conditions is usually necessary, in order for narrowing of such entity to cause nerve root compression to occur.

REFERENCES

ARNOLDI C.C., BRODSKY A.E., CAUCHOIX J., CROCK H.V., DOMMISSE G.A. et al.: Lumbar spinal stenosis and nerve root entrapment syndromes. Definition and classification. *Clin. Orthop.* **115:** 4, 1976.

EISENSTEIN S.: Measurements of the lumbar spinal canal in 2 racial groups. *Clin. Orthop.* **115:** 42, 1976.

EISENSTEIN S.: The morphometry and pathological anatomy of the lumbar spine in South African Negroes and Caucasoids with specific reference to spinal stenosis. *J. Bone and Joint Surg.* **59-B:** 173, 1977.

KIRKALDY-WILLIS W.H., PAINE K.W.E., CAUCHOIX J., MCIVOR G.: Lumbar spinal stenosis. *Clin. Orthop.* **99:** 30, 1974.

PERUGIA L., POSTACCHINI F.: Le stenosi lombari. *Giorn. Ital. Ortop. Traumatol.* Suppl. 2, **6:** 47, 1980.

POSTACCHINI F.: Lumbar spinal stenosis and pseudostenosis. Definition and classification of pathology. *Italian Journal of Orthopaedics and Traumatology* **9:** 339, 1983.

POSTACCHINI F., RIPANI M., CARPANO S.: Morphometry of the lumbar vertebrae. An anatomic study in two Caucasoid ethnic groups. *Clin. Orthop.* **172:** 296, 1983.

SCHATZKER J., PENNAL G.F.: Spinal stenosis. A cause of cauda equina compression. *J. Bone and Joint Surg.* **50-B:** 606, 1968.

VERBIEST H.: Neurogenic intermittent claudication in cases with absolute and relative stenosis of the lumbar vertebral canal (ASLC and RSLC), in cases with narrow lumbar intervertebral foramina, and in cases with both entities. *Clin. Neurosurg.* **20:** 204, 1973.

VERBIEST H.: Pathomorphologic aspects of developmental lumbar stenosis. *Orthop. Clin. North Am.* **6:** 177, 1975.

VERBIEST H.: *Neurogenic intermittent claudication. Lesions of the spinal cord and cauda equina, stenosis of the vertebral canal, narrowing of intervertebral foramina and entrapment of peripheral nerves.* In «*Clinical Neurology*», vo. 20, cap. 19, 1976.

Chapter IV
Epidemiology

INCIDENCE

The various forms of lumbar stenosis represent, after disc herniations, the most frequent cause of compression of the caudal nerve roots. However, the absolute incidence of stenosis and its frequency with respect to disc herniations remain to be well defined. Verbiest (1977) reported on 147 patients with stenosis of the spinal canal who were treated surgically in a 27-year period and Getty (1980) on 35 cases observed in a period of 10 years, whereas Robertson *et al.* (1973) found 35 cases of lumbar stenosis in a series of 2000 lumbar myelograms. Reale *et al.* (1978), in a three-year period, observed 61 patients with stenosis of the spinal canal and 71 with disc herniation in a normally sized spinal canal. Of the 455 patients in the series of Paine (1976), 31% had only a disc herniation and 69% a stenosis, either isolated or associated with a herniated disc; similarly, in the series of Kirkaldy-Willis and McIvor (Kirkaldy-Willis *et al.*, 1974), only 25% of the patients had a herniated disc, whereas 75% had a stenosis, associated or not with a disc herniation. The incidence of the single forms of stenosis of the spinal canal is also extremely variable in the various series reported. According to Verbiest, stenosis of the spinal canal is almost consistently developmental or combined (according to the definition of the present author). In contrast, in the series of Tile *et al.* (1976), Paine (1976), Dick *et al.* (1977), Hasue *et al.* (1977) and Getty (1980) the incidence of primary stenosis ranges from 10% to 31%, that of degenerative forms from 53% to 94% and that of combined stenosis from 0 to 26%.

As far as concerns isolated stenosis of the nerve root canal, Epstein *et al.* (1972) found 15 cases of this condition in a series of 400 patients submitted to surgery for suspected lumbar disc herniation, whereas Choudhury and Taylor (1977), in a two-year period, observed 28 cases compared with 9 cases of stenosis of the spinal canal. Venner and Crock (1981), on the other hand, in about two years, observed 50 cases of stenosis of the nerve root canal of L_5 and/or S_1 in patients with an L_5-S_1 disc resorption.

The considerable difference in the absolute incidence reported for the various forms of lumbar stenosis and their frequency with respect to the disc herniations is to be attributed, to a large extent, to the different criteria used to define the term stenosis. A definition not adequately delimiting the concept of stenosis may lead to a considerable and misleading increase in the number of cases, particularly if strict criteria are not followed in the diagnosis of the condition. Other factors, however, may also be involved, such as the variations in the size of the spinal canal and the different predisposition to spondylotic changes related to ethnic factors. In the African negro population, for example, the incidence of lumbar stenosis seems to the significantly lower than in the Indoeuropean and Asian races (Eisenstein, 1977; 1985).

SEX

Developmental stenosis and, to a lesser extent, combined stenosis show a considerably higher incidence in males (Verbiest, 1976; Reale *et al.*, 1978; Paine, 1976). In degenerative stenosis, particularly when associated with spondylolisthesis, the proportion of females is increased with respect to the other forms (Cauchoix, 1976; Epstein *et al.*, 1976); even in combined stenosis, however, females are less frequently affected than males.

No definite explanation has yet been found for the greater incidence of developmental stenosis in males. In degenerative and combined stenosis, the reason for the male predominance is likely to be attributed, at least in part, to the greater exposure of males to physical stresses and, thus, to the greater predisposition to degenerative changes of the intervertebral discs and apophyseal joints.

AGE

The mean age at which lumbar spinal stenosis is usually diagnosed varies in relation to the definition that is given of this condition, as well as to the pathological type of stenosis. If conditions characterized by a *narrow* spinal canal, associated or not with disc herniation, are considered forms of stenosis, the mean age is about 30 years (Paine, 1976), an age very similar to, or even lower than, that of the patients with disc herniation in a spinal canal of normal size. If only those conditions characterized by a «constriction of the spinal canal by hypertrophic laminal arches, pedicles and/or osteophytic ridges» (Teng and Papateodorou, 1963), with or without degenerative spondylolisthesis are considered, the mean age lies somewhere between 50 and 70 years of age (Epstein, 1976; Teng and Papateodorou, 1963; Surin, 1982). Lastly, if only stenosis of the nerve root canal is considered, the mean age at the time of diagnosis is 30 to 40 years (Epstein *et al.*, 1972; Choudhury and Taylor, 1977).

Personal experience, based upon the above-mentioned definition of stenosis, had shown that developmental stenosis of the spinal canal is usually observed between 30 and 50 years, and only exceptionally in the second and third decade, since a developmentally narrow canal does not usually determine compression of the caudal nerve roots in the absence of spondylotic changes, the occurrence of which is strictly related to the ageing process. Degenerative and combined stenoses, on the other hand, are usually observed after 50 years and, only exceptionally, before 40. Post-traumatic and post-infectious stenoses, as well as stenoses related to systemic bone diseases, although independent of age, are usually diagnosed between 40 and 60 years, probably because, even in these forms, degenerative vertebral changes favour the occurrence or the clinical manifestations of compression of the nerve roots of the cauda equina.

Isolated stenosis of the nerve root canal usually tends to occur between 30 and 50 years on account of the important role played by degenerative disc changes in the etiology of nerve root compression.

Regardless of the type of stenosis, males tend to be affected earlier than females. The entity of compression of the nervous structures and the number of levels involved do not, however, show any significant relationship to the age of onset of the symptoms.

PHYSICAL CHARACTERISTICS

It might be assumed that developmental and combined stenosis, on account of the smaller dimensions of the spinal canal, would be more frequently observed in subjects with a very low stature. There does not seem, however, to be any significant relationship between statural values and size of the spinal canal, except in achondroplastic dwarfs, in whom the narrow vertebral canal, as well as the statural defect, are due to peculiar changes in the cartilage growth plates.

Similarly, there is no definite relationship between obesity and frequency or entity of vertebral degenerative changes and, more generally, between the type of physical structure and incidence of lumbar stenosis syndromes.

OCCUPATION

Lumbar stenosis, since it is, in part or entirely, caused by degenerative vertebral changes, tends to occur more often in individuals, such as manual workers, in whom the lumbar spine is exposed to higher functional stresses. This is consistent with the observation that the incidence of lumbar spinal stenosis is higher in males. This occupational predisposition appears, however, to be somewhat generic, as there are no exhaustive statistical data indicating a higher incidence of lumbar spinal stenosis in specific work categories.

FAMILIARITY

Verbiest (1976) reported on the cases of two brothers and two sisters, in two different families, showing developmental stenosis of the lumbar vertebral canal. In the two brothers, the lumbar levels involved were the fourth and fifth in one, and the fourth in the other. The two sisters, on the other hand, both presented stenosis from the second to the fifth lumbar level and both showed a disc protrusion at L_2-L_3 level. Another patient with lumbar spinal stenosis observed by Verbiest reported that one of his brothers, who had died ten years earlier, had complained of low back pain and intermittent claudication, which had not apparently a vascular aetiology. Verbiest obtained permission to dig up the skeleton in order to measure the dimensions of the vertebral canal, but the grave was found to be empty. The series reported by Scapinelli (1973) included two bicorial twins aged 43 years, who complained of lumbo-radicular intermittent claudication; one of the two underwent surgical treatment, whereas it is not stated whether diagnosis, in the other, was only clinical or also myelographic. Varughese and Quartey (1979) described the cases of four brothers with disc herniation at one or more levels presenting myelographic evidence of narrowing of the vertebral canal in the sagittal diameter. At surgery, three brothers had a stenosis of the spinal canal and two had a sequestered herniated disc.

CASES OBSERVED BY THE AUTHOR

Postacchini *et al.* (1985) have observed three siblings, two brothers and a sister, with stenosis of the lumbar vertebral canal (Fig. 4.1). Furthermore, at least one other member of the same family probably had a developmental narrowing of the vertebral canal.

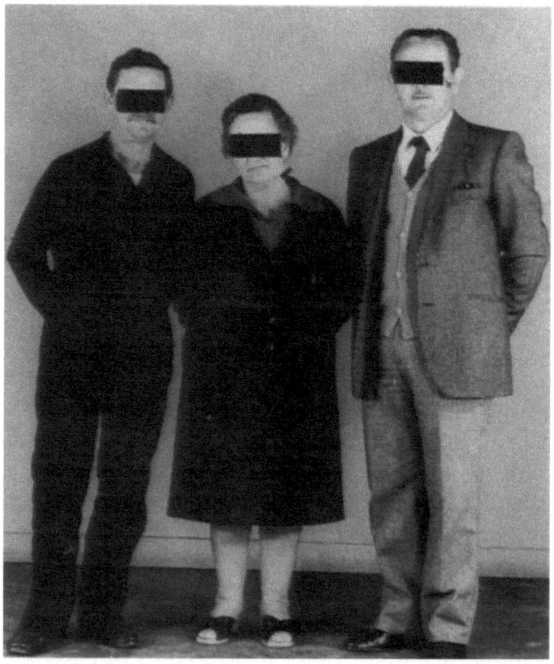

Fig. 4.1 - Three siblings with lumbar spinal canal stenosis.

Case reports

The three siblings.

Case 1. A forty-six-year-old man, a bricklayer, was admitted to Orthopaedic Clinic of the University of Rome with a nine-month history of low-back pain, hypoesthesia in the anteromedial aspect of the right thigh and leg, and weakness of the quadriceps muscle on the right. Both the lumbar and radicular symptoms were exacerbated by any increase in lumbar lordosis and were relieved by flexion. The patient also presented progressive weakness in the lower limbs during walking. The walking capacity was about 100 meters.

Physical examination revealed mild restriction of motion of the lumbar spine, marked exacerbation of the radicular pain during flexion of the knee with the hip extended, hyphalgesia in the right fourth lumbar dermatome, weakness and wasting of the quadriceps muscle, and absence of the patellar reflex on the right.

Radiographs of the spine revealed markedly short pedicles, narrow interlaminar spaces, and mild degenerative changes of the articular processes in all of the lumbar vertebrae. Myelo-

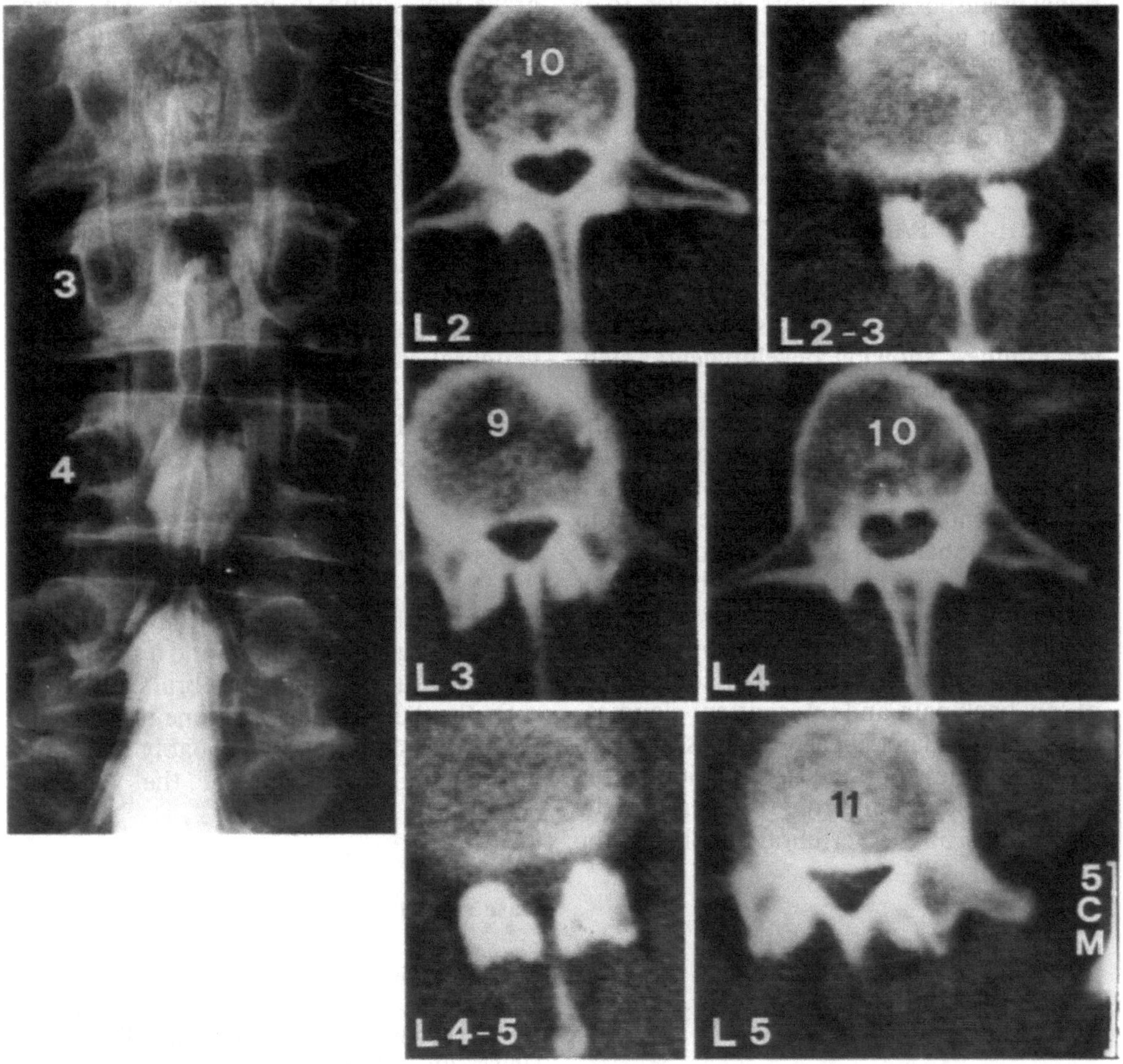

Fig. 4.2 - Case 1. The anteroposterior myelogram shows a complete block of the dye column at L_2-L_3 and L_3-L_4 levels and a subtotal block at L_4-L_5. Low resolution CT scans reveal short midsagittal dimensions of the spinal canal at L_2 (10 mm), L_3 (9 mm) and L_4 (10 mm) levels. At L_4-L_5 level, the articular processes appear to be hypertrophic.

graphy showed multiple constrictions of the column of contrast medium from the first to the fourth lumbar level (Fig. 4.2). Computed tomography of the lumbar spine with eight millimeter-thick transverse sections revealed markedly short midsagittal diameters of the spinal canal and mildly hypertrophic articular processes (Fig. 4.2). A diagnosis of developmental lumbar stenosis from the second to the fourth lumbar level was made.

Bilateral laminectomy and partial facetectomy was performed from the lower half of the second lumbar vertebra to the upper half of the fifth lumbar vertebra. Exploration of the second, third, and fourth lumbar interspaces revealed bulging of the discs but no herniation. Therefore, the discs were not removed. Postoperatively, the patient was completely relieved of the radicular pain. The strength of the quadriceps muscle on the right and the patient's walking capacity gradually improved. At the last follow-up examination, six years postoperatively, the patient was free from pain and leading a normal active life.

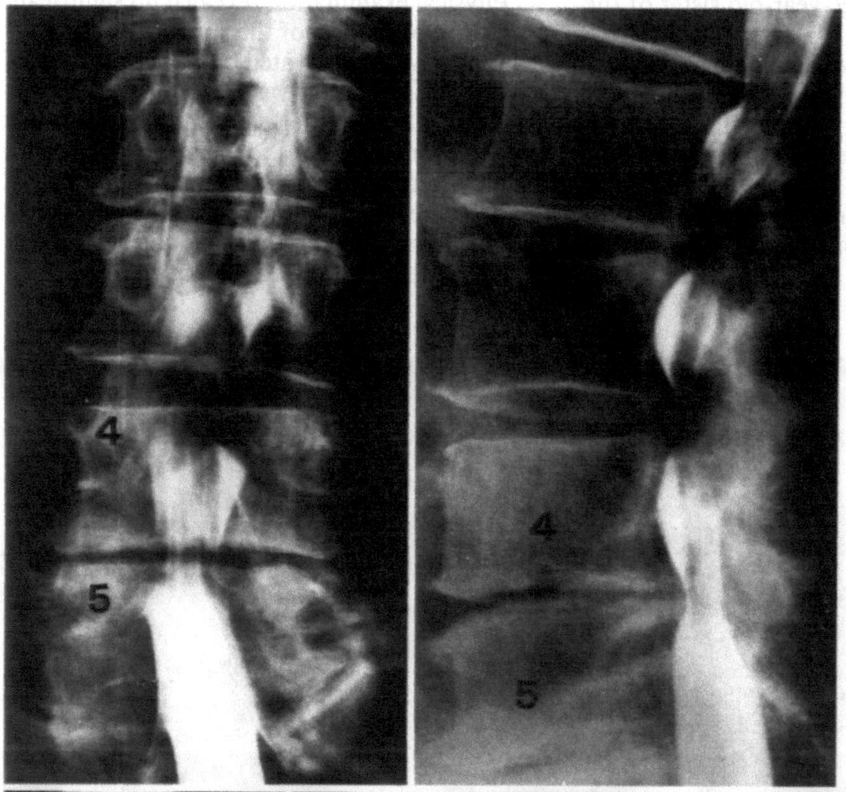

Fig. 4.3 - Case 2. Lumbar myelograms show, as in case 1, a complete block of the dye column at L_2-L_3 and L_3-L_4 levels, and less severe compression of the nervous structures at L_4-L_5 level. On CT scans, the vertebral canal appears developmentally narrow, the midsagittal diameters ranging from 9 to 11 mm at L_2, L_3 and L_4 levels. The articular processes, which present marked degenerative changes, encroach on the central portion of the spinal canal and/or the nerve root canals at L_2-L_3 and L_3-L_4 levels.

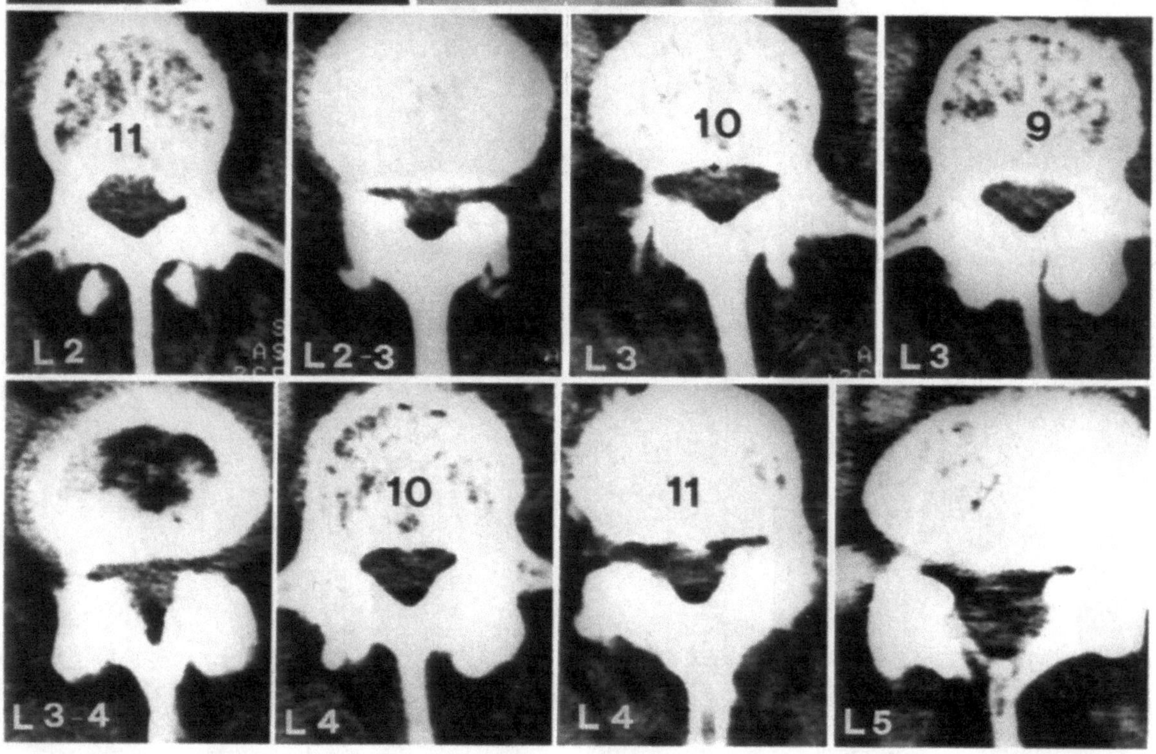

Case 2. The sixty-three-year-old sister of the patient described in Case 1 was admitted with a twenty-year history of low-back pain and a two-year history of pain in the anteromedial aspect of the left thigh and the posterolateral area of the lower limbs, with more severe pain in the right lower limb. She also had decreased sensation in the right fifth-lumbar dermatome, impaired dorsiflexion of the right foot, and progressive loss of strength in the lower limbs.

Physical examination revealed no significant restriction of motion of the spine. The patient's symptoms were aggravated by hyperextention of the lumbar spine, but were not relieved by spinal flexion. Straight leg-raising was moderately restricted on both sides, and knee flexion with the hip extended exacerbated the pain in the left thigh. There was decreased sensation in the fifth lumbar dermatome on the right and, to a lesser extent, on the left. Severe weakness of the tibia-

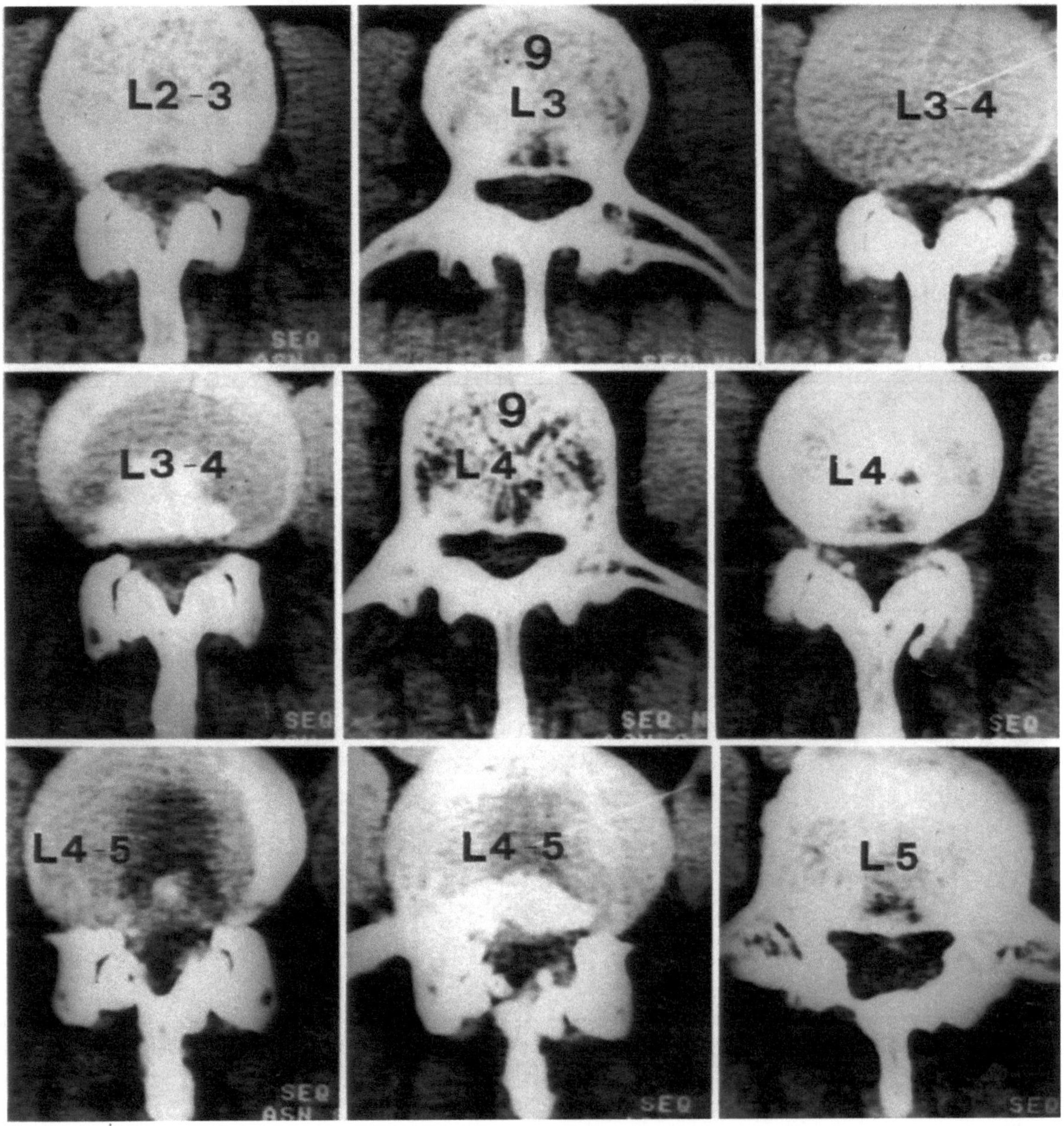

Fig. 4.4 - Case 3. The transpedicular CT scans at L_3 and L_4 levels show markedly narrow (9 mm) midsagittal diameters of the spinal canal. The nerve root canals and the central spinal canal are narrowed by hypertrophic articular processes at L_3-L_4 and L_4-L_5 levels.

lis anterior, peronei, and extensor hallucis proprius was evident on the right. The Achilles' reflex was absent on both sides.

Radiographs of the lumbar spine revealed short pedicles, very narrow interlaminar spaces, degenerative changes of the articular processes, which were particularly severe at the fourth lumbar level, and a bone ridge arising from the posterosuperior margin on the body of the fifth lumbar vertebra.

Myelography showed multiple constrictions of the column of the contrast medium from the second to the fourth lumbar level (Fig. 4.3). High resolution computed tomography revealed a developmentally narrow spinal canal from the second to the fourth lumbar level, hypertrophic articular processes encroaching on the spinal canal at the lowest four lumbar levels, and marked narrowness of the nerve root canals of the lowest three lumbar vertebrae (Fig. 4.3). A diagnosis of combined stenosis of the lumbar spinal canal from the second to the fourth lumbar level and stenosis of the nerve root canals of the fifth lumbar vertebra was made.

Bilateral laminectomy and unroofing of the nerve root canals was performed at the lowest four lumbar levels. No significant lesions of the discs were found. A few days after the operation the patient was free from radicular pain, and she remained thus for the thirteen-month period of follow-up. Recovery of the preoperative motor deficit, was, however, only partial.

Case 3. The fifty-six-year-old brother of the two patients described, a gardner, presented with a history of several years of low-back pain and a seven-month history of pain in the posterolateral aspect of both thighs and legs, which was more severe on the right.

Physical examination revealed local tenderness in the lumbar spine, but no restriction of movement in the right limb. There was hypalgesia in the right fifth-lumbar dermatome.

Plain radiographs of the lumbar spine showed short pedicles and laminae, degenerative changes of the articular processes and vertebral bodies, and loss of height of the fifth lumbar disc. High resolution CT scan of the lumbar spine revealed very short midsagittal diameters of the spinal canal at the third and fourth lumbar levels (Fig. 4.4). Moderate hypertrophy of the articular processes, and narrowing of the nerve root canals of the lowest two lumbar vertebrae were also evident. A diagnosis of combined stenosis at the third and fourth lumbar levels and narrow lateral recesses of the fifth lumbar vertebra was made. Myelographic studies were not performed due to refusal on the part of the patient.

Bilateral laminectomy and partial facetectomy of the third, the fourth, and the proximal half of the fifth lumbar vertebra was carried out. The third and fourth intervertebral discs, which were slightly bulging but not herniated, were not excised. Postoperatively, the patient was completely relieved of radicular pain. At a six-month follow-up examination, the patient complained only of mild back pain, which, however, had completely disappeared at the last follow-up, three years later.

The other members of the family. The parents of the three siblings had also had another son who had died while in good health, in an automobile accident at the age of thirty-eight years.

The father had died, at the age of seventy-two years, of lung cancer. During the last two decades of life he had complained of mild chronic low-back pain and, in his last few years, presented symptoms in the lower limbs, such as pain and weakness in walking, suggesting the presence of lumbar spinal stenosis. The mother was still alive. She also complained of low-back pain, but had no significant symptoms in the lower limbs. Plain radiographs of the lumbar spine revealed no abnormalities except for mild degenerative changes of the facet joints at the lowest three lumbar levels. Two of the three siblings with lumbar stenosis had married and had had, respectively, two children (Case 1) and one child (Case 3). The two children of Case 1, who were twenty-two and twenty-four years old, had no complaint and presented normal neurological examination as well as apparently normal plain radiographs. The only child of the patient described in Case 3, a thirty-four year old, complained of recurrent low-back pain but had no radicular symptoms.

Plain radiographs of the lumbar spine showed some abnormalities — short pedicles, narrow interlaminar spaces, and sagittally oriented articular facets — suggesting developmental narrowing of the lumbar spinal canal. He refused, however, to undergo CT scan of the lumbar spine. This member of the family had two children, aged six and four years, who showed no evidence of disease or congenital abnormalities.

CONCLUSIONS

In the cases reported in the literature and in those described here stenosis was developmental or combined, i.e. the lumbar spinal canal in all patients was abnormally narrow in the midsagittal diameter at one or more levels. These findings suggest that the dimensions of the vertebral canal may be regulated by genetic factors and that for developmental and combined stenosis a familial predisposition, although not a strictly hereditary transmission, might exist.

REFERENCES

CAUCHOIX J., BENOIST M., CHASSAING V.: Degenerative spondylolisthesis. *Clin. Orthop.* **115:** 122, 1976.

CHOUDHURY A.R., TAYLOR J.C.: Occult lumbar spinal stenosis. *J. Neurol. Neurosurg. Psych.* **40:** 506, 1977.

DICK P., PHEASANT H.C., DOYLE J.B., RIEDER J.J.: Intermittent cauda equina compression syndrome. Its recognition and treatment. *Spine* **2:** 75, 1977.

EISENSTEIN S.: The morphometry and pathological anatomy of the lumbar spine in South African Negroes and Caucasoids with specific reference to spinal stenosis. *J. Bone and Joint Surg.* **59-A:** 173, 1977.

EISENSTEIN S.: Personal communication, 1985.

EPSTEIN J.A., EPSTEIN B.S., ROSENTHAL R.C., LEVINE S.L.: Sciatica caused by nerve root entrapment in the lateral recess: the superior facet syndrome. *J. Neurosurg.* **36:** 584, 1972.

EPSTEIN J.A., EPSTEIN B.S., LEVINE L.S., CARRAS R., ROSTENTHAL A.D.: Degenerative lumbar spondylolisthesis with an intact neural arch (pseudospondylolisthesis). *J. Neurosurg.* **44:** 139, 1976.

GETTY C.J.M.: Lumbar spinal stenosis. The clinical spectrum and the results of operation. *J. Bone and Joint Surg.* **62-B:** 481, 1980.

HASUE M., KIDA H., INOUE K., AWANO N.: Lumbar spinal stenosis. A clinical study of symptoms and therapeutic results. *Intern. Orthop. (SICOT)* **1:** 133, 1977.

KIRKALDY-WILLIS W.H., PAINE K.W.E., CAUCHOIX J., MCIVOR G.: Lumbar spinal stenosis. *Clin. Orthop.* **99:** 30, 1974.

KIRKALDY-WILLIS W.H., WEDGE J.H., YONG-HING K., REILLY J.: Pathology and pathogenesis of lumbar spondylosis and stenosis. *Spine* **3:** 319, 1978.

PAINE K.W.: Results of decompression for lumbar spinal stenosis. *Clin. Orthop.* **115:** 96, 1976.

POSTACCHINI F., MASSOBRIO M., FERRO L.: Familial lumbar stenosis. Case report of three siblings. *J. Bone and Joint Surg.* **67-A:** 321, 1985.

REALE F., DELFINI R., GAMBACORTA D., CANTORE G.P.: Congenital stenosis of lumbar spinal canal: comparison of results of surgical treatment for this and other causes of lumbar syndrome. *Acta Neurochir.* **42:** 199, 1978.

ROBERTSON G.H., LIEWELLYN H.J., TAVERAS J.M.: The narrow lumbar spinal canal syndrome. *Radiology* **107:** 89, 1973.

SCAPINELLI R.: Sindromi da stenosi del canale vertebrale lombare. *La Clin. Ortop.* **24:** 79, 1973.

SURIN U., HEDELIN E., SMITH L.: Degenerative lumbar spinal stenosis. *Acta Orthop. Scand.* **53:** 79, 1982.

TENG P., PAPATEODOROU C.: Myelographic findings in spondylosis of the lumbar spine. *Br. J. Radiol.* **36:** 122, 1963.

TILE M., MCNEIL S.R., ZARINS R.K., PENNAL G.F., GARSIDE H.: Spinal stenosis. Results of treatment. *Clin. Orthop.* **115:** 104, 1976.

VARUGHESE G., QUARTEY G.R.C.: Familial lumbar spinal stenosis with acute disc herniations. Case reports of four brothers. *J. Neurosurg.* **51:** 234, 1979.

VENNER R.M., CROCK H.V.: Clinical studies of isolated disc resorption in the lumbar spine. *J. Bone and Joint Surg.* **63-B:** 491, 1981.

VERBIEST H.: *Neurogenic intermittent claudication. Lesions of the spinal cord and cauda equina, stenosis of the vertebral canal, narrowing of intervertebral foramina and entrapment of peripheral nerves.* In «Handbook of Clinical Neurology» ed. by Vinken P.J.; and Bruyn G.W., vol. 20, pp. 678-679, New York, Acad. Elsevier, 1976.

VERBIEST H.: Results of surgical treatment of idiopathic developmental stenosis of the lumbar vertebral canal. *J. Bone and Joint Surg.* **59-B:** 181, 1977.

Chapter V

Aetiopathogenesis

AETIOPATHOGENETIC FACTORS

ACHONDROPLASIA

Achondroplasia, the most common cause of dwarfism, is a developmental abnormality caused by a defective enchondral bone formation, in the presence of normal intramembranous ossification, which becomes apparent towards the end of the second month of foetal life. In most cases the disease is due to gene mutation, which seems to be related to increasing maternal age (Bailey, 1973). The gene abnormality is transmitted with a dominant autosomic pattern.

The impaired skeletal development is related to abnormalities of the growth plate cartilage of the long bones. Changes in cell and intercellular matrix have been observed in all the areas of the growth plate, but particularly in the hypertrophic zone, which shows a considerable decrease in height in the achondroplastic dwarf, and in the proliferative zone (Ponseti, 1970; Maynard *et al.*, 1981). In these areas, the cells may be arranged in columns, as in normal growth or, less frequently, may show a clustered arrangement. At the cartilage-metaphyseal bone junction numerous osteoclasts are present, which may be responsible for an abnormal metaphyseal resorptive mechanism (Maynard *et al.*, 1981).

The structural abnormalities of the growth plates result in a reduced length of the long bones, which, however, are of normal width due to the normal pattern of perichondral ossification. In the vertebrae, the defective bone formation mainly affects the pedicles, which have a growth plate similar to that of the long bones. The most characteristic feature of achondroplastic vertebrae is the reduced length, often associated with an abnormal width, of the pedicles. These changes are responsible for an abnormal shortness of the midsagittal and/or the transverse diameter of the vertebral canal. Another morphologic characteristic of the achondroplastic vertebrae, particularly in the lumbar region, is the marked concavity of the posterior surface of the body. The abnormal concavity may be related to defective enchondral ossification of the vertebral end-plates and/or the pressure exerted by the nervous structures on the vertebral body during skeletal growth.

Unlike the bony components, the nervous structures of the achondroplastic dwarf develop normally. Thus, at the end of skeletal growth, there is very little or no reserve space for the spinal cord and the nerve root of the cauda equina within the vertebral canal and there is, therefore, a condition of potential stenosis. The latter occurs if and when the disc and osteoligamentous structures of the vertebral canal undergo, with advancing age, degenerative changes responsible for a reduction, even mild, of the dimensions of the spinal canal.

DEVELOPMENTAL NARROWING OF THE SPINAL CANAL

Abnormal narrowing of the osteoligamentous vertebral canal may be related to genetic or environmental factors.

The dimensions of the vertebral canal, as other somatic characteristics, are very likely to be regulated by genetic factors. Variation of the genetic pool, therefore, may produce considerable oscillation in the size of the vertebral canal, which in most individuals remains within normal limits but may, in a few subjects, exceed these limits. The genetic interpretation is supported not only by the cases of familial stenosis, but also, and particularly, by the finding that the dimensions of the spinal canal (mean values and limits of normal) vary in males and females in a same population, as well as in different races and in different ethnic groups of the same race (Eisenstein 1977; Postacchini *et al.* 1983).

The possibility that environmental factors may play a significant role in the morphogenesis of the spinal canal has been suggested by Clark *et al.* (1985), who have examined skeletons from a genetically homogeneous prehistoric American-Indian population, which changed its lifestyle, over a few centuries, from hunting and gathering (Pre-Mississipian) to maize growing (Mississipian). This led to a distinct change in diet from protein rich to protein poor food. The content of food protein did not presumably decrease with change in diet. However, maize is known to lack some of the aminoacids essential for the formation of proteins in infants. Thus, Mississipian infants, who were fed essentially maize, presumably had a deficient protein metabolism. Measurements of the diameters of the spinal canal have shown that canal size was significantly smaller in Mississipian, compared to Pre-Mississipian, skeletons. Since the development of the vertebral canal occurs almost entirely in infancy, it is reasonable to hypothesize that subclinical defects in skeletal growth, related to nutritional or other factors, may irreparably compromise the morphogenesis of the spinal canal, thus influencing the morphometry of the canal at the end of skeletal growth.

The aetiopathogenetic role of developmental narrowing of the vertebral canal (in the central portion and/or the lateral portions) is that of a predisposing factor to lumbar spinal stenosis. In itself, in fact, developmental narrowing of the spinal canal is not sufficient to produce a stenotic condition. Indeed, if this were not the case, developmental stenosis would be observed with a high frequency in teenagers and young adults. Conversely, stenosis usually develops in the middle years of life, when degenerative vertebral changes become apparent, which, in a narrow spinal canal, may considerably alter the precarious equilibrium between the capacity of the canal and the volume of the spinal nervous structures. This interpretation is supported by the observation that, even in patients with developmental stenosis of the vertebral canal, as in those with degenerative or combined stenosis, compression of the dural sac and the caudal nerve roots usually occurs only in the intervertebral portions of the spinal canal, when structures, such as intervertebral disc, vertebral end-plates, articular processes and ligamenta flava, may undergo degenerative changes.

The lowest mean values of the midsagittal dimensions of the vertebral canal are found at the third and fourth lumbar level. Similarly, in the majority of cases, the vertebrae with midsagittal dimensions of the spinal canal below the lower limits of normal are the third, fourth or fifth lumbar vertebra. These findings may explain why in developmental and combined stenosis of the spinal canal the lowest three lumbar levels are usually involved; at these levels, in fact, the spinal canal, being tendentially narrower or «irregular», i.e. with the highest oscillation of the mean values, presents the greatest predisposition to undergo stenosis.

SPONDYLOTIC CHANGES

The comprehensive term of spondylosis is used to indicate the complex series of degenerative changes affecting the intervertebral disc, the zygohypophyseal joints and the vertebral body.

Intervertebral disc

Degenerative changes of the intervertebral disc start with decrease in the amount of proteoglycans, and subsequent decrease in water content of the nucleus pulposus, which gradually becomes fibrous in nature due to the simultaneous increase in amount of the collagen fibers. These changes make the boundaries and the structural differences between the nucleus pulposus and the annulus fibrosus progressively less distinct. In the annulus, circumferential tears may become apparent, which may be associated with radial tears from the centre to the peripheral area, mostly posterior or posterolateral, of the disc. These tears may subsequently coalesce to form cavities in the context of the nucleus pulposus and/or the annulus fibrosus (Schmorl and Junghanns, 1932). The result is a loss of disc height, which may be associated, or not, with bulging of the annulus fibrosus in all or part of its circumference. In the very advanced stages, the nucleus pulposus has almost completely disappeared and the disc is reduced to a crevice delimited by a thin layer of annulus fibrosus, largely disrupted in its lamellar structure.

These changes, though an expression of the ageing process of the intervertebral disc, differ in entity at the different vertebral levels. In the lumbar spine, the discs which most frequently undergo degenerative changes are the lowest two, probably because of the greater mechanical stress to which they are submitted compared with the upper three. Furthermore, the two lowest discs are those more often presenting extensive changes (Lewin, 1964).

Degenerative disc disease may play a multiple role in the aetiology of stenosis. Degenerative changes, modifying the mechanical properties of the disc, may produce segmental instability, which exposes the posterior joints to abnormal mechanical stress, thus favouring degenerative changes of the joints. Disc resorption not only causes a decrease in height of the intervertebral foramen, but also produces subluxation in a cranio-caudal direction of the articular facets, which are more exposed to degenerative changes owing to abnormal mechanical stress.

Facet joints

The degenerative changes which apophyseal joints may undergo are similar to those seen in diarthrodial joints in the limbs.

Initially the articular cartilage, normally smooth and whitish, becomes wrinkled and yellowish. Subsequently, the cartilage shows necrotic areas and erosions at the level of which the subchrondral bone may appear necrotic or be replaced by necrotic tissue. In many areas, between the subchondral bone and the basal portion of articular cartilage, a layer of fibrocartilagineous tissue is present, from which newly formed bone originates. Areas of newly formed bone are often seen also at the insertion of the articular capsule. In a more advanced stage, large areas of articular cartilage are replaced by connective tissue, fibrocartilage, or newly formed bone.

In some areas, subchondral bone consists of large trabeculae separated by thin narrow spaces, whereas in others it is replaced by connective tissue. In the zones of insertion of the articular capsule, which are, at times, markedly thickened, osteophytic outgrowths of varying size may be seen, whereas in the areas of insertion of the ligamentum flavum large zones of chondroid or bony metaplasia may be visible. At this stage, the apophyseal joint appears enlarged and variously deformed due to hypertrophy of the articular processes, marginal osteophytes and bony metaplasia in the juxta-articular portion of the ligamenta flava.

Degenerative abnormalities of the zygohypophyseal joints are mainly related to the ageing process. Marked osteoarthrotic changes are rarely observed before 45 years of age, whereas after that age 50% to 90% of individuals show evident degenerative changes at one or more lumbar levels, which tend to increase in severity with advancing age (Guntz, 1934; Putti and Logroscino, 1937; Lewin, 1964).

Osteoarthrotic changes in the apophyseal joints, however, appear to depend not only on age but also on other factors, such as vertebral level, degenerative disc changes and orientation of the articular facets.

The facet joints of the three lower lumbar levels show earlier and more marked degenerative abnormalities than the two upper lumbar levels. Of the lower three lumbar levels, the L_4-L_5 level presents, overall, the greatest tendency to osteoarthrotic changes (Putti and Logroscino, 1937; Ingelmark, 1956, 1959; Lewin 1964).

Degenerative changes, even marked, of the intervertebral disc are not generally associated, below 45 years, with osteoarthrotic changes in the zygoapophyseal joints; arthrotic changes, on the other hand, may not be associated, at any age, with degenerative disc changes. Over 45 years of age, however, degenerative disease of the intervertebral disc is very often associated with arthrotic changes, of varying entity, in the facet joints. These observations suggest that the degenerative changes in the disc and facet joints are related from a pathogenetic point of view, even if there is no strict cause-effect relationship between these two pathological conditions.

Vertebral body

The formation of marginal osteophytes in the vertebral body is strictly related to the ageing process. Osteophytes, in fact, are rarely seen before 45 years, whereas, after this age, they are observed more and more frequently, until they become an almost constant finding in old age (Lewin, 1964). Furthermore, their dimensions also show an age-related increase.

Marginal osteophytes may form in the entire circumference of the vertebral end-plate. In the majority of cases, however, they develop in the anterior or anterolateral portion of the vertebral body. Osteophytes of the posterior border are fairly rare and usually small in size. Posterior osteophytes, in a single vertebra, are generally associated with anterior osteophytes, compared to which the posterior bony spurs are almost consistently less prominent. In an attempt of offer an explanation for the formation of marginal osteophytes of the vertebral body two pathogenetic mechanisms have been proposed, both of which, however, have been specifically formulated for anterolateral osteophytic outgrowths.

According to a pathogenetic hypothesis, osteophytes of the vertebral body form as a result of degenerative changes of the annulus fibrosus in the zone of insertion of the latter on the vertebral body (Schmorl and Junghanns, 1932). In this zone, annular clefts become apparent, into which portions of the nucleus pulposus may penetrate and protrude beneath the posterior longitudinal ligament. Mechanical stress, to which the ligament is submitted, stimulates the development, within the latter, of foci of reactive bone formation. According to another theory, the formation of osteophytic outgrowths results from degeneration of the entire intervertebral disc and subsequent loss of disc height. This may involve an anterior protrusion of the nucleus pulposus, which thus exerts marked pressure effects on the annulus fibrosus. In its central portion, which is thicker and reinforced by the anterior longitudinal ligament, the annulus is able to resist the pressure exerted by the nucleus. In contrast, in the marginal portions, nuclear tissue may rise and stretch the vertebral periosteum, which reacts with the gradual formation of new bony tissue (Collins, 1949). Neither of these two pathogenetic mechanisms would appear to completely explain the development of posterior marginal osteophytes of the vertebral body. The latter hypothesis, however, appears more plausible considering that posterior osteophytes are almost consistently observed in the presence of a significant narrowing of the intervertebral space and/or marked posterior bulging of the annulus fibrosus.

Anterolateral osteophytes do not play any direct role in the pathogenesis of stenosis. Posterior osteophytes, conversely, may narrow the central spinal canal and/or the nerve root canal. The former is very rarely narrowed, to a significant extent, by osteophytes arising from the central portion of the posterior vertebral border. The nerve root canal is narrowed, in the portion corresponding to the lateral recess, by posterolateral osteophytes of the superior vertebral end-plate and, in the portion corresponding to the intervertebral foramen, by osteophytes of both vertebral end-plates, when they develop at the level of the pedicle. However, osteophytic outgrowths of the superior end-plate of the vertebra delimiting inferiorly the foramen are usually of little clinical importance, as the nerve root occupies only the superior portion of the neuroforamen.

Degenerative spondylolisthesis

This condition — termed in the past pseudospondylolisthesis (Junghanns, 1930) or spondylolisthesis with an intact neural arch (McNab, 1950) — is usually observed in individuals over 50 years of age and, only exceptionally, before 40 years. Females are affected three times more often than males; the black race appears to be more prone than the white (Rosenberg, 1975). For the vertebra to be considered olisthetic, the amount of slipping, as evaluated on plain radiographs, must be at least equal to 5% of the sagittal diameter of the lower vertebral end-plate (Fig. 5.1). At the time of the initial clinical observation, the majority of patients have an olisthesis of 10% to 20% (Fig. 5.2). A slipping of 20% to 30% is fairly unusual (Fig. 5.4). In most cases, the olisthetic vertebra is the fourth lumbar vertebra (McNab, 1950; Potter and Narcross, 1954; Rosenberg, 1975; Fitzgerald and Newman, 1976). The third and fifth lumbar vertebrae are affected in similar proportions and often in association with the fourth (Figs. 5.3 and 5.4). The fifth lumbar is the vertebra showing the greatest degree of slipping.

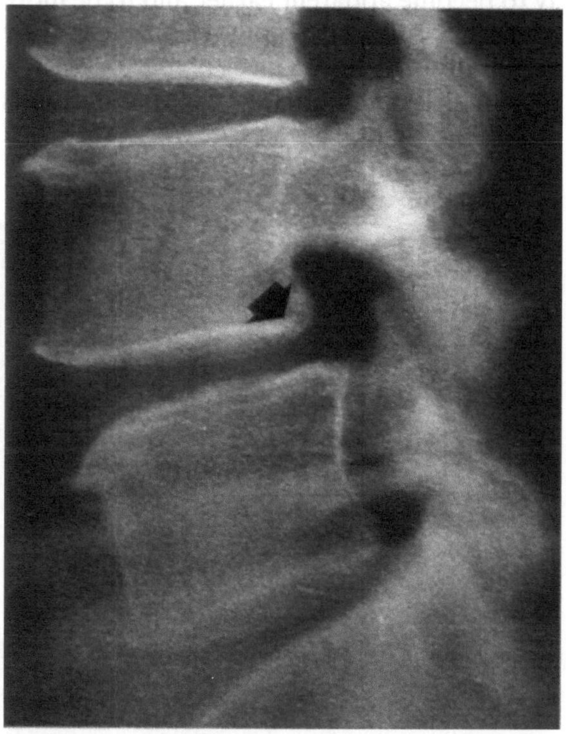

Fig. 5.1 - Degenerative spondylolisthesis of L_4. Although mild (7%) the olisthesis of L_4 (arrow) is clearly visible, when compared with the normal alignement of the posterior corners of the vertebral bodies at L_3-L_4 and L_5-S_1 levels.

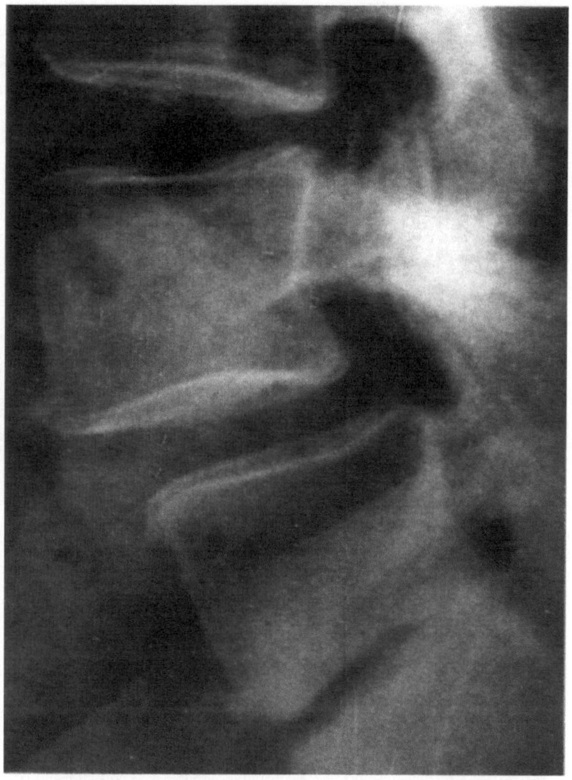

Fig. 5.2 - Moderate degenerative spondylolisthesis (18%) of the fourth lumbar vertebra. Note the marked disc resorption at L_5-S_1.

The pathogenesis of degenerative spondylolisthesis is, to a large extent, unknown. Some observations, however, may help to delineate the mechanism of occurrence of the vertebral slipping, particularly that of L_4, which is the most frequently affected vertebra:

a) In the series of Rosenberg (1975), spondylolisthesis of L_4 was found to be four times more frequent in patients with unilateral or bilateral sacralization of the fifth lumbar vertebra than in those with a mobile L_5 vertebra. Moreover, in all patients, the degree of lumbar lordosis was less, and the L_5 vertebral body less trapezoidal, than in normal subjects. These vertebral characteristics — compared with the completely opposite characteristics (more marked lordosis and more trapezoidal L_5 vertebra than normal) of patients with a typically unstable condi-

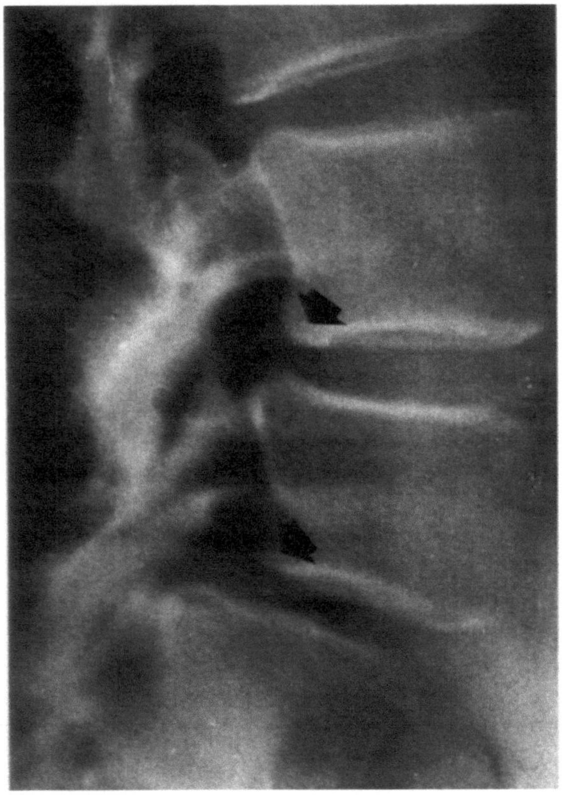

Fig. 5.3 - Severe, and mild, degenerative spondylolisthesis (arrows) of L_5 and L_4, respectively. Slipping of L_5 is 27%.

tion, such as isthmic spondylolisthesis of the fourth lumbar vertebra — suggest that, in patients with degenerative spondylolisthesis of L_4, the fifth lumbar vertebra is more stable than normal, even in the absence of sacralization.

b) It has been observed that in the majority of patients with degenerative spondylolisthesis of L_4, this vertebra is abnormally high with respect to the iliac crests (Fitzgerald and Newman, 1976). In fact, while in most normal individuals the tangent line through the iliac crests intersects the lumbar spine approximately at the level of the lower half of the L_4 vertebra, in patients with degenerative spondylolisthesis this line usually intersects the L_4-L_5 intervertebral disc or the fifth lumbar vertebra (Fig. 5.5). Due to this high position, the protection to the L_4 vertebra normally given by the soft tissues present between the iliac crests is probably decreased, thus exposing the L_4-L_5 level to excessive mobility.

c) The intervertebral disc below the olisthetic vertebra is rarely normal in height. In most cases, it is decreased in height, but to a relatively mild extent; marked resorption of the intervertebral disc is usually associated with moderate or slight slipping.

d) The zygoapophyseal joints, at the level of spondylolisthesis, consistently show prominent degenerative changes (Fig. 5.6). The severity of the latter, however, is not related to the degree of vertebral slipping. Severe degenerative changes, in fact, are often observed in the presence of a relatively mild vertebral slipping, whereas, equally frequently, relatively mild osteoarthrotic alterations may be found associated with a pronounced vertebral olisthesis.

e) Anatomical studies on skeletons from individuals aged over forty years of age have shown that the interspinous ligament between the fourth and fifth lumbar vertebra is almost consistently degenerated or even interrupted (Rissanen, 1964). These changes are likely to become apparent earlier and to be more marked in subjects who have an excessively mobile fourth lumbar vertebra.

These observations suggest that olisthesis occurs in the presence of intrinsic vertebral

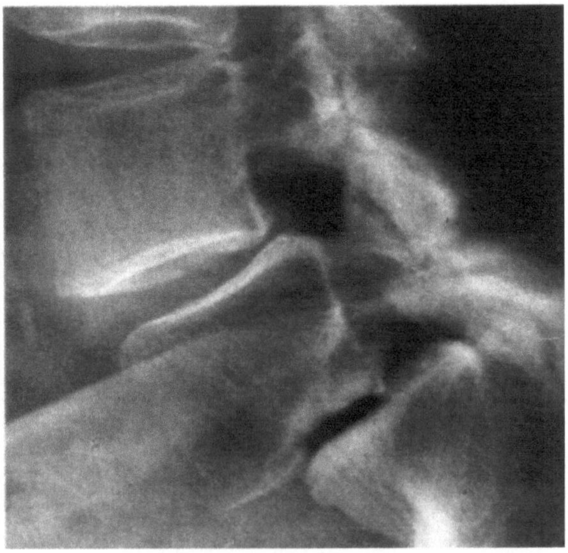

Fig. 5.4 - Degenerative spondylolisthesis of L_5, with 43% slipping. Degenerative olisthesis of such severity is exceptional. The L_4 vertebra also shows anterior slipping of mild entity.

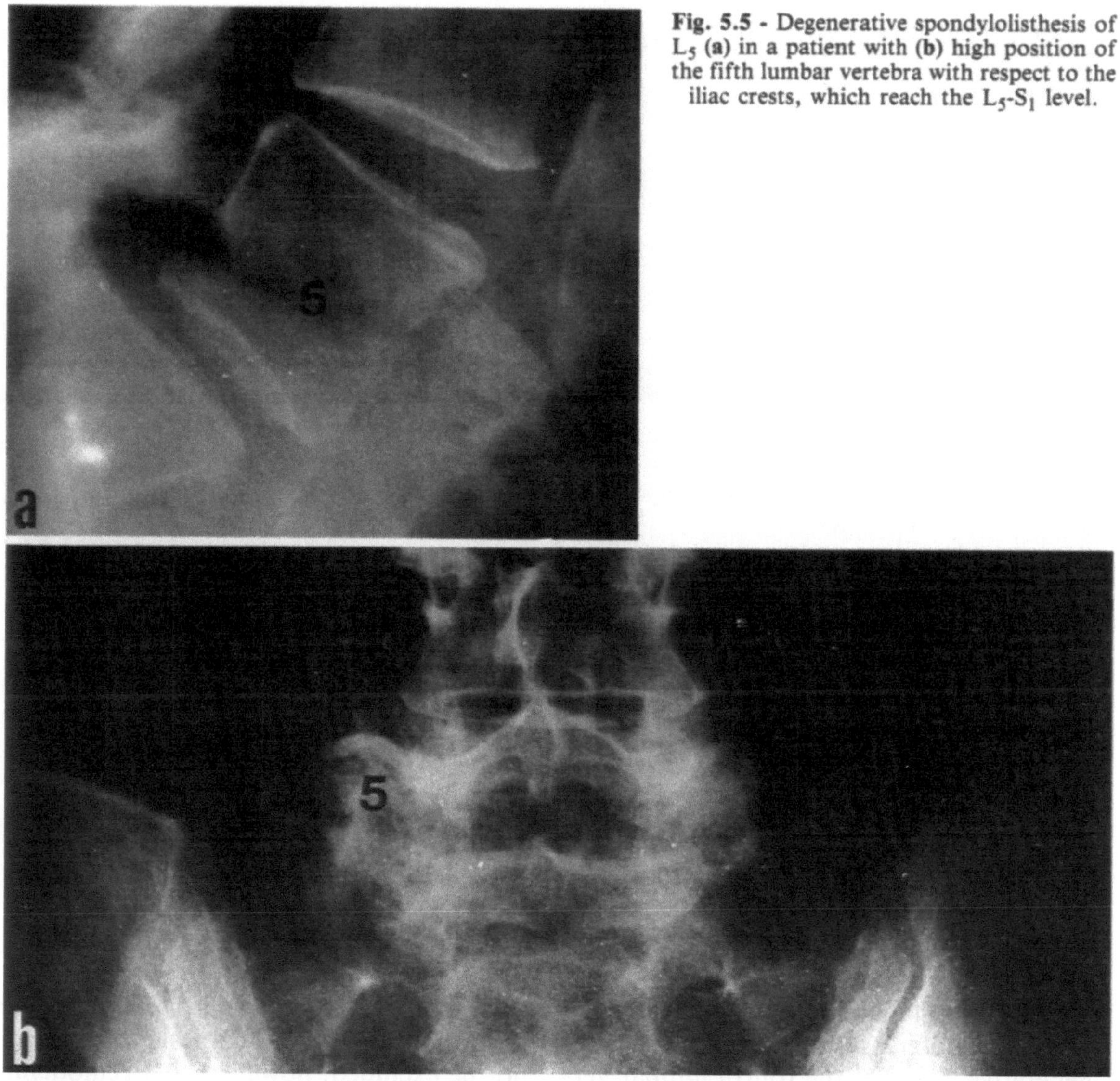

Fig. 5.5 - Degenerative spondylolisthesis of L_5 (a) in a patient with (b) high position of the fifth lumbar vertebra with respect to the iliac crests, which reach the L_5-S_1 level.

instability associated with severe degenerative changes of the posterior stabilizing structures.

The L_4 vertebra is the most mobile of the lumbar vertebrae, probably becoming more mobile than normal when it is located at an abnormally high level with respect to the tangent plane through the iliac crests. The same occurs when the fifth lumbar vertebra is more stable than normal, because in this event the functional stress is concentrated on the L_4-L_5 level, instead of being distributed over the lowest two lumbar levels. As a result of the abnormal mobility of the L_4 vertebra, the facet joints of the L_4-L_5 level are submitted to excessively high functional stress, which is responsible, with time, for osteoarthrotic changes in these joints. At the same time, the articular capsule of the facet joints and the posterior ligamentous structures (legamenta flava and interspinous ligament), which are submitted to undue stress in traction, undergo structural changes which progressively reduce their stabilizing function of two adjacent vertebrae. This function is then essentially or esclusively performed by the L_4-L_5 intervertebral disc. The latter, whilst intact, is able to prevent the fourth lumbar vertebra from slipping ventrally. When the intervertebral disc also looses, even

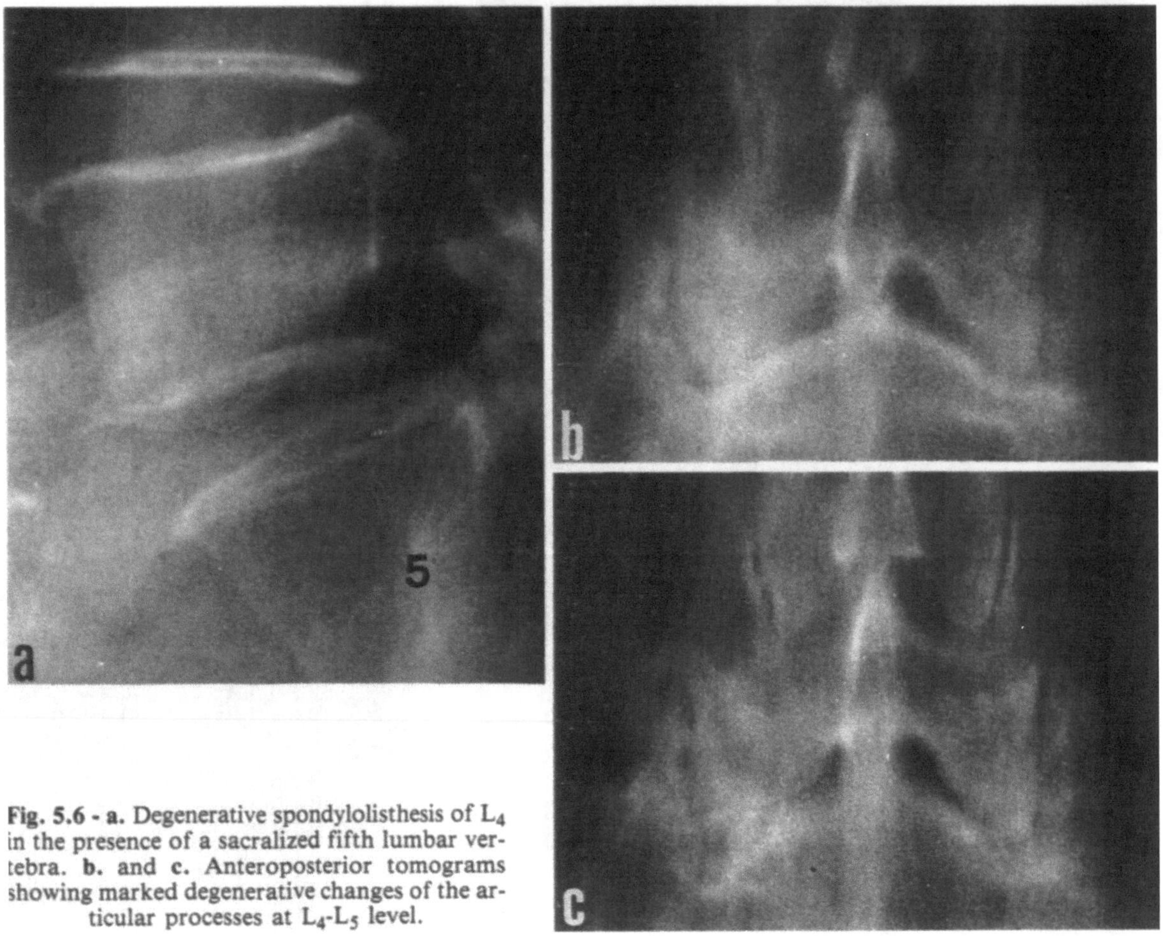

Fig. 5.6 - a. Degenerative spondylolisthesis of L_4 in the presence of a sacralized fifth lumbar vertebra. b. and c. Anteroposterior tomograms showing marked degenerative changes of the articular processes at L_4-L_5 level.

partially, its stabilizing capacity due to excessive functional stress and consequent degenerative changes, the fourth lumbar vertebra starts to slip forward. Slipping may increase until the disc is elastic and mobile, but halts when, in the presence of marked disc resorption, intervertebral mobility considerably decreases until it is completely exhausted (Fig. 5.7). Considerable vertebral instability is associated with even partial disc integrity. Gradually, as slipping proceeds, the zygoapophyseal joints undergo osteoarthrotic changes which become progressively more marked. These changes are associated, in the most advanced stages, with a sort of remodeling of the facet joints, the anteromedian portion of which becomes hypertrophic and can be placed on an almost transverse plane. These changes are probably related to the abnormal anatomical relationship in which the articular processes are found as a result of vertebral slipping. It cannot be excluded, however, that remodeling of the articular processes represents a compensating mechanism aimed at limiting vertebral olisthesis.

The presence of degenerative spondylolisthesis results in a narrowing of varying entity of the spinal canal and/or the nerve root canals. This narrowing is caused, in part, by the osteoarthrotic changes of the zygoapophyseal joints and, in part, by the vertebral olisthesis. Osteoarthrotic changes of the superior articular processes of the vertebra below the olisthetic one are responsible for narrowing of the nerve root canals of the slipped vertebra and sometimes even of the intervertebral foramen that the articular process contributes to delimit. Narrowing may be slight and not cause compression of

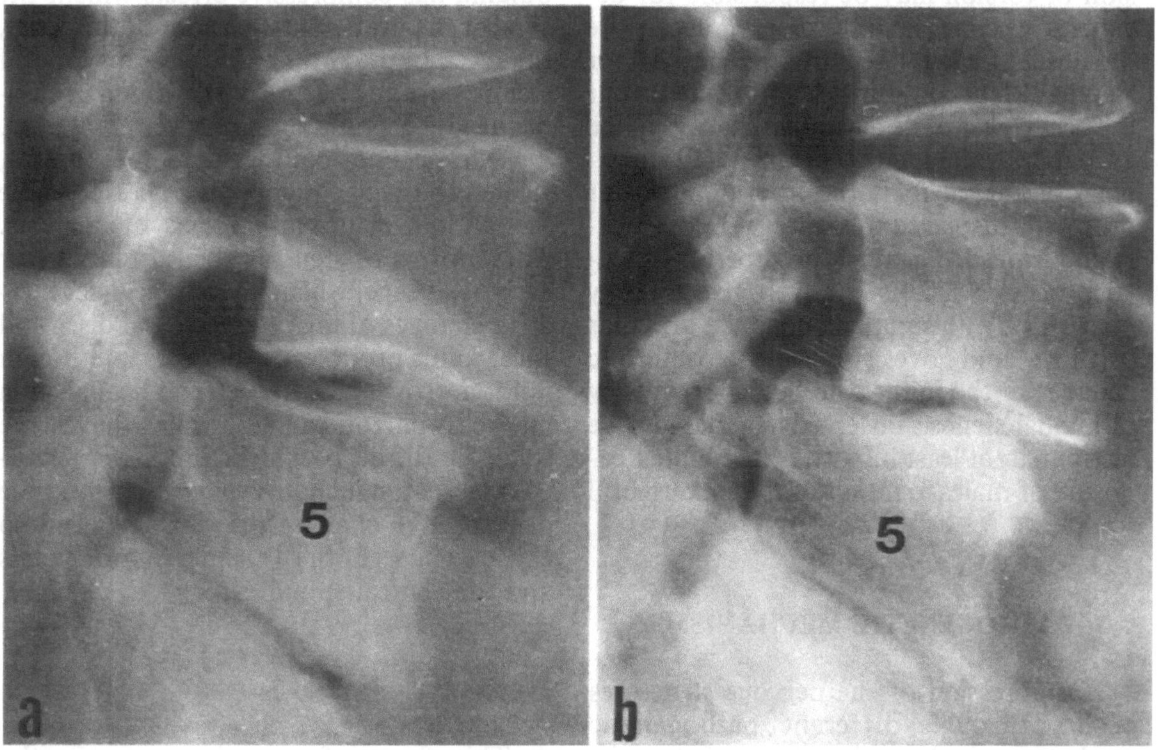

Fig. 5.7 - Degenerative spondylolisthesis of L_4. **a.** The L_4-L_5 disc is well preserved (1978). **b.** Five years later (1983), the olisthesis had increased, with a loss in the disc height. In subsequent follow-ups, the amount of slipping has remained unchanged.

the spinal nerve roots or may produce stenosis of varying entity of the nerve root canal and the neuroforamen. Degenerative disease (hypertrophy and osteophytosis) of the inferior articular processes of the olisthetic vertebra causes narrowing of the central spinal canal, which is further constricted, to a significant extent, by vertebral slipping. In fact, due to the integrity of the posterior vertebral arch, which follows the vertebral body in the slipping, the dural sac is as if it were guillottined between the laminae and inferior articular processes of the slipped vertebra and the posterosuperior border of the underlying vertebra. The pathological effects of these two anatomical changes (hypertrophy of the inferior articular processes and olisthesis) are, however, strictly related to the original width of the vertebral canal. If the latter is wide and vertebral slipping of slight entity, compression of the nervous spinal structures may not occur. In the presence of a normally sized spinal canal, the dural sac is usually encroached upon at the level of its lateral portions which are in direct contact with the inferior articular processes. If the dimensions of the spinal canal are at the lower limits of normal or below, marked compression of the dural sac occurs even in the presence of mild degenerative changes of the articular processes or moderate vertebral slipping.

TRAUMAS

Traumas may play multiple roles in the aetiopathogenesis of stenosis. A single trauma may cause: a vertebral fracture responsible for narrowing and segmental deformation of the vertebral canal; tears in the annulus fibrosus, in which the nucleus pulposus may become wedged; partial fractures or clefts of the cartilagineous end-plates, which may produce or accentuate degenerative changes of the intervertebral disc. Repeated minor traumas in flexion, compression or torsion may be responsible for degenerative changes in the disc, or accelerate the onset of age-related disc changes. Minor traumas in torsion, furthermore, may favour the occurrence of degenerative changes in the zygoapophyseal joints (Farfan, 1969). In axial rotation, in fact, the inferior articular process is displaced medially and posteriorly and is pushed against the superior articular process, which is relatively fixed (Lamy *et al.*, 1975); this may damage the articular cartilage and give rise to osteoarthrotic changes in the joint. The higher frequency of lumbar stenosis observed in males may be attributed, at least in part, to the higher exposure of males to minor or major vertebral traumas.

PATHOGENETIC MECHANISMS

Compression of the nervous structures occurs through different pathogenetic mechanisms in the various types of stenosis. Schematically, two main pathogenetic sequences may be distinguished, one for the primary forms of stenosis (achondroplastic and developmental) and the other for degenerative stenosis. In combined stenosis, there is an association of the two pathogenetic mechanisms, which may prevail one over the other, according to the case.

PRIMARY FORMS OF STENOSIS

Achondroplastic or developmental narrowing of the spinal canal does not cause compression of the nervous structures unless vertebral degenerative changes occur. The latter may be of two types: changes in the intervertebral disc in the form of a protrusion of the annulus fibrosus; and abnormalities in the disc and facet joints related to the ageing process.

Posterior bulging of the annulus fibrosus — caused by traumas and/or an individual predisposition to degenerative disease of the intervertebral disc — does not produce significant compression of the nervous spinal structures in a wide spinal canal. In a narrow vertebral canal, on the other hand, disc bulging has compressive effects which, the smaller the primary dimensions of the canal, the more marked they will be. This type of stenosis usually occurs in the young or middle-aged, generally at a single vertebral level.

The second pathogenetic mechanism, related to the ageing process, is responsible for multilevel primary forms of stenosis. These forms of stenosis occur in middle or early senile age, when physiological degenerative changes of the intervertebral discs and facet joints produce a progressive, although mild, narrowing of the vertebral canal. In a markedly narrow canal, in which the reserve space for the nervous structures is very limited or absent, mild narrowing caused by senile degenerative changes may be sufficient to cause stenosis both of the nerve root canals and the central spinal canal.

DEGENERATIVE STENOSIS

This form of stenosis occurs in the presence of marked spondylotic changes, which consistently involve both the intervertebral disc and facet joints.

The pathogenetic sequence leading to stenosis may start with degenerative changes of either the disc or the posterior joints (Kirkaldy-Willis *et al.*, 1978). Degenerative changes of the disc, when primary, may put abnormal functional stress on the facet joints due to segmental instability and/or the decrease in height resulting from the degenerative modifications. The zygopophyseal joints, as a consequence, may undergo marked degenerative changes, especially at those vertebral levels submitted to the greatest static-dynamic stress and in those subjects presenting a spondylotic predisposition or who are particularly exposed to vertebral traumas or microtraumas. If the facet joints lose their vertebral stabilizing function as a result of the osteoarthrotic changes, the disc will be submitted to greater functional stress, which then increases the articular degenerative changes. Finally, if the disc also loses its stabilizing function, spondylolisthesis may occur of the vertebra below the disc involved. The same events occur, with an inverse sequence, when degenerative changes involve primarily the facet joints. This series of disc-joint changes may cause stenosis of the nerve root canal associated, or not, with narrowing of the central portion of the spinal canal.

The last stage of the disc degeneration process is resorption of the nucleus pulposus, leading to marked loss of disc height. This reduction in height has two effects: subluxation of the articular processes, which not only contributes to narrow the nerve root canal and the neuroforamen, but also further increases the degenerative changes of the zygoapophyseal joints; and an approximation of the two adjacent vertebrae, which produces an increase in thickness of the ligamenta flava and a prominence of the latter in the spinal canal. A further possible effect of disc resorption is development of posterior marginal osteophytes of the vertebral body. As a result of these degenerative changes, the whole spinal canal and the intervertebral foramen undergo a varying degree of narrowing, which may be responsible, or not, for compression of the nervous structures, depending upon the extent of the degenerative changes and the primary width of the various canalar structures in the spine.

Two- or multilevel stenosis may develop either when degenerative changes involve simultaneously two or more vertebral levels, or as a result of marked degenerative changes at a single vertebral level. Disc resorption at a single level, in fact, leads to a decrease or a loss of segmental mobility and, as a result, to a greater functional stress on the motion segments above and/or below, which may undergo progressive disc and articular changes (Kirkaldy-Willis *et al.*, 1978).

REFERENCES

BAILEY J.A.: *Disproportionate short stature. Diagnosis and management.* W.B. Saunders, Philadelphia-London, Toronto, 1973.

CLARK G.E., PANJABI M.M., WETZEL F.J.: Can infant malnutrition cause adult vertebral stenosis? *Spine* **10:** 165, 1985.

COLLINS D.H.: *The pathology of articular and spinal diseases.* Edward Arnold, London, 1949.

FARFAN H.F.: Effect of torsion on the intervertebral joints. *Can J. Surg.* **12:** 336, 1969.

FITZGERALD J.W.A., NEWMAN P.H.: Degenerative spondylolisthesis. *J. Bone and Joint Surg.* **58-B:** 184, 1976.

GUNTZ E.: Die Erkrankungen der Zwischenwirbelgelenke. *Arch. Orthop. Unfallchir.* **34:** 333, 1934.

INGELMARK B.E.: De funktionelle anatomiska furhallandema: ryggraden mes sarskild hansyn Eill dess smaleder. *Acta Univ. Gotheburg* **62:** 1, 1956.

INGELMARK B.E.: Spinal joint changes and dental infections. *Acta Anat.* (Basel) **38:** suppl. 36, 1959.

KIRKALDY-WILLIS W.H., WEDGE J.H., YONG-HING K., REILLY J.: Pathology and pathogenesis of lumbar spondylosis and stenosis. *Spine* **3:** 319, 1978.

LAMY C., BAZERGNI A., KRANS H., FARFAN H.F.: The strength of the neural arch and the etiology of spondylosis. *Orthop. Clin. North Am.* **6:** 215, 1975.

LEWIN T.: Osteoarthritis in lumbar synovial joints. A morphologic study. *Acta Orthop. Scand.* suppl. 73, 1964.

MARCHETTI P.G., BARTOLOZZI P.: *Le spondiloliste-si.* Aulo Gaggi Editore, Bologna, 1985.

MAYNARD J.A., IPPOLITO E., PONSETI I.V., MICKELSON M.R.: Histochemistry and ultrastructure of the growth plate in achondroplasia. *J. Bone and Joint Surg.* **63-A:** 969, 1981.

MCNAB I.: Spondylolisthesis with an intact neural arch. The so-called pseudo-spondylolisthesis. *J. Bone and Joint Surg.* **32-B:** 325, 1950.

PONSETI I.V.: Skeletal growth in achondroplasia. *J. Bone and Joint Surg.* **52-A:** 701, 1970.

POSTACCHINI F., RIPANI M., CARPANO S.: Morphometry of the lumbar vertebrae. An anatomic study in two Caucasoid ethnic groups. *Clin. Orthop.* **172:** 296, 1983.

POTTER R.M., NARCROSS J.R.: Spondylolisthesis without isthmus defect. *Radiology* **63:** 678, 1954.

RISSANEN P.M.: Comparison of pathologic changes in intervertebral disc and interspinous ligament of the lower part of the lumbar spine in the light and autopsy findings. *Acta Orthop. Scand.* **34:** 54, 1964.

ROSENBERG N.J.: Degenerative spondylolisthesis. Predisposing factors. *J. Bone and Joint Surg.* **57-A:** 467, 1975.

SCHMORL G., JUNGHANNS H.: *Die gesunde und kranke Wirbelsäule im Roentgenbild.* Leipzig, 1932.

Chapter VI

Pathomorphology

F. Postacchini, W. Rauschning

INTRODUCTION

The pathomorphology of the stenotic vertebral canal has been the subject of several anatomical studies, which have described the pathological changes typical of primary stenosis and, particularly, the effects of spondylosis and osteoarthrosis of the facet joints on the vertebral canal and the neuroforamen (Crock, 1975; Yong-Hing *et al.*, 1976; Kirkaldy-Willis *et al.*, 1978; Schneck, 1985). Over the last few years cryomicrotomy, which in fresh autopsy specimens allows a detailed visualization of both the vertebral canal and its contents, has significantly contributed to our knowledge of the normal spinal anatomy, the morphological characteristics of the stenotic vertebral canal and, in particular, the static and dynamic effects of loading and movement of the stenotic spine on the vertebral nervous and vascular structures (Rauschning, 1985; Tajima and Kawano, 1986).

VERTEBRAL CANAL AND INTERVERTEBRAL FORAMEN

PRIMARY STENOSIS

The stenotic vertebral canal in achondroplastic dwarfs shows pathological features very similar to those of the most typical forms of idiopathic developmental stenosis. In both forms of stenosis, the pedicles and laminae are abnormally short and the articular processes are often orientated in a sagittal direction. The posterior surface of the vertebral bodies may be considerably concave in the sagittal plane (Figs. 6.1a and 6.1b). The intervertebral discs are frequently normal in height and, in some instances, appear to be higher than normal due to reduced height of the vertebral bodies (Figs. 6.1a and 6.1b). The posterior surface of the lumbar discs normally bulges slightly into the vertebral canal (Figs. 6.1a and 6.1b). This posterior bulge may be determined by degenerative changes of the disc, but may also be observed in the absence of structural disc pathology. In the most typical forms of developmental stenosis, in fact, the intervertebral discs are not, or are only very slightly, degenerated. Bulging, in these cases, seems to be a peculiar morphologic feature, possibly related to the posterior prominence of the vertebral end-plates.

When examined in transverse section the vertebral canal shows an abnormally short interarticular diameter due to the shortness of the laminae and the sagittal orientation of the articular processes. A true nerve root canal is frequently detectable not only at the lowest two lumbar levels, but also at L_3-L_4, and sometimes L_2-L_3, level. The intervertebral portion of the nerve root canals and the lateral recesses are narrow as a result of the shortness of the pedicles and the sagittal orientation of the superior articular processes. In developmental stenosis the articular processes show mild degenerative changes and the ligamenta flava are normal in thickness or appear only slightly thicker than normal.

Posterior disc bulging and prominence of the vertebral end-plates, associated or not with thickening of the ligamenta flava, produce a segmental narrowing of the vertebral canal, which increases in width at the level of the superior and inferior vertebral bodies. The presence of a narrow area between wider areas gives the sagittal section of the vertebral canal a characteristic hourglass appearance (Fig. 6.1b).

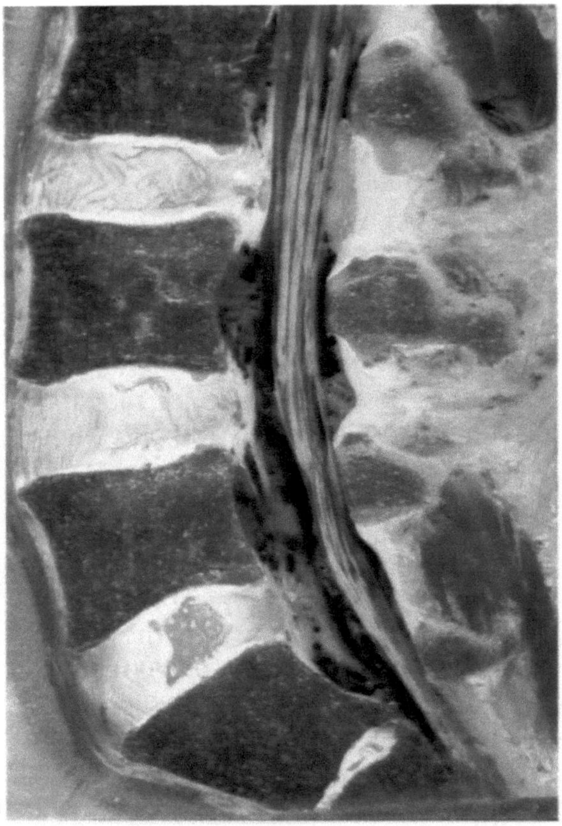

a

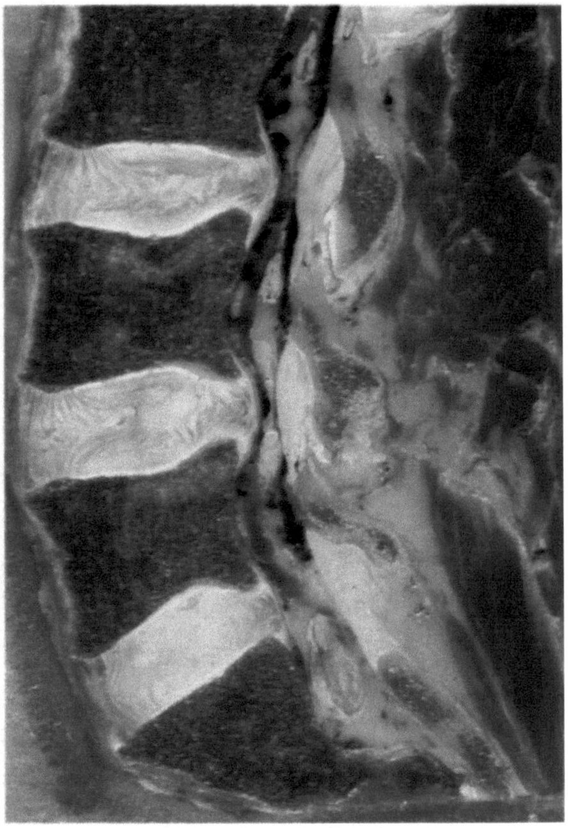

b

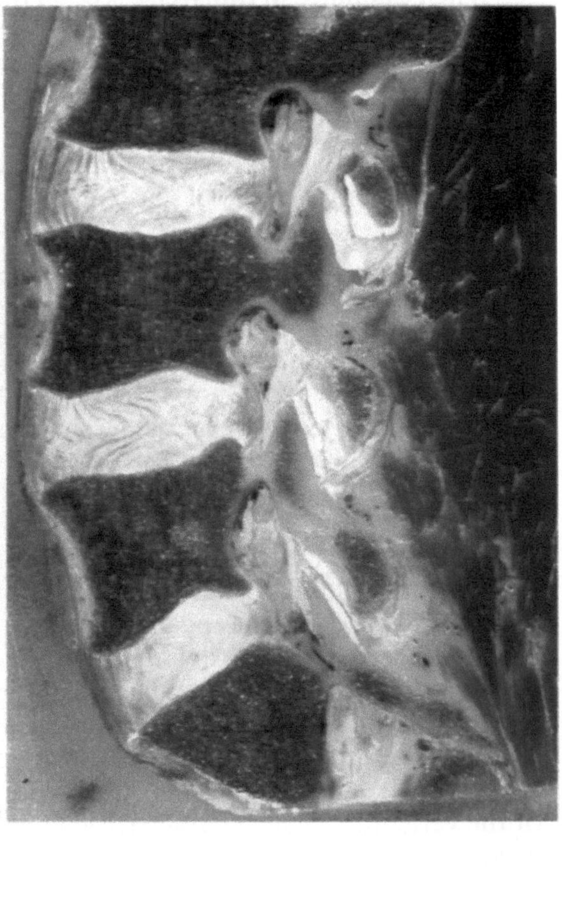

c

Fig. 6.1 - Sagittal sections of a lumbo-sacral spine with developmental stenosis. **a.** Midsagittal section. The intervertebral discs are higher than normal and bulge into the spinal canal. The posterior aspect of the vertebral bodies show a marked concavity, occupied by fat tissue and epidural vessels. The dural sac is narrow and is in contact, at L_3 level, with the disc anteriorly and the ligamentum flavum posteriorly. **b.** Sagittal section through the nerve root canals. The nerve roots have emerged from the dural sac, but have not yet entered into the intervertebral foramen. The L_3-L_4 and L_4-L_5 discs show mild degenerative changes and bulge markedly into the spinal canal. The ligamenta flava are thick. Due to disc bulging and slight ventral buckling of the ligamenta flava, the spinal canal appears sinusoidal in shape with segmentary narrowing at the level of the intervertebral spaces. **c.** Sagittal section at the level of the entrance of the intervertebral foramina. The latter, due to the shortness of the pedicles, display short sagittal dimensions and, on account of posterior concavity of the vertebral bodies, have a definite inverted tear-drop shape, particularly at L_4-L_5 level. At this level, the caudal portion of the neuroforamen appears to be obliterated.

Due to the shortness of the pedicles, the intervertebral foramina are narrow and slit-shaped in the sagittal plane, whereas the vertical dimensions are generally normal on account of the normal height of the intervertebral discs (Fig. 6.1c). The middle and caudal portions of the neuroforamina may be abnormally narrow due to posterolateral bulging of the intervertebral discs, but the nerve roots are rarely compressed, since they occupy the cranial portion of the foramina.

DEGENERATIVE STENOSIS

Disc degeneration and osteophytosis of the vertebral body

At a stenotic intervertebral level, the disc usually shows degenerative changes, which may be related to the physiologic ageing process or may be clearly pathological. The degenerative changes may consist in bulging of the annulus fibrosus or disc resorption. An individual may present only one of the two types of changes or even both types at different vertebral levels.

Posterior protrusion of a degenerated disc, unlike that usually occurring in the presence of disc herniation, may involve either the entire circumference, or the anterior or posterior hemicircumference, of the disc. The nucleus pulposus has a fibrous appearance and may show radial and circumferential tears. Clefts, usually arranged in a concentric fashion, may also be present in the annulus fibrosus, which bulges to a varying extent into the vertebral canal and the intervertebral foramina. The disc bulge in the vertebral canal reduces the sagittal dimensions of the central portion of the canal and the width of the intervertebral portion of the nerve root canal. The bulge in the intervertebral foramen results in narrowing or obliteration of the middle and caudal portions of the neuroforamen, which is occupied by fat tissue and blood vessels.

Disc resorption, when marked, is generally associated with sclerosis of the cancellous bone adjacent to the vertebral end-plates and, often, with posterior marginal osteophytes of the vertebral bodies (Figs. 6.2a and 6.2b). The osteophytes produce similar effects, on the spinal canal and the nerve root canal, as disc protrusion; that is, they narrow the central portion of the vertebral canal and the nerve root canal at the level of both the intervertebral portion (osteophytes of both the vertebral end-plates) and the lateral recess (osteophytes of the superior vertebral end-plate). Disc resorption involves a narrowing of the intervertebral portion of the nerve root canal and a decrease in size of the intervertebral foramen. Narrowing of the nerve root canal is caused by the subluxation of the articular processes, due to disc resorption and the consequent nearing of the medial border of the superior articular process to the anterior wall of the vertebral canal. However, a reduction in width occurring only by this mechanism is relatively mild. Narrowing of the neuroforamen is related to resorption of the disc both directly (reduction in height) and indirectly due to subluxation of the articular processes (reduction in width). The amount and pathological effects of the reduction in width of the intervertebral foramen depend on the extent of loss of disc height and the volume of the marginal osteophytes possibly present. Marked disc resorption results in considerable decrease in height of the neuroforamen and an upward displacement of the superior articular process, which invades the cranial portion of the foramen, thus impinging on the spinal nerve root in its intraforaminal course. The nerve root, in the presence of a large osteophyte of the inferior vertebral end-plate, may be entrapped between the osteophyte and the superior articular process of the vertebra below (Fig. 6.2b).

Compression of the nerve root, on the other hand, does not occur if loss of disc height is not marked and/or the osteophytes of the vertebral body are not prominent (Fig. 6.3).

Osteoarthrotic changes of the facet joints

Degenerative hypertrophy of the inferior articular processes is responsible, at intervertebral level, of a transverse narrowing of the central portion of the vertebral canal. The

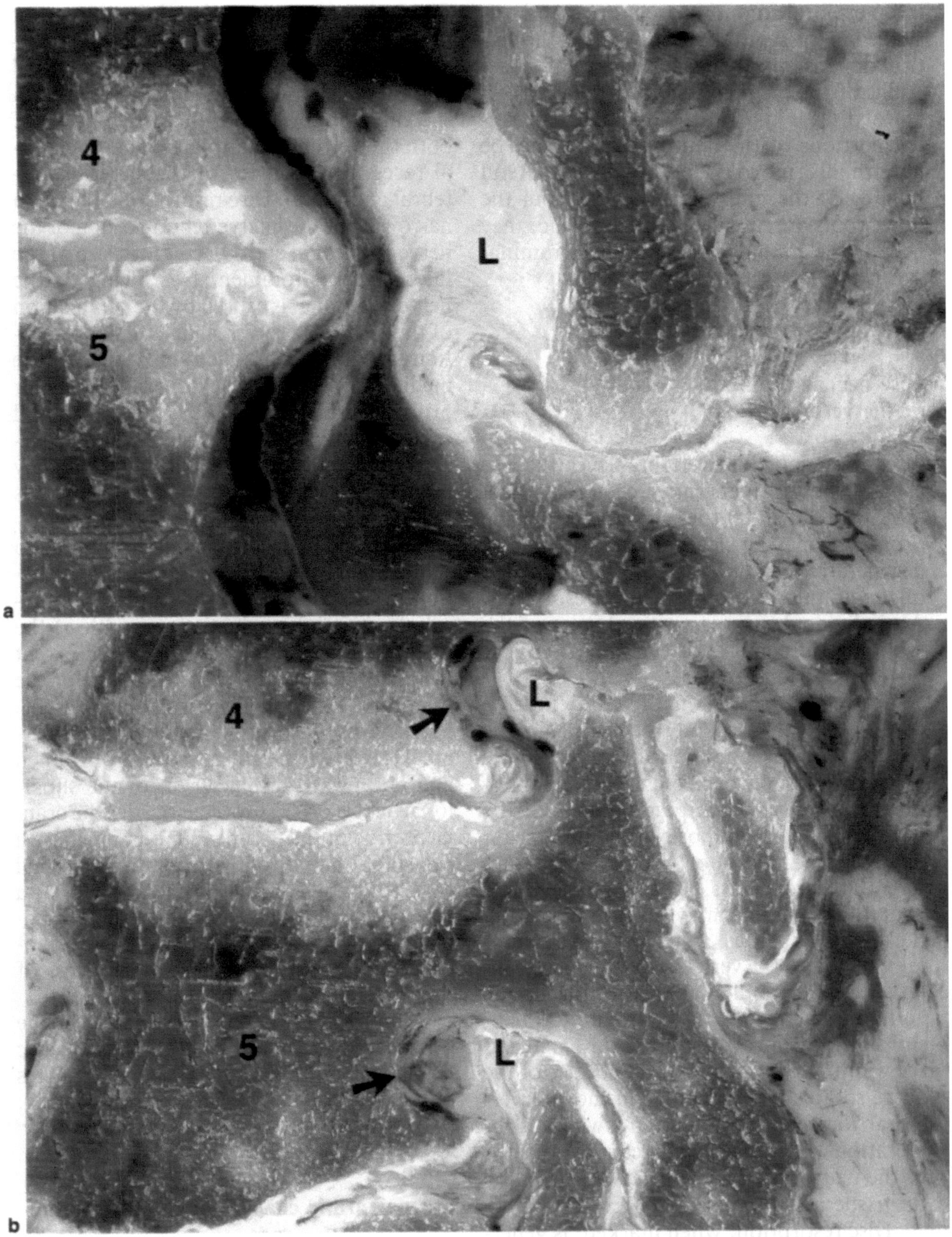
4
5
L
a
4
L
5
L
b

Fig. 6.2 - 65-year-old male. **a.** Sagittal section through the lateral portion of the spinal canal at L_4-L_5 level. Complete resorption of the intervertebral disc and posterior osteophytosis of the bony end-plates, which appear sclerotic. The ligamentum flavum (L) buckles markedly into the spinal canal. A nerve root (arrow) still contained in the dural sac is visible, which is entrapped between the end-plate osteophyte and the ligamentum flavum. **b.** Sagittal section through the L_4-L_5 and L_5-S_1 intervertebral foramina. Buckling of the capsular ligamenta flava (L) narrows, at both levels, the cranial portion of the neuroforamen, which is occupied by the nerve root (arrow). At L_4-L_5 level, the nerve root appears to be entrapped between the vertebral body and the ligamentum flavum.

◄

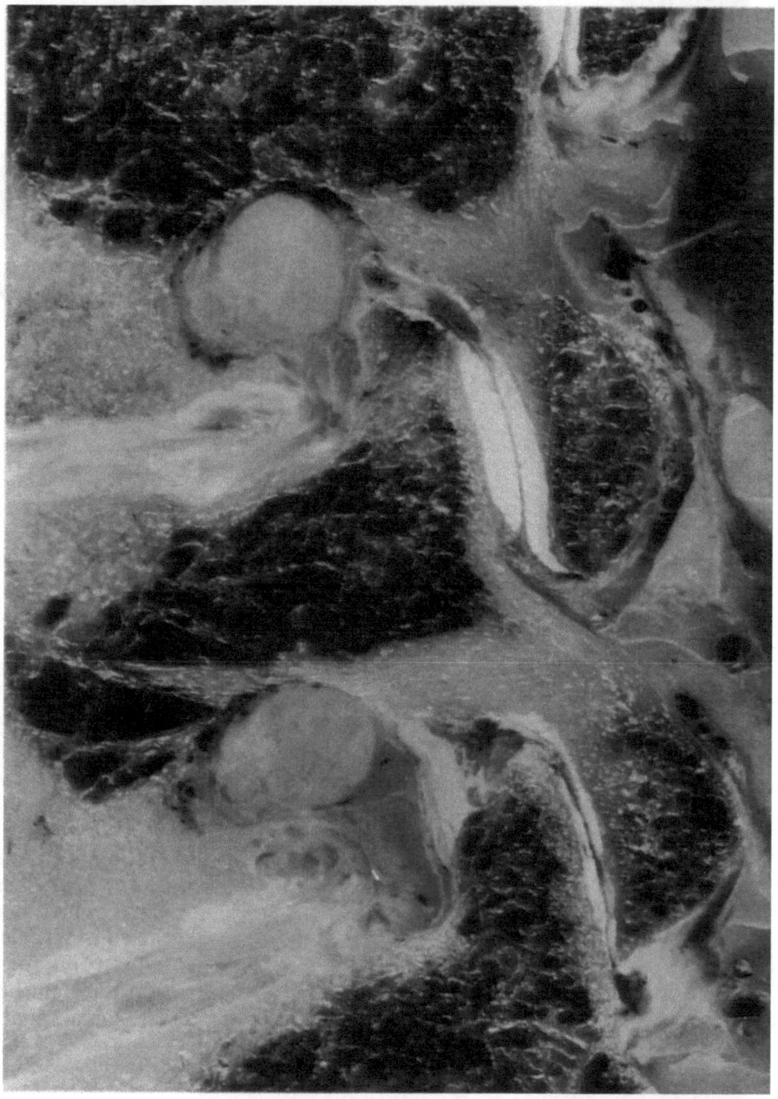

Fig. 6.3 - Sagittal section through the lower two lumbar intervertebral foramina. Despite disc resorption, the nerve roots are not compressed. The upper intervertebral foramen is narrowed by an end-plate osteophyte, which occludes the distal portion of the neuroforamen, not occupied by the nerve root.

latter, seen in axial sections, tends to assume, at the upper lumbar levels, the shape of a triangle with more or less convex sides and, at the lower two lumbar levels, a trefoil shape (Figs. 6.4a and 6.5b). Distally and proximally to the intervertebral space, the spinal canal increases in width and regains, depending upon the vertebral level, a roundish or triangular shape (Figs. 6.4b and 6.5b). In a multilevel stenosis, these changes produce a continuous alternation of narrow and deformed areas with larger areas of normal shape. Hypertrophy of the superior articular processes, associated or not with osteophytosis of the anteromedial border, contributes to the deformation of the central portion of the vertebral canal and narrows the intervertebral portion of the nerve root canal (Fig. 6.6b). Degenerative changes in the base of the superior articular process cause a narrowing of the cranial portion of the lateral recess. Finally, the superior articular process, when hypertrophic, produces a narrowing of the intervertebral foramen in the sagittal diameter and may impinge, with its apical portion, on the nerve root running in the foramen (Figs. 6.2a and 6.6a).

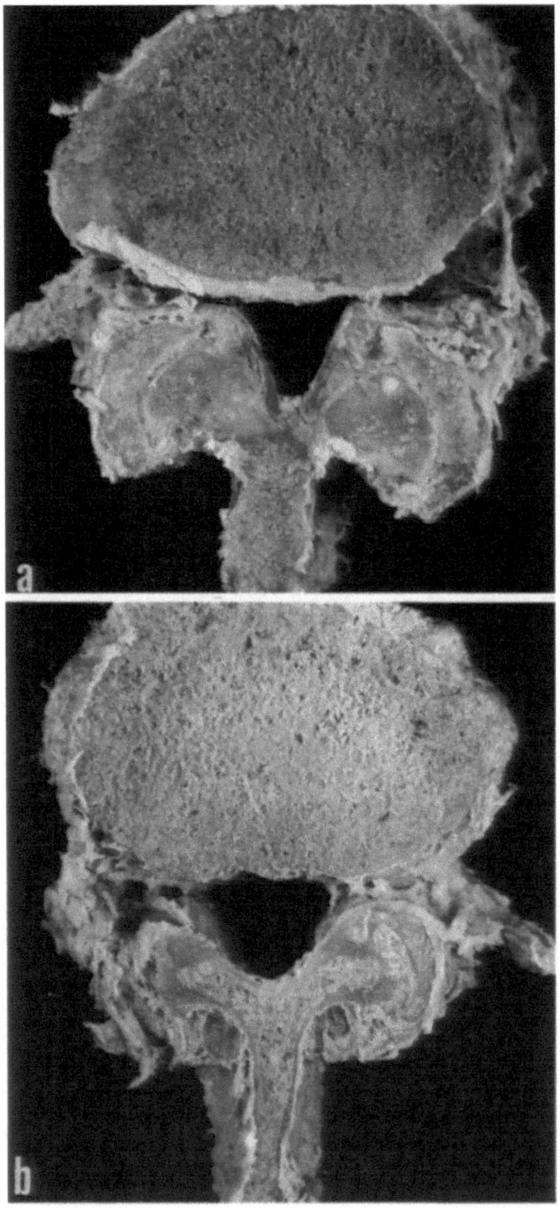

Fig. 6.4 - a. Axial section of L_3 vertebra, 3 mm proximally to the L_3-L_4 disc. Degenerative hypertrophy of the inferior articular processes and thickening of the ligamenta flava give the spinal canal a triangular shape. **b.** Section of the same vertebra 1.5 cm proximally to the L_3-L_4 disc (middle portion of the vertebral body). The spinal canal, delimited posterolaterally by the laminae, is roundish in shape.

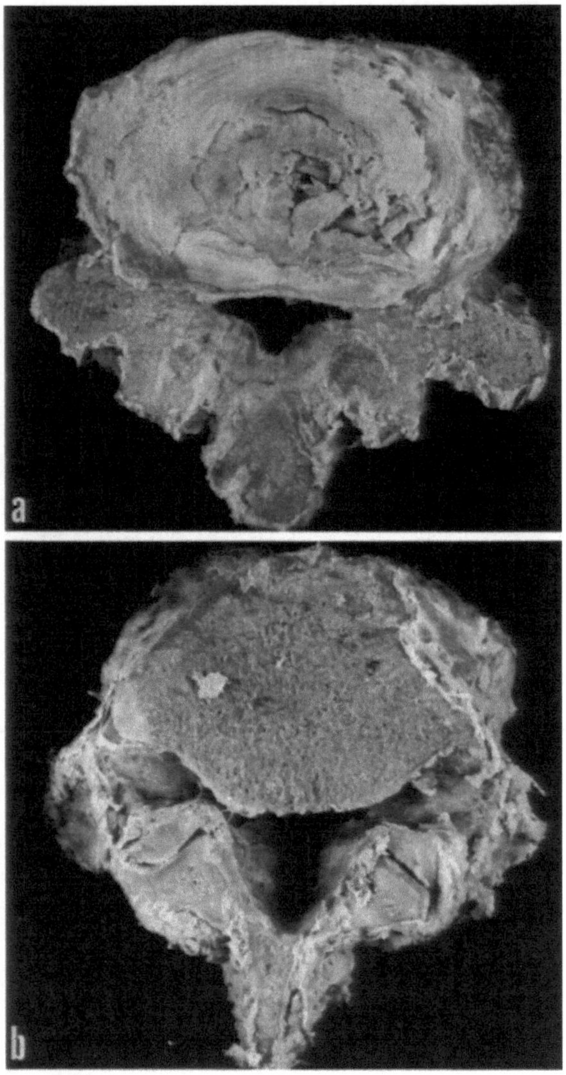

Fig. 6.5 - a. Axial section through the distal portion of the L_4-L_5 disc. Marked narrowing of the spinal canal, which is trefoil in shape. Narrowing is due to the considerable thickness of the ligamenta flava and hypertrophy of the articular processes. **b.** Axial section through the lower half of the L_5 vertebral body. The spinal canal is considerably increased in width and shows a triangular shape.

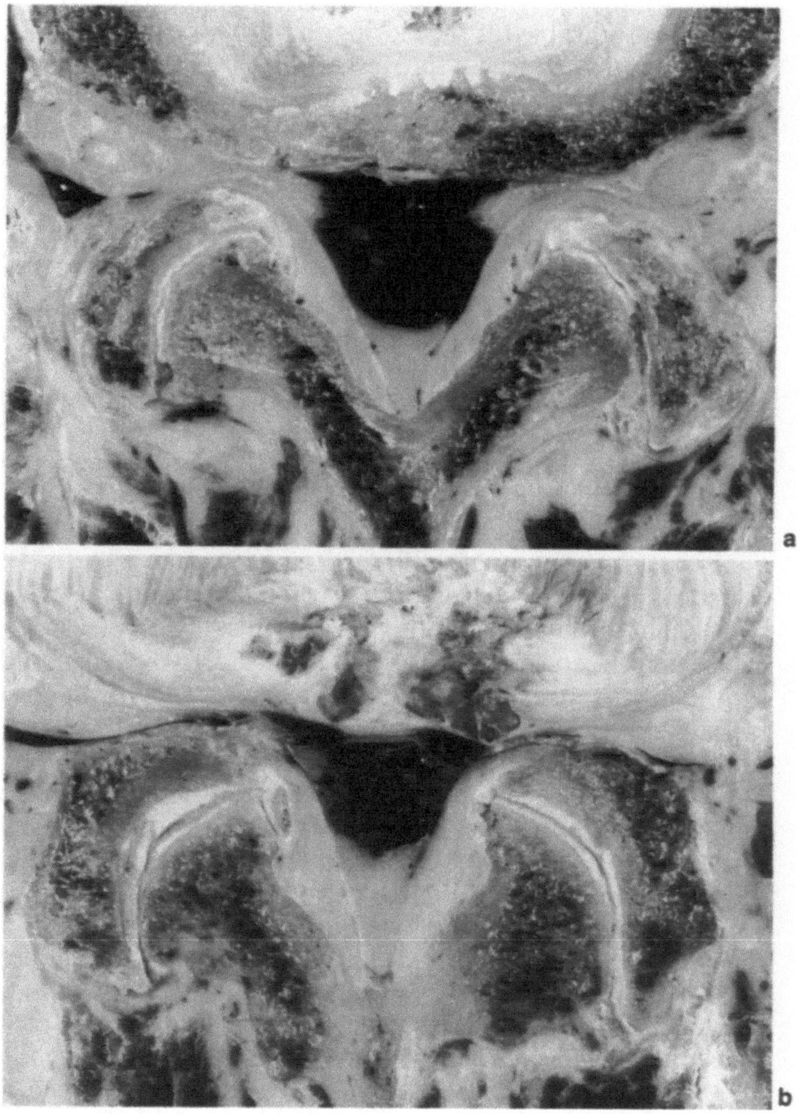

Fig. 6.6 - a. Axial section through the lower end-plate of L_4. The intervertebral foramen, occupied by the L_4 nerve root, is delimited posteriorly by the superior articular process of L_5, covered by the ligamentum flavum. It is clear that the superior articular process, when hypertrophic, may compress the spinal nerve root in the neuroforamen. **b.** Section through the proximal portion of the L_4-L_5 disc. The disc is degenerated and protrudes posteriorly. The articular processes, showing arthrotic changes, and the thickened ligamenta flava constrict the spinal canal; note the reduced cross-sectional area of the dural sac compared with the upper section (**a**), which is only a few millimeters higher up. The hypertrophy and medial prominence of the superior articular processes narrow the lateral portions of the spinal canal (not occupied by the spinal nerve roots, which have not yet emerged from the dural sac).

Thickening of the laminae

It has often been reported that the laminae, in stenosis of the spinal canal, may be sclerotic and thickened. Indeed the laminae are often sclerotic in degenerative and combined stenosis, but no more so than the other bony vertebral structures. Thickening, on the other hand, is more likely to be due to calcification and/or ossification of the portion of the ligamenta flava located ventrally to the caudal half of the laminae, than to a true bony hypertrophy. This is consistent with the findings of Verbiest (1980), who did not observe any histological abnormality in the bony structure of the laminae in patients submitted to surgery for lumbar stenosis.

Changes of the ligamenta flava

Ligamenta flava are generally shortened in the vertical plane, narrowed in the transverse plane, and thickened up to as much as double their normal thickness. Shortening is due to loss of disc height and consequent approaching of the two contiguous vertebrae. Transverse narrowing is caused by hypertrophy of the inferior articular processes, which is responsible for the closing-in of the medial border of these processes to the spinous process. A significant role in the aetiology of these two changes in the ligamenta flava may also be played by ossification of the insertions of the ligaments on the laminae and articular processes. Thickening seems to be caused essentially by shortening of the ligaments, which involves retraction and an increase in thickness of the elastic fibers; the latter, in fact, as well as the collagen fibers, do not show degenerative changes, which may be responsible for a significant thickening of the ligamenta flava (Ramsey, 1966; Ramani *et al.*, 1975). The increase in thickness of the portion of the ligamenta flava attached to the laminae narrows the central posterior part of the vertebral canal, thus contributing to a significant extent to compression of the dural sac (Fig. 6.6b). Approximation of the ligamenta flava of the two sides reduces the width of the posterior angle of the vertebral canal.

Thickening of the portion of the ligamentum flavum covering the anterior part of the zygoapophyseal joint capsule narrows the central anterior portion of the vertebral canal and the intervertebral portion of the nerve root canal (Fig. 6.6b). The increase in thickness and infolding of this portion may contribute to narrow the intervertebral foramen and compress the spinal nerve root, when the apex of the superior articular process approaches the pedicle of the vertebra above (Fig. 6.2b).

DYNAMIC STENOSIS

Normally, the sagittal dimensions of the lumbar spinal canal increase in flexion of the spine and decrease in extension (see page 42). If the vertebral canal has a large reserve space for the nervous structures, the decrease in size caused by extension of the spine has no pathologic effect. If, however, the reserve space is limited, or the spinal nerve roots and/or the dural sac are already compressed, further narrowing, caused by functional modifications, determines a compression or an increase of compression of the nervous structures. Changes in size and shape of the vertebral canal occurring in flexion-extension, and particularly those caused by the ligamenta flava, essentially affect the dural sac (Fig. 6.7). Dynamic changes in the nerve root canal are less marked than those of the central vertebral canal and are almost exclusively caused by the intervertebral disc.

Torsion of a vertebra with respect to the subjacent vertebra results in a posterior displacement of the lateral portion of the proximal vertebra and the intervertebral disc on the side towards which torsion occurs. On this side, the nerve root canal decreases in width and this may be responsible for compression of the nerve root or may increase compression if the canal is narrow or stenotic (Fig. 6.8).

DEGENERATIVE SPONDYLOLISTHESIS

Degenerative spondylolisthesis causes narrowing of varying extent of the vertebral canal and/or the nerve root canals. This narrowing is produced, in part, by osteoarthrotic changes in the articular processes and, in part, by vertebral olisthesis. Osteoarthrotic changes in the superior articular processes of the vertebra below the olisthetic one produce a narrowing of the nerve root canals of the slipped vertebra and, sometimes, even of the intervertebral foramina, which the articular processes contribute to delimit. Narrowing may be slight and not determine compression of the spinal nerve root or may be responsible for stenosis, of varying severity, of the nerve root canal and the neuroforamen (Fig. 6.9). Degenerative changes (hypertrophy and osteophytosis) of the inferior articular processes of the olisthetic vertebra cause a narrowing of the central spinal canal, which is further constricted to a significant extent by vertebral slipping. In fact, due to the integrity of the posterior vertebral arch, which follows the vertebral body in the slipping, it is as if the dural sac were guillotined between the laminae and the inferior articular processes of the olisthetic vertebra and posterosuperior border of the vertebral body below.

The pathological effects of these two changes — hypertrophy of the inferior articular processes and olisthesis — are,

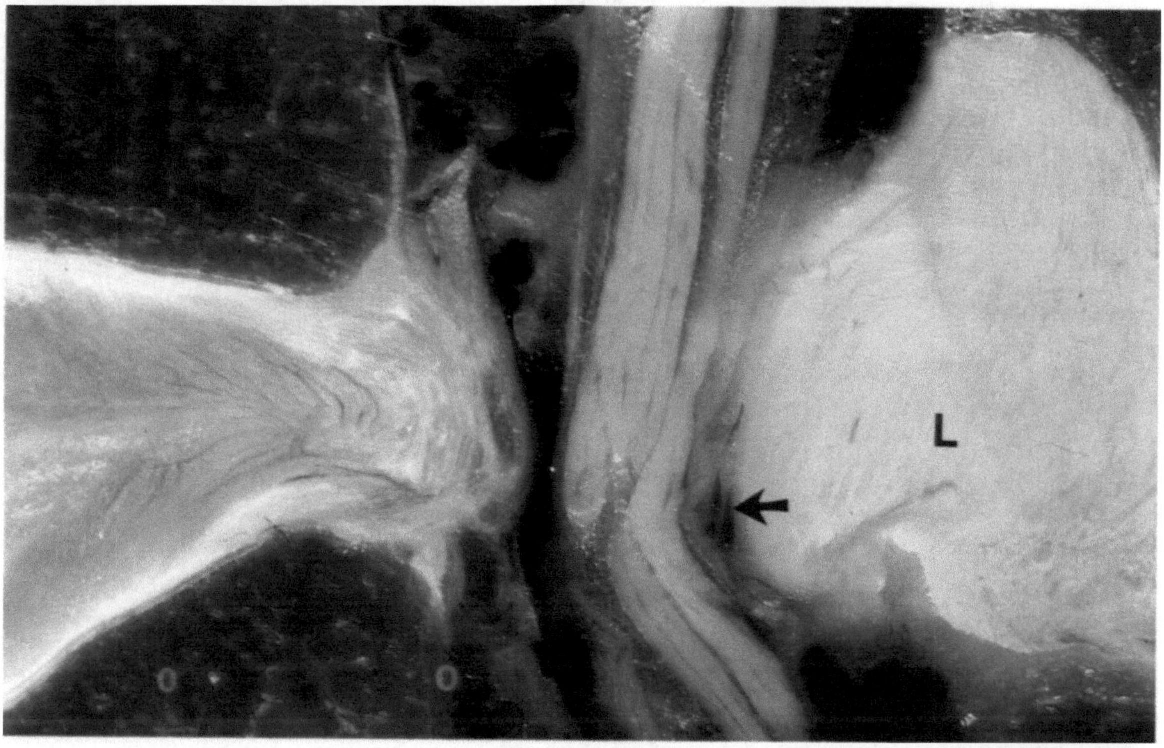

Fig. 6.7 - Sagittal section 1 cm lateral to the midline of a spine frozen in moderate extension. The disc shows degenerative changes and a posterior radial cleft. Both the annulus fibrosus and the ligamentum flavum (L) bulge markedly into the spinal canal. The result is compression, essentially posterior, of the lateral portion of the thecal sac and caudal nerve roots (arrow).

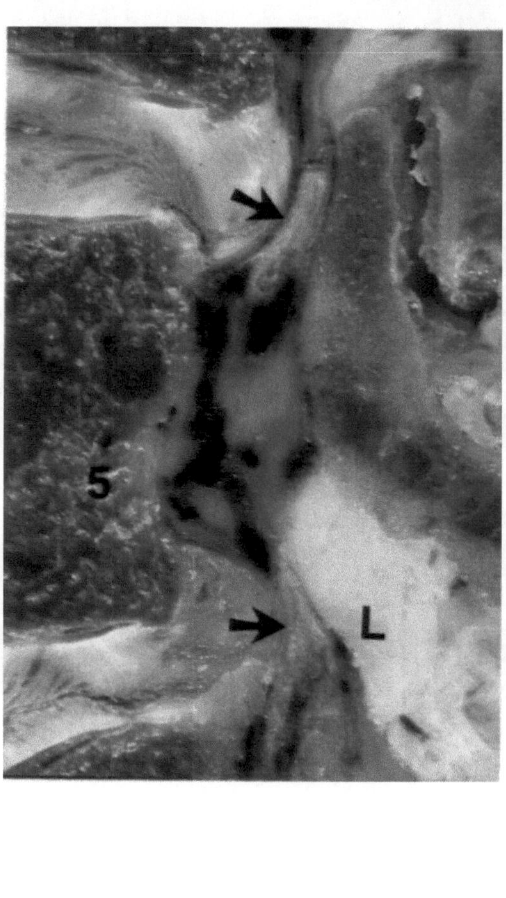

however, related to the original width of the vertebral canal. If the latter is wide and slipping is mild, the spinal neurovascular structures may not undergo significant compression. If, on the other hand, the vertebral canal is of normal size, compression usually occurs of the lateral portions of the dural sac, which are in contact with the inferior articular processes. If the dimensions of the spinal canal are at the lower limits of normal or even below, marked compression of the dural sac occurs, also in the presence of mild degenerative changes of the articular processes or a slight vertebral slipping (Fig. 6.10).

Fig. 6.8 - Sagittal section through the nerve root canals in a spine frozen in moderate rotation. The L_5 vertebral body is visible, with the adjacent discs bulging into the spinal canal. As a result of rotation, the L_4-L_5 facet joint gapes and the L_5 nerve root (arrow) is compressed between the disc and the superior articular process of L_5. At L_5-S_1 level, the S_1 root (arrow) is entrapped between the disc and the buckling ligamentum flavum (L).

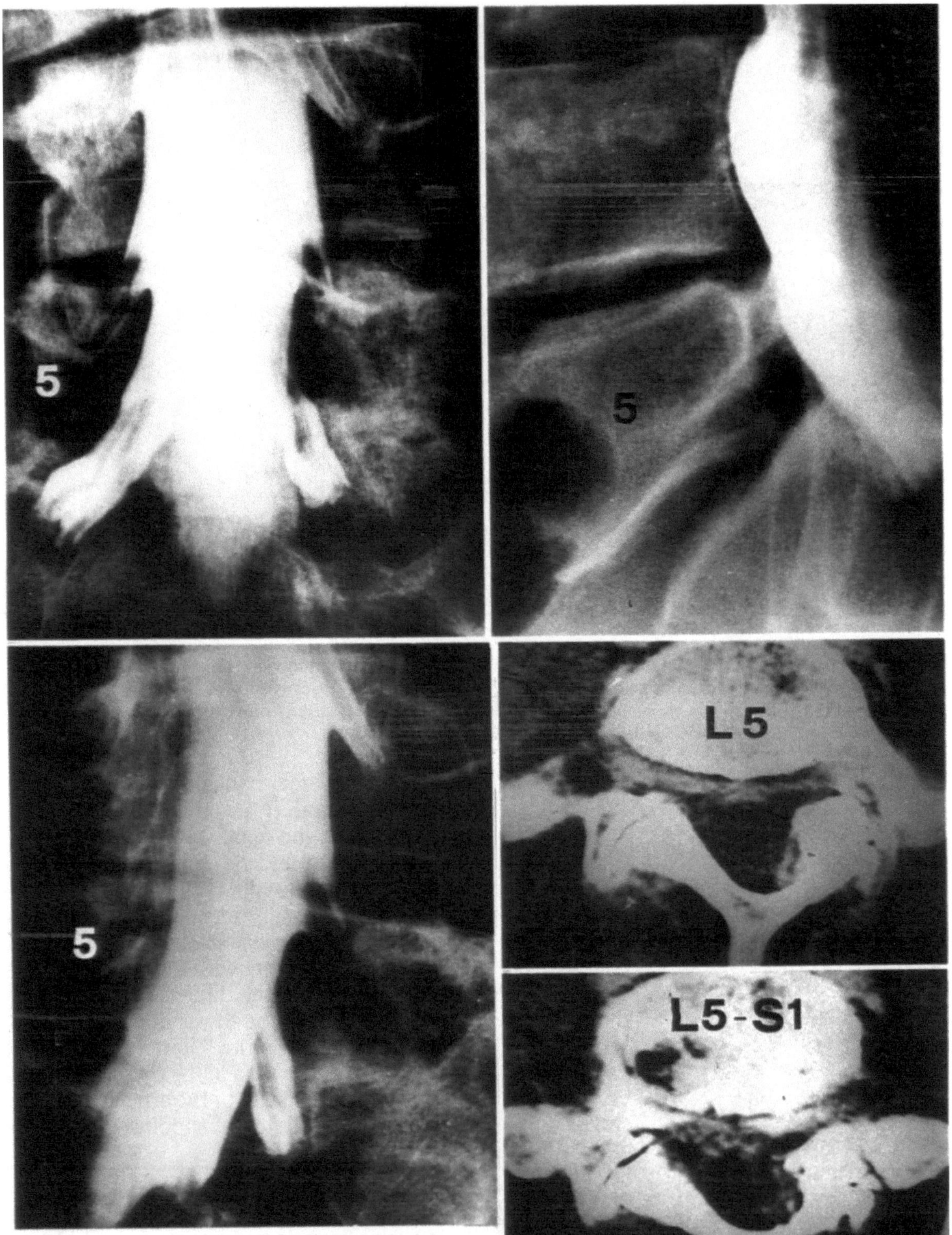

Fig. 6.9 - Degenerative spondylolisthesis of L_5. Myelograms show evidence of compression of the left L_5 and S_1 nerve roots, in the absence of compression of the thecal sac. CT scans display narrowing of the left L_5 and S_1 nerve root canals due to hypertrophy of the superior articular processes of S_1.

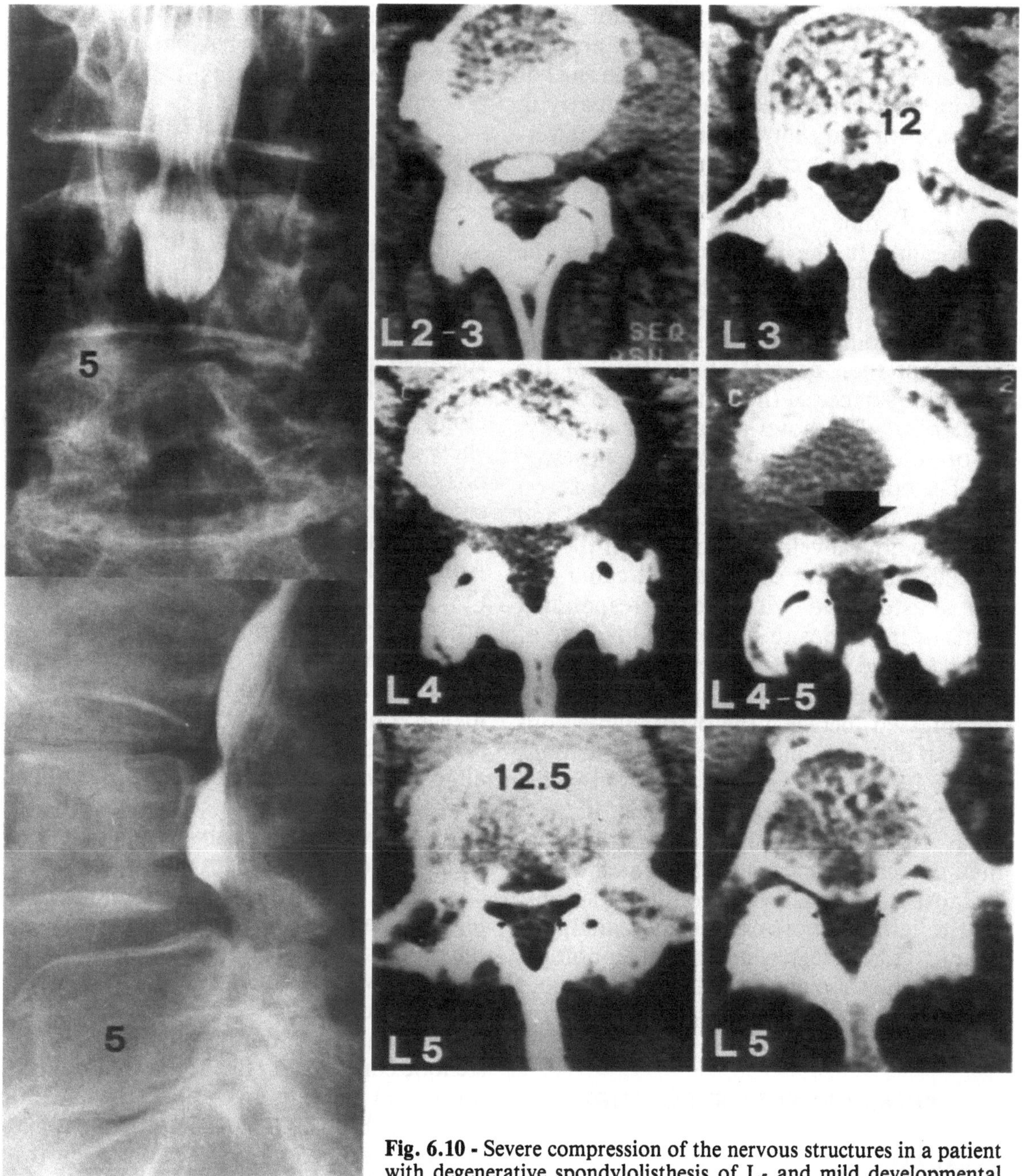

Fig. 6.10 - Severe compression of the nervous structures in a patient with degenerative spondylolisthesis of L_5 and mild developmental narrowing of the spinal canal. Myelograms display a complete block of the dye column at the level of the spondylolisthesis, which is mild. CT scans show marked arthrotic changes of the articular processes in the sections through the lower end-plate of L_4 and the L_4-L_5 disc. The arrow in the latter scan points to the body of L_5, which is visible due to the olisthesis of L_4. The sagittal dimensions of the spinal canal, marked on the scans through L_3 and L_5, are at the lower limits of normal.

EPIDURAL TISSUE

The dural sac and spinal nerve roots are normally surrounded by a layer of fat tissue; the greater is the calibre of the container — vertebral canal and neuroforamen — in relation to the size of the nervous structures, the thicker is the epidural tissue layer.

In a stenotic spinal canal, the epidural fat tissue initially decreases and even disappears in the areas in which the osteoligamentous walls of the canal compress the nervous structures. This usually occurs at the level of the intervertebral space and particularly in the anterior and central portions of the vertebral canal, whereas in the posterior interlaminar angle, not occupied by the dural sac, a variable amount of fat is almost consistently present. In the laminar portion of the canal, in which the dural sac is usually not compressed, adipose tissue reappears in a normal amount; sometimes it is even more abundant than normal at the level of the posterior surface of the vertebral body, particularly if this shows a marked concavity, as often is the case in primary stenoses.

The epidural venous plexus consists, on each side, of two venous trunks (medial and lateral epidural veins) which run in the anterolateral portion of the spinal canal and are anastomosed with the corresponding veins of the opposite side by a convolute of veins located behind the vertebral body. In a stenotic spinal canal the epidural veins are compressed, between the osteoligamentous walls of the canal and the nervous structures, at the level of the stenotic areas, that is, usually, at the intervertebral levels. In these areas, the veins may show a constricted lumen, which is sometimes obliterated due to collapse of the walls or thrombotic lesions. In the laminar portions of the canal, the venous vessels regain normal morphology, but they may also appear dilated and tortuous due to impaired venous drainage.

SPINAL NERVOUS STRUCTURES

DURAL SAC

In developmental stenosis, the sagittal and transverse dimensions of the dural sac, in non compressed areas, may be normal or less than normal due to primary narrowing. In degenerative stenosis, the size of the dural sac is normal in non constricted areas, whereas in the constricted areas it may be less than half the normal size. The dura mater may be very thin or, occasionally, opaque and sclerotic. The arachnoid membrane may, at times, be thickened; a true arachnoiditis, however, is extremely rare, at least in subjects who have not been submitted to repeat myelographies or surgical treatment.

SPINAL NERVE ROOTS IN THE INTRATHECAL COURSE

Within the dural sac, the nerve roots of the cauda equina normally have a rectilinear or slightly undulated course. It is not infrequent, in stenosis of the spinal canal, to find so-called redundancy of the caudal nerve roots. In these cases, the nerve roots appear elongated and sometimes thickened, and show a slightly sinuous to markedly tortuous course. In some instances, they form a serpiginous coil and, as soon as the arachnoid membrane is incised, they gush out from the dural tube as if this were too tight (Tsuji *et al.*, 1985). Redundant nerve roots are most frequently observed in patients with severe stenosis, usually degenerative or combined in nature. In most cases, this pathological condition is present proximally to the stenotic, or the more stenotic, area and almost always at the level of the second and third lumbar vertebra. Redundancy of the caudal nerve roots is probably due to several factors: a) excessive length of the nerve roots, compared to the length of the lumbar vertebral canal; this discrepancy is the result of the progressive reduction in height of the spinal canal with advancing age, particularly in the presence of marked resorption of the intervertebral disc at multiple levels; b) chronic stenotic compression of the dural sac and the intradural nerve roots; since the stenotic levels are those in the mid-lumbar area, lumbosacral nerve roots lengthen particularly in their proximal portion, immediately below the conus medullaris; c) attrition occurring, during movements of the spine, both between the individual redundant nerve roots, and the latter and the dural tube and/or the osteoligamentous walls of the spinal canal; this may result in a chronic inflammatory process of the radicular pia mater and the interfascicular connective tissue, with consequent thickening of the nerve root (Tsuji *et al.*, 1985).

Radicular arteries usually remain patent

at the level of the stenotic areas, since they may resist even marked compression on account of the thickness of their walls. In contrast, radicular veins, which have thinner walls and lower blood pressure, may be occluded in a stenotic area, and dilated and congested proximally and distally to the zone of compression (Parke and Watanabe, 1985).

SPINAL NERVE ROOTS IN THE EXTRATHECAL COURSE

Compressed spinal nerve roots sometimes appear thickened and fibrous in consistency. These changes, which are present particularly in degenerative and combined forms of stenosis, are probably due to thickening of the dural sheath and/or intraradicular venous stagnation and increase in amount of the perifascicular and interfascicular connective tissue.

REFERENCES

CROCK H.V.: Isolated lumbar disk resorption as a cause of nerve root canal stenosis. *Clin. Orthop.* **115:** 109, 1975.

KIRKALDY-WILLIS W.H., WEDGE J.H., YONG-HING K., REILLY J.: Pathology and pathogenesis of lumbar spondylosis and stenosis. *Spine* **3:** 3/9, 1978.

PARKE W.W., WATANABE R.: The intrinsic vasculature of the lumbosacral spinal nerve roots. *Spine* **10:** 508, 1985.

RAMANI P.S., PERRY R.H., TOMLINSON B.E.: Role of ligamentum flavum in the symptomatology of prolapsed lumbar intervertebral discs. *J. Neurol. Neurosurg. Pshychiat.* **38:** 550, 1975.

RAMSEY R.H.: The anatomy of the ligamenta flava. *Clin. Orthop.* **44:** 129, 1966.

RAUSCHNING W.: *Detailed sectional anatomy of the lumbar spine.* In «*Multiplanar CT of the spine*». Ed. by Rothman S.L.G. and Glenn W.V., University Park Press, Baltimore, 1985.

SCHNECK C.: The anatomy of lumbar spondylosis. *Clin. Orthop.* **193:** 20, 1985.

TAJIMA N. and KAWANO K.: Cryomicrotomy of the lumbar spine. *Spine* **11:** 376, 1986.

TSUJI H., TAMAKI T., TATSUO I., YAMADA H., MOTOE T., TATEZAKI S., NOGUCHI T., TAKANO H.: Redundant nerve roots in patients with degenerative lumbar spinal stenosis. *Spine* **10:** 72, 1985.

VERBIEST H.: *Stenosis of the bony lumbar vertebral canal.* In «*The narrow lumbar canal. Radiologic signs and surgery*». Ed. by Wackenheim Babin, Springer-Verlag, Berlin-Heildelberg-New York 1980.

YONG-HING K., REILLY J., KIRKALDY-WILLIS W.H.: The ligamentum flavum. *Spine* **1:** 226, 1976.

Chapter VII

Clinical features

CLINICAL SYNDROMES

Lumbar spinal stenosis can present clinically with three different types of radicular or lumboradicular syndrome: a continuous syndrome, an intermittent syndrome (intermittent claudication), and a combined syndrome in which continuous and intermittent symptoms are associated (Postacchini, 1983).

CONTINUOUS RADICULAR SYNDROME

This syndrome is characterized by the presence, at rest, of lumbar and/or radicular pain associated or not with sensory disturbances. On walking, the radicular symptoms can remain unchanged or worsen, but in the latter instance there is no modification of their clinical characteristics or dermatomal distribution. The progressive worsening of symptoms during walking can sometimes force the patient to stop. It is not, however, a true intermittent claudication because the symptoms responsible for claudication are also present at rest and, on walking, they only increase in severity, as often occurs even in patients with a disc herniation in a normally sized spinal canal. This syndrome can present in two distinct clinical patterns, acute and chronic.

The *acute syndrome* is characterized by severe radicular symptoms of less than three months' duration, which are usually sudden in onset, either when in good health or in the presence of back pain of varying duration. This syndrome, which is generally not distinguishable from that produced by a disc prolapse, is dominated by back and/or radicular pain. It is frequently characterized by signs of compression of a single nerve root or, less frequently, of two nerve roots of the same level or different levels. Spinal range of motion can be decreased and nerve root tension signs are generally positive. Slight sensory and motor deficits can, sometimes, be present, showing a metameric distribution which does not coincide with the area of radiation of pain. In rare cases, the clinical presentation can be that of a cauda equina syndrome (Scapinelli, 1978).

The *chronic syndrome*, which may have a slow onset or be subsequent to an acute syndrome, is characterized by continuous or intermittent radicular pain, associated or not with low-back pain. The clinical picture may be dominated by pain or, more often, by pain and paraesthetic disturbances. In most cases, the symptoms have a monoradicular or biradicular distribution and in the latter instance one leg or, less frequently, both lower limbs can be affected in symmetrical or asymmetrical metamers. More rarely the pain and paraesthesiae are dissociated, affecting different metamers in one or both limbs. Sometimes the symptoms are vague, with no precise radicular distribution, or may alternate between the two lower limbs.

The objective clinical picture is characterized by a normal or slightly reduced spinal range of motion and signs of nerve root compression at one level or multiple levels. Sensory and motor deficits usually dominate the clinical presentation, while nerve root tension signs are negative or only weakly positive. When symptoms are monoradicular there may be signs of compressions of the symptomatic root alone or, less frequently, marked signs of compression of this root and mild signs of involvement of other nerve roots. When the symptoms are pluriradicular, also the clinical examination will usually reveal involvement of multiple roots. In the majority of patients marked signs of compression of one nerve root are observed, together with minimal signs of involvement of another root (or two roots) on the same or the opposite side.

INTERMITTENT RADICULAR SYNDROME

Lumbo-radicular intermittent claudication is characterized by the appearance, on walking, of radicular or lumbo-radicular symptoms which are not present at rest. The symptoms worsen progressively with walking, to a point where the patient is forced, in most instances, to stop or sit. With rest, symptoms decrease in severity, allowing the patient to walk again. The walking distance before symptoms appear can vary from only some, to a few hundred, metres. This distance can remain constant over time or, especially in the initial phases of disease, vary widely from day to day. Radicular claudication can be of three types: algic, paraesthetic, or asthenic.

The algic form is characterized by back pain and/or deep muscular pain affecting one or more metamers in one or both lower limbs. When bilateral, pain can have a symmetrical or an asymmetrical radicular distribution.

The paraesthetic form is characterized by paraesthesiae (pins and needles, burning, numbness, stiffness) in one or more dermatomes.

In the asthenic form there is weakness of one or more muscular groups or the whole limb on one or both sides.

All these forms of intermittent claudication can manifest separately or in association with each other. In the majority of cases, the presentation is mixed and displays an association of two of the three types of symptoms, most commonly weakness and paraesthesiae.

Frequently, the symptoms responsible for claudication tend to become more rapidly apparent if the patient walks with the trunk erect or in hyperextension and improve on flexion of the spine. This phenomenon is related to two functional changes: in flexion, the vertebral canal lengthens and the spinal roots stretch, whilst in extension the canal shortens and the roots acquire a winding course, thus undergoing an increase in their total volume (Breig, 1960; Breig and Marions, 1963); in addition, trunk extension increases the bulging of the ligamenta flava and the intervertebral discs into the spinal canal, which, therefore, becomes narrower opposite the intervertebral spaces (Ehni, 1965). The onset of symptoms in the lower limbs after prolonged standing and their improvement with sitting are due to the same mechanisms. These orthostatic disturbances — of algic, paraesthetic or asthenic type — can be associated with a typical intermittent claudication or, more rarely, can represent the only clinical manifestation of a stenotic condition.

In the intermittent syndrome, the patient does not have radicular symptoms at rest but may complain of back pain of varying severity. Neurological examination at rest can be normal or show sensory and motor deficits, which can worsen with walking.

COMBINED RADICULAR SYNDROME

This syndrome is characterized by radicular or lumbo-radicular symptoms at rest, and intermittent symptoms differing in quality and metameric distribution to those present at rest. The most common clinical presentation is of radicular pain at rest, mostly monometameric in distribution, which, on walking, tends to worsen and become associated with weakness in one or both lower limbs. In other instances, pain and paraesthesiae may appear with walking in metamers which are asymptomatic at rest. The objective findings at rest are similar to those of the continuous radicular syndrome, particularly of the chronic type. On walking, the radicular deficits present at rest may worsen and signs of compression of other nerve roots may become apparent.

Illustrative case reports

Case 1. A fifty-four-year-old man, self employed, presented with a five-year history of occasional back pain, often radiating to the right buttock and the posterior aspect of the right thigh. The

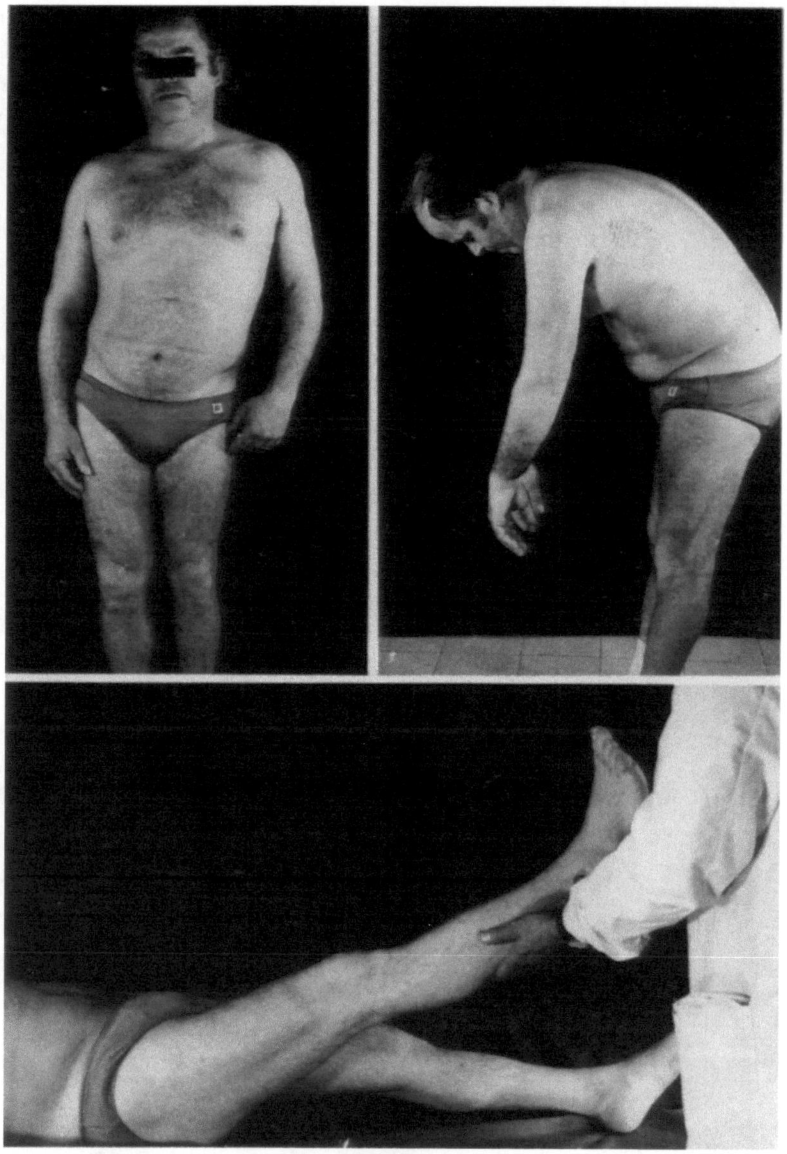

Fig. 7.1 - Case 1. This patient, complaining of acute low-back pain and radicular pain on the right side, had spinal canal stenosis at L_4-L_5 level (Fig. 7.2). There was evidence of marked sciatic scoliosis, decreased spinal flexion and, on the right, severe restriction of the straight leg raising.

patient reported one or two episodes of pain per year, each lasting two to three weeks. In between these episodes he had been completely asymptomatic. Three months prior to admission, there had been a spontaneous sudden onset of back pain, which, a few days later, had begun to radiate to the posterior aspect of the thigh and the posterior and lateral aspect of the right leg. A month later, the pain had also appeared in the posterior aspect of the left thigh. On this side, however, the symptoms were much less severe. In the last two weeks, the pain had been associated with paraesthesiae in the posterior aspect of the leg extending down to the heel. The back and leg pain was improved by lying down, but made worse by standing and, especially, walking. This was not restricted, but made difficult by the pain.

On examination, a marked sciatic scoliosis with left-side trunk list was noted (Fig. 7.1). Forward flexion was markedly restricted and any attempt of extension of the lumbar spine immediately increased the right leg pain. Straight leg raising was limited to 40° to the right and 70° to the left. The extensor hallucis longus muscle power was graded four bilaterally and foot dorsiflexion was four on the right and five on the left. The patient was unable to stand on tip toe on the right leg. The right ankle jerk was absent and

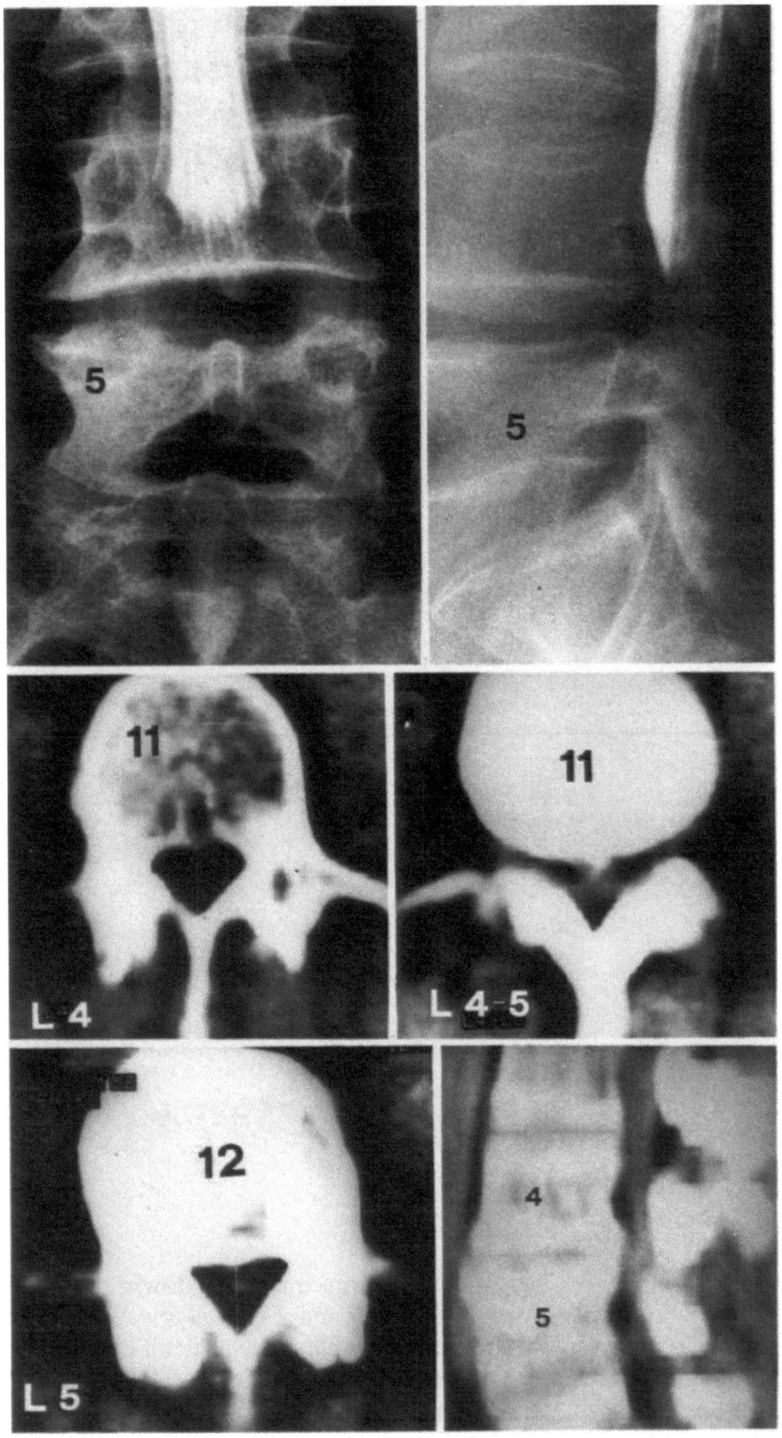

Fig. 7.2 - Case 1. Myelograms show a complete block of the contrast medium at the level of the inferior end plate of L_4, with a fringed (AP view) and pointed (lateral view) aspect of the extremity of the dye column. Axial CT scans show short midsagittal dimensions of the spinal canal at L_4 and L_4-L_5 levels (11 mm); at L_5 level, instead, the midsagittal diameter of the vertebral canal is within normal limits (12 mm). Sagittal reconstruction displays narrowing of the spinal canal at L_4-L_5 due to posterior prominence of the L_4 and L_5 vertebral bodies.

there was light hypoaesthesia on the lateral aspect of the dorsum of the right foot.

Plain radiographs showed short pedicles and an abnormal prominence of the posteroinferior corner of the L_4 vertebral body.

Myelography showed a complete block at the level of the distal half of L_4 and a decreased sagittal diameter (14 mm on the radiograph) of the contrast column proximal to the block (Fig. 7.2). CT scan of the lumbar spine revealed a narrow spinal canal in the transpedicular section at L_4 level, a marked narrowing of the canal in the subpedicular sections of L_4, and normal dimensions of the canal in the transpedicular sections of L_5 (Fig. 7.2). Sagittal reconstruction showed a marked narrowing of the spinal canal at L_4-L_5 level, due to posterior prominence of the inferior and superior corners of the vertebral bodies of L_4 and L_5, respectively, (Fig. 7.2).

At surgery, the vertebral canal appeared markedly narrowed at the L_4-L_5 level. The fourth lumbar intervertebral disc was bulging into the spinal canal, but was hard in consistency and not herniated.

Case 2. A-sixty-three-year-old woman had been complaining for many years of continuous back pain, with periodic exacerbations of the symptoms. In the last three years the patient had begun to complain of pain in the posterior and lateral aspect of both lower limbs, more marked on the right. There were no associated sensory changes. The radicular pain, which had worsened significantly in the last year, was also present at rest and was made worse by walking. The patient was often forced to stop after a distance varying from 100 to 300 metres. The inability to continue to walk was exclusively due to the progressive worsening of the back and leg pain, which only partially improved with rest.

On physical examination, forward flexion of the lumbar spine was within normal limits, whereas extension was almost abolished and made the back and leg pain worse. Straight leg raising test was mildly positive bilaterally, particularly on the right. Muscle power of the tibialis anterior, foot everters, and extensor hallucis longus was graded four bilaterally. The patient had difficulty in standing on tip toe on one leg on either side and was unable to repeat this more than four times. Light touch sensation was decreased in the dorsum of the right foot and the ankle jerk was absent bilaterally.

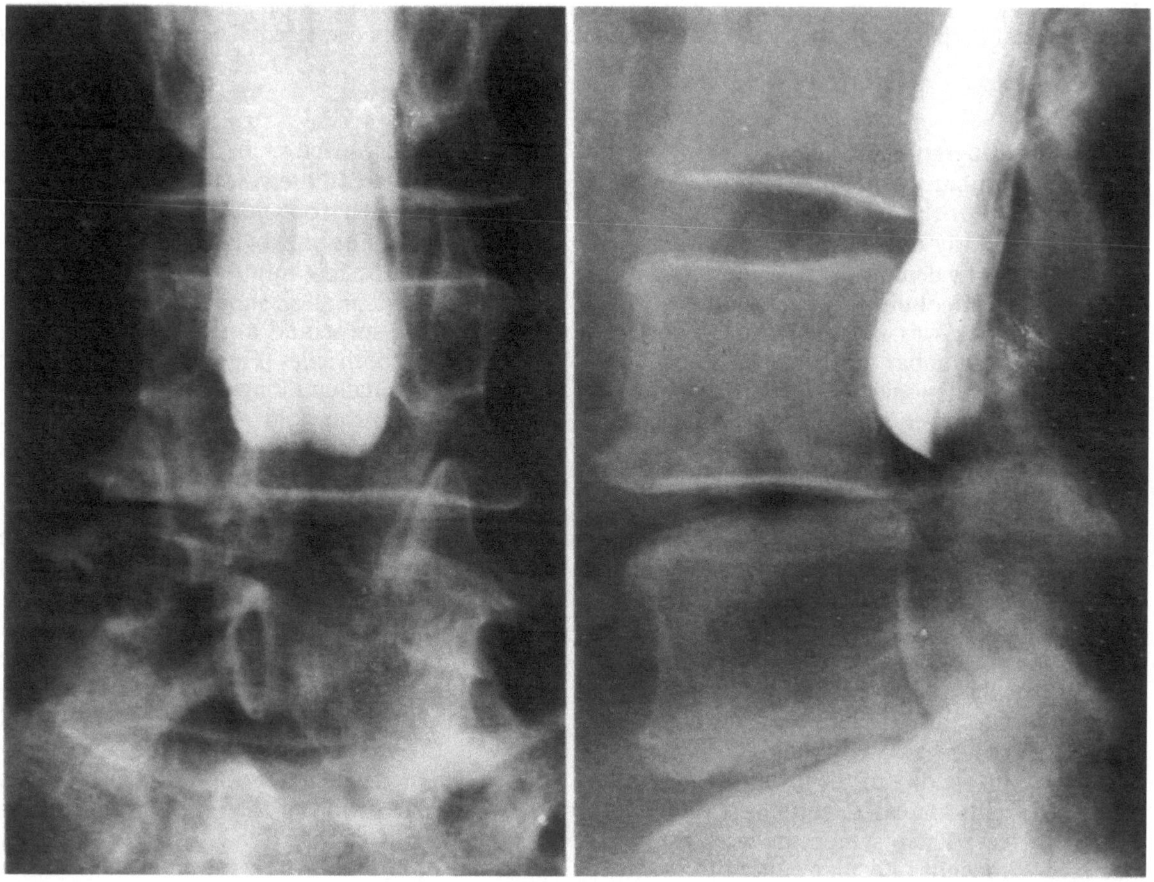

Fig. 7.3 - Case 2. Complete block of the dye column at L_4-L_5 level. At this level, the interapophysolaminar space is markedly narrow (anteroposterior view) and the intervertebral disc almost completely resorbed (lateral view).

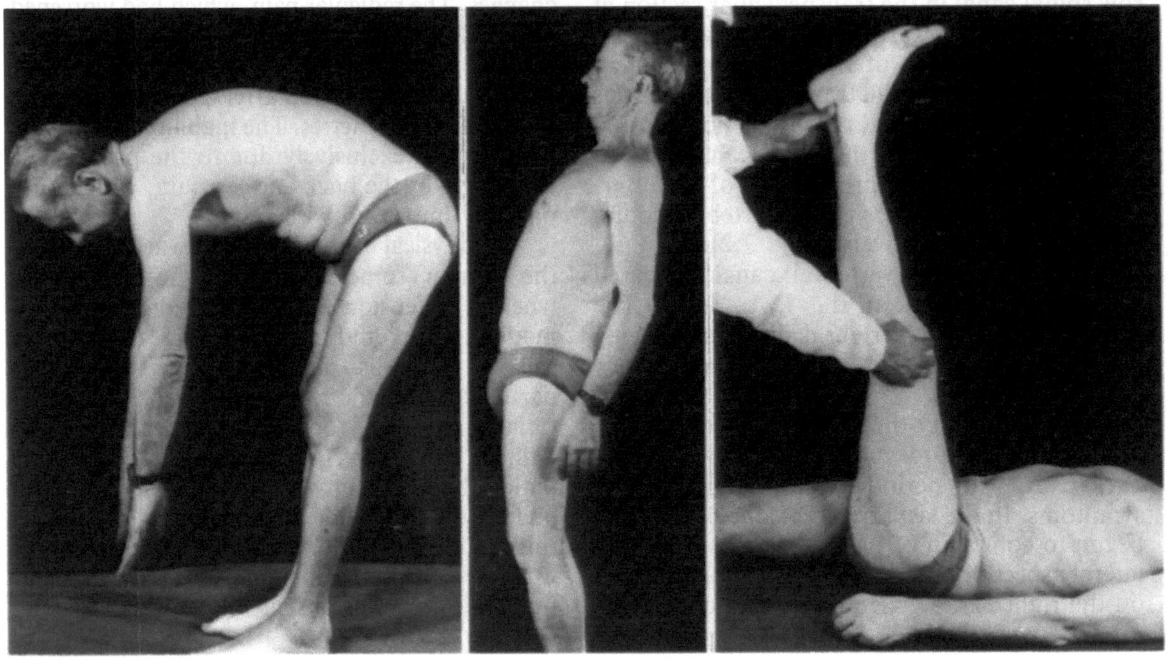

Fig. 7.4 - Case 3. This patient complained of a bilateral intermittent radicular syndrome. There was no restriction of spinal flexion, whereas extension of the lumbar spine was mildly decreased. The straight leg raising test was negative on both sides.

Plain radiographs showed narrowing of the lower two lumbar intervertebral discs, degenerative changes of the apophyseal joints at L_4-L_5 level, particularly on the right.

Myelography demonstrated a complete block of the contrast column at the L_4-L_5 level (Fig. 7.3). The block was not modified by forward flexion of the lumbar spine.

Case 3. A fifty-seven-year-old driver with a past history of infrequent episodes of back pain. During the last four years the patient had complained of symptoms in the lower limbs, which had slowly and progressively increased in intensity, limiting his walking ability. These symptoms consisted of weakness of the lower limbs, numbness in the anteromedial aspect of the legs and the dorsal and plantar aspect of the feet, and mild pain in the posterior aspect of the right thigh and leg. At rest, the patient was completely asymptomatic apart from some numbness in both feet, particularly the right. On walking, a sense of weakness and rigidity of the lower limbs rapidly appeared, with increased numbness in the legs and both feet. These symptoms were often associated with right radicular pain mild in entity and generally well tolerated. Until a year prior to admission the patient had been able to walk for about 200 metres, while in the last two months his walking distance had progressively decreased. This varied from day to day, but was rarely more than 50 metres, after which the patient was forced to stop and, if possible, sit. With rest, the symptoms improved gradually and disappeared after a few minutes.

Clinical examination showed a good range of flexion of the spine and a negative straight leg raising test on both sides (Fig. 7.4). Muscle power of the extensor hallucis longus and foot dorsiflexors was two on the right and three on the left. The patient, when asked to walk on his heels, was unable to lift his forefeet off the ground. Moreover, he was unable to stand on tip toe on one leg, but was just able to do so on both. The knee jerk was present only on the right, whereas the ankle jerk was absent on both sides. Light touch sensation was reduced in the big toe and the lateral half of the foot bilaterally, but more on the right. Plain x-rays showed an almost complete resorption of the third lumbar intervertebral disc with the «vacuum phenomenon» of Knutsson, a slight degenerative spondylolisthesis at L_3-L_4 and narrowing of the interapophysolaminar spaces, particularly at L_3-L_4 and L_4-L_5 levels. At L_3-L_4 level there was, on myelograms, a complete block of the contrast medium (Fig. 7.5). CT scan demonstrated normal dimensions of the vertebral canal at L_2 and L_3, degenerative narrowing of the spinal canal (which suggested less

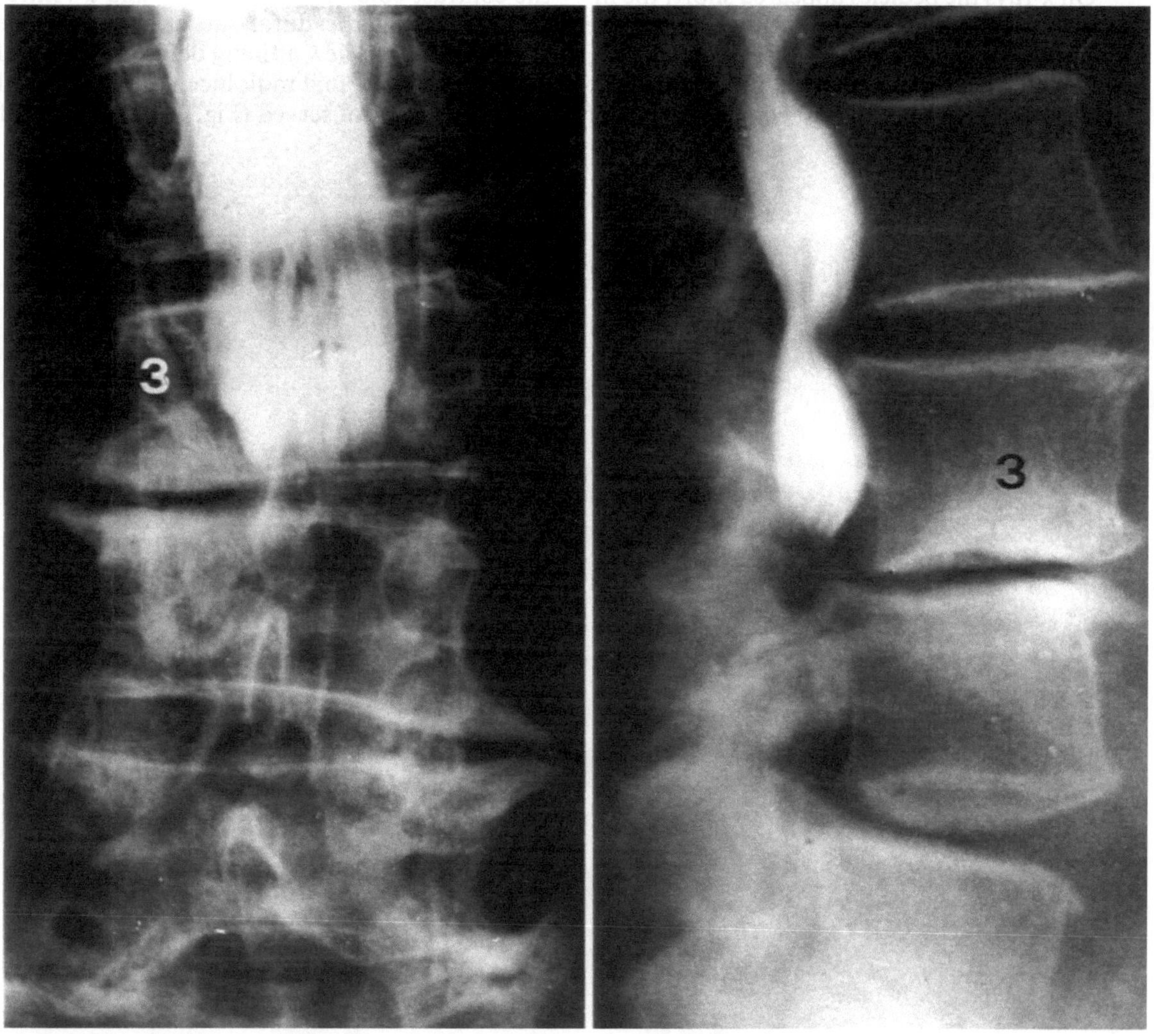

Fig. 7.5 - Case 3. Complete block of the dye column at L_3-L_4 level and anterior and posterior compression of the dural sac at L_2-L_3 level. The second and, to a greater extent, the third lumbar vertebra show a degenerative spondylolisthesis.

marked compression of the neural structures than shown by myelography) at L_3-L_4 and L_4-L_5 and bilateral nerve root canal stenosis at the L_5-S_1 level.

Case 4. A forty-seven-year-old labourer with no significant past history of back pain. Two years prior to presentation, he had started to complain of pain in the left buttock, radiating down the posterior aspect of the thigh and lateral aspect of the leg. During the last year he had been complaining of back pain, which was, however, much less severe than the leg pain. The latter was present at rest and was made only slightly worse by walking, during which the pain was associated with weakness of the left limb and pins and needles and numbness in the lateral aspect of the left thigh and leg. These symptoms appeared after a distance of approximately 100 metres and continued to worsen with walking, but disappeared when the patient stopped. Only rarely, however, was the patient forced to stop.

On physical examination there was a good range of motion of the lumbar spine both in flexion and extension. Straight leg raising on the left was restricted to about 50°, and knee flexion on the left with the patient prone was modestly positive. Muscle power of the extensor hallucis longus on the left was three and that of the left tibialis anterior was four, whereas there was no detectable motor deficit on the right. The knee and ankle jerks were present but decreased on both sides. There was some hypoaesthesia in the left big toe.

On x-rays the pedicles appeared short, the interapophysolaminar spaces narrowed, and the apophyseal joints were sagittally orientated and, at the L_4-L_5 level, moderately hypertrophic. The myelograms showed an almost complete block of the contrast column at L_4-L_5 level and a ventral indentation on the dural sac at L_3-L_4. In the antero-posterior view a filling defect of the dural sac with an abnormal radiolucency of the spinal nerve roots was observed (Fig. 7.6). CT scan of

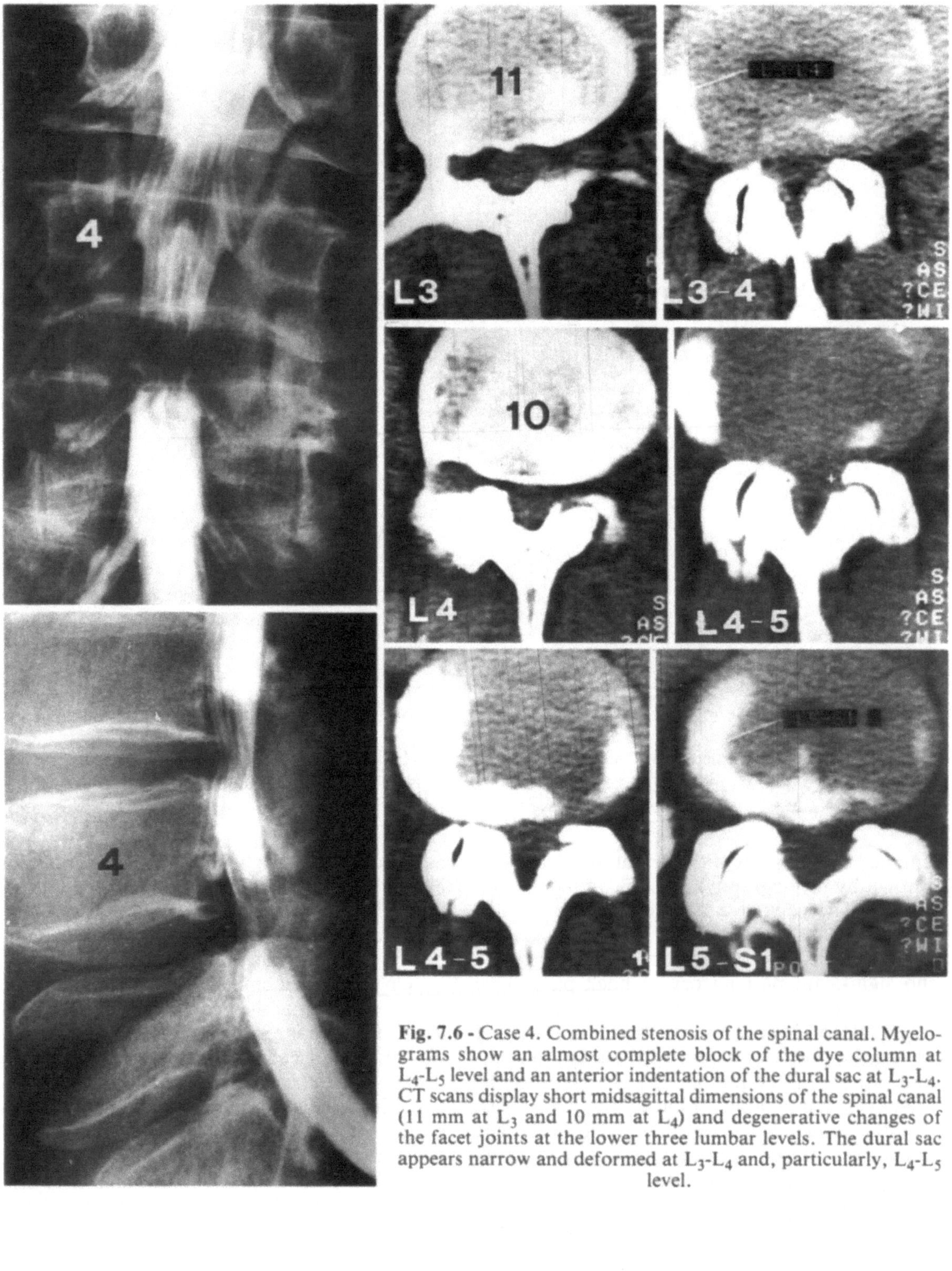

Fig. 7.6 - Case 4. Combined stenosis of the spinal canal. Myelograms show an almost complete block of the dye column at L_4-L_5 level and an anterior indentation of the dural sac at L_3-L_4. CT scans display short midsagittal dimensions of the spinal canal (11 mm at L_3 and 10 mm at L_4) and degenerative changes of the facet joints at the lower three lumbar levels. The dural sac appears narrow and deformed at L_3-L_4 and, particularly, L_4-L_5 level.

the lumbar spine showed a developmental narrowing of the spinal canal from L_2 to L_4 and hypertrophy of the apophyseal joints at L_3-L_4 and, more markedly, at L_4-L_5. At the latter level, a deformation of the dural sac was seen (Fig. 7.6).

Case 5. A forty-six-year-old woman, with a four-year history of occasional back pain of mild severity, had begun to complain in the last two years of pain in the posterior aspect of the left thigh and leg, and hypoaesthesia of the left heel and the lateral half of the dorsum of the foot. The leg symptoms had been of gradual onset and initially had been treated with anti-inflammatory

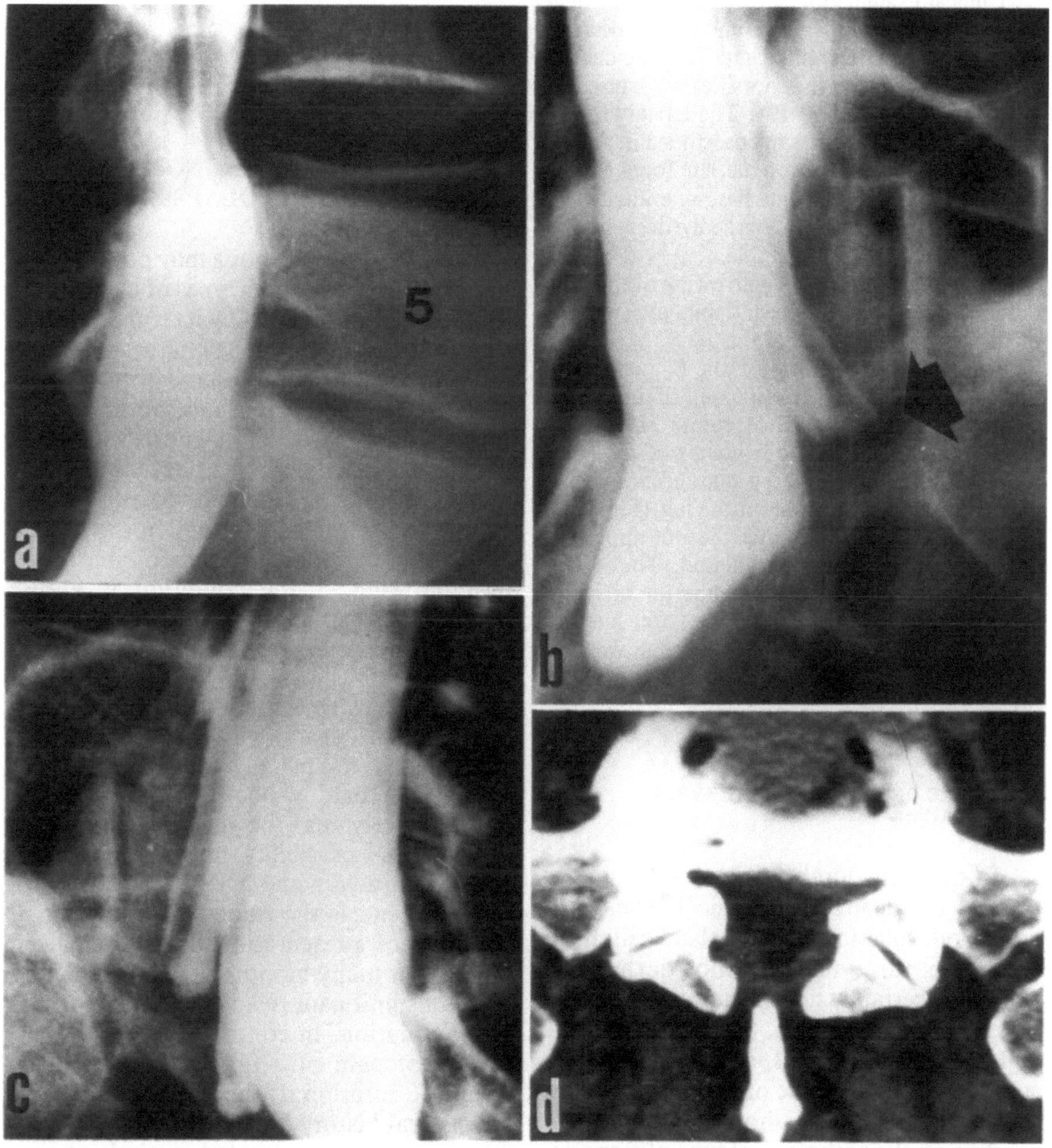

Fig. 7.7 - Case 5. Isolated stenosis of the left S_1 nerve root canal. Myelograms show marked resorption of the L_5-S_1 disc (**a**) and a filling defect of the left S_1 nerve root sheath (**b**), which is dilated proximally to the site of compression (arrow). Conversely, the right S_1 nerve root shows no evidence of compression (**c**). CT scan (**d**) at L_5-S_1 level reveals a lateral recess stenosis, particularly on the left.

drugs, which had improved both the pain and paraesthesiae for three months. Subsequently, the leg pain had reappeared and had become resistant to medical and physical therapy. The leg pain, relatively mild at rest, was quite severe on prolonged walking and was often, but not always, associated with an increased hypoaesthesia in the heel and foot. The patient, however, had no restriction in her walking capacity.

Clinical examination showed a normal range of motion of the lumbar spine and a slight decrease of straight leg raising on the left. This manoeuvre, when associated with foot dorsiflexion, caused severe leg pain at around 50°. The left ankle jerk was absent and there was hypoaesthesia in the lateral half of the dorsum of the left foot. Muscle strength of the left calf muscles, as evaluated by standing on tip toe, was markedly decreased in comparison with the right side.

X-rays showed marked narrowing of the lumbosacral intervertebral disc and mild hypertrophy of the apophyseal joints at this level. Myelography showed a non-filling of the S_1 nerve root sheath on the left, which appeared slightly dilated proximally to the site of compression (Fig. 7.7). CT scan showed no evidence of disc protrusion, but demonstrated a marked narrowing of the S_1 nerve root canal on the left (Fig. 7.7).

At surgery, the L_5-S_1 disc did not appear to be herniated and was not excised. The left S_1 root was compressed by the superior articular process of the first sacral vertebra. After surgery, there was complete relief of the leg pain, whereas the hypoaesthesia, although improved, was still present at the eight-month follow-up.

INCIDENCE OF THE DIFFERENT TYPES OF SYNDROME

In the past, lumbar spinal stenosis has often been identified in clinical terms with lumbo-radicular intermittent claudication. In actual fact this syndrome, though the most typical, is certainly neither unique nor, in its pure clinical expression, the most frequent, at least in the whole spectrum of lumbar stenoses. The incidence of the various types of clinical syndromes, however, varies depending on the pathological type of stenosis.

In stenosis of the spinal canal, the most common clinical syndrome is the combined, followed by the pure intermittent, syndrome. The continuous acute syndrome, which is rare but not exceptional, is seen especially in the presence of disc disease in the form of annular disc bulge or true disc prolapse. In isolated stenosis of the nerve root canal, the most frequent syndrome is the continuous, generally in the chronic form, followed by the combined. The intermittent syndrome is rare and almost never as typical as that found in spinal canal stenosis. In the rare case of isolated stenosis of the intervertebral foramen the syndrome most commonly observed is the continuous, followed by the combined.

DIFFERENTIAL DIAGNOSIS WITH DISC PROLAPSE

Lumbar spinal stenosis may present schematically with two main types of clinical syndromes; one dominated by intermittent claudication and the other characterized by lumbo-radicular continuous symptoms, associated or not with claudication. In the former, the differential diagnosis with a disc prolapse is generally easy, because it is very rare for a pure disc herniation to cause a typical intermittent claudication. In the second type, it may be difficult or impossible to determine whether the condition is a disc prolapse or a spinal stenosis. Some clinical features, however, may be helpful to orient the diagnosis (Fig. 7.I).

Patients with lumbar stenosis are generally over 50 years, while those showing a disc prolapse are usually younger. This does not exclude that low-back and radicular pain in the elderly may be due to a pure disc prolapse; this possibility, however, grows less likely with advancing age. In patients with lumbar stenosis the radicular symptoms at the time of presentation have often been present for many months or years, generally without significant relapses. Patients with a disc herniation, in contrast, usually have a history of pain of a few weeks', to a few months', duration. If the duration is longer, the clinical history is almost always characterized by, even protracted, periods of partial or complete relapse of symptoms. In patients with stenosis, the symptoms in the lower limbs tend to be more marked than those in the low back, which are often com-

Table 7.I

MAIN DIFFERENCES BETWEEN THE TYPICAL CLINICAL PATTERNS OBSERVED RESPECTIVELY IN DISC PROLAPSE AND STENOSIS

	Disc prolapse	**Stenosis**
Age	<50	>50
Duration of symptoms	short	long
Relapse of symptoms	yes	no
Low back pain	yes	poor or absent
Claudication	no	yes
Radicular bilateral symptoms	no	yes
Radicular sensory deficits	+	+ +
Spinal motion	reduced	normal
SLRT and Lasègue	+ +	—(+)*

* In brackets alternative less frequent possibilities.

pletely absent. Patients with prolapse do not have a constant clinical presentation, but in the majority of cases complain of back pain of similar or only slightly less severity than the radicular symptoms. In stenoses, peripheral symptoms are commonly bilateral and sensory deficits are frequent and sometimes very prominent in the history, whereas in disc herniations there is generally a monoradicular symptomatology, represented mainly or exclusively by pain.

On physical examination, patients with lumbar stenosis usually have a normal or only slightly decreased range of spinal motion with no, or minor, nerve root tension signs, in the presence of even marked motor deficits; these, moreover, can be bi- or multiradicular, especially in central spinal stenosis. In contrast, patients with disc prolapse mostly have a reduced spinal motion, with moderate or marked nerve root tension signs and monoradicular motor deficits.

LUMBO-RADICULAR INTERMITTENT CLAUDICATION

PATHOGENESIS

Three theories have been put forward to explain the pathogenesis of intermittent claudication; the compressive theory, the ischaemic theory, and the theory of stagnant anoxia.

According to the *compressive theory* (Wilson, 1969; Nelson, 1973) lumbo-radicular intermittent claudication is due to disturbances of the neural function as a result of compression of the spinal nerve roots by the osteoligamentous structures of the spinal canal and/or the intervertebral discs. This hypothesis has been especially advanced to explain the so-called postural pseudo-claudication, that is, the appearance of radicular symptoms on standing. The increase in lumbar lordosis which standing implies, in fact, increases the buckling of the ligamenta flava and the intervertebral discs into the spinal canal, which, therefore, is further narrowed. At the same time, the spinal nerve roots tend to increase in volume as a result of the reduction in length of the vertebral canal — and of the roots — caused by the increase in lumbar lordosis. Both of these effects are responsible for the increase in compression of the dural sac and nerve roots and cause the appearance or worsening of the lumbo-radicular symptoms.

The *ischaemic theory* (Blau and Logue, 1961; Evans, 1964) attributes intermittent claudication to an insufficient blood flow in the lumbosacral spinal roots during walking. This theory implies a physiological increase of the arterial blood flow in the nerve root during exercise. In patients with lumbar stenosis, or lumbo-radicular claudication, the compression of the caudal nerve roots prevents the radicular vasodilatation, which normally occurs during walking. This causes a nerve roots ischaemia, which is responsible for the sensory and motor deficits that appear on walking.

The theory of *stagnant anoxia* suggests that the increase in cerebrospinal fluid pressure, which occurs distally to the site of a marked compression of the dural sac, could oppose the radicular venous drainage in this area with subsequent hypoxia of the spinal roots (Kavanaugh *et al.*, 1968).

The compressive theory can explain the postural pseudoclaudication but not the typical intermittent claudication, because the entity of compression of neural structures presumably remains constant as walking progresses. The theory of stagnant anoxia could explain the appearance of radicular symptoms in both static and dynamic conditions, but does not explain why a typical claudication is not observed in other conditions, such as caudal neurinomas, characterized by an increase in cerebrospinal fluid pressure. The ischaemic theory is based on the experimental observation of an increased vascularization of the lumbar spinal cord and caudal nerve roots in animals undergoing prolonged muscular stimulation of the rear limbs (Blau and Ruthworth, 1958). Although the latter investigation is not free from criticism, it seems reasonable to conceive that exercise would imply an increase in metabolic activity, and consequently in blood flow, in the nerve roots and spinal cord. A marked compression of the caudal nerve roots — especially if at multiple levels, as is often the case in lumbar stenosis — may prevent the increase in arterial blood flow normally occurring during walking and this may be responsible for an ischaemic neuritis, which would manifest exclusively during exercise.

Recently, the ischaemic theory has been reformulated by Parke and Watanabe (1985) in a more articulate and convincing fashion on the basis of a better understanding of the intrinsic vasculature and the microstructure of the spinal roots and the surrounding pial sheaths. Both the main and the collateral radicular arteries have a well developed tunica media, while veins have thin walls without a tunica media which cause them to be more vulnerable to the effects of mechanical obstruction. The latter may be caused by the osteoligamentous structures of the spinal canal or the intervertebral discs, or, even more easily, by an excessive stretching of the root. Investigations on peripheral nerves have demonstrated that stretching a nerve beyond 8% of its length will arrest the intraneural microcirculation (Lundborg, 1975). Since the epinevrium and perinevrium of peripheral nerves are thicker and more resistant than the corresponding structures of the nerve roots, it is reasonable to presume that even a mild traction may compromise the radicular microcirculation. Under physiological conditions, the nerve root can tolerate a certain amount of traction because of the presence, in the interfascicular arterial branches, of compensating coils which elongate with traction, thus allowing a continued intraneural arterial blood flow (see Chapter 2). In the presence of a stenosis, however, the relative fixity and angulation of the root at the site of compression may prevent interfascicular micromovements and cause excessive root traction during spinal movements. The effect of the excessive traction, as well as the direct compression and angulation of the root, will affect only, or mostly, the thin-walled radicular veins. The resulting stagnation of venous blood will obstruct the arterial blood flow and reduce the nutritional supply to the root. This reduction of nutrition will be more noticeable during the increased metabolic needs produced by walking.

The radicular circulation is not the only source of nutrition of the root. An important exchange of metabolites also occurs with the cerebrospinal fluid (Rydevik *et al.*, 1984). Stagnation of cerebrospinal fluid distally to a marked compression of the thecal sac may cause a reduction in the metabolic exchanges in the radicular tissue. Such exchanges, on the other hand, can be further reduced in the presence of a chronic inflammation of the pial sheaths caused by compression, and consequent microtraumas, to which the root is submitted. Thickening of the radicular pia mater that inflammation involves, in fact, will reduce the number and width of the sheath micropores which allow percolation of cerebrospinal fluid and thus reduces the nutritional supply to the root.

In light of this interpretation, it is possible to explain radicular symptoms at rest and those occurring during walking. The former are likely to be due to a marked nerve root compression, while the latter are caused by ischaemia of roots which are not markedly compressed, but are deviated in their course or less mobile than normal. Even ischaemic theory, however, leaves somewhat unexplained a number of the multiple aspects of lumbo-radicular claudication, such as: the multiplicity of symptoms (weakness, pain or paraesthesiae) responsible for claudication; the unilateral involvement in patients with bilateral nerve root compression or the monometameric characteristics of claudication in patients with multiple root compression; and the appearance of sphintheric disturbances with walking. It is possible that these clinical characteristics of claudication are due to different degrees of resistance to ischaemia of the various nerve fibres (large myelinated, small myelinated, and non-myelinated fibres), different mode of expression of ischaemia depending on the severity of nerve root compression (Gilliat and Wilson, 1954), or an associated ischaemia of spinal cord or dorsal root ganglia. A thorough explanation of these clinical features may provide a more complete pathogenetic interpretation of this form of claudication, the ischaemic origin of which, although convincing, is still based, at least in part, on inductive elements.

DIFFERENTIAL DIAGNOSIS WITH OTHER TYPES OF CLAUDICATION AND PSEUDOCLAUDICATION

Medullary intermittent claudication

Neurogenic claudication can be observed in cervical or thoracic spinal stenosis and in thoracic disc prolapses. In cervical stenosis, it is extremely rare to observe the typical presentation of intermittent claudication; the patient with cervical myelopathy will usually complain of a constant weakness of the lower limbs, which would be present from the beginning of walking and limit his walking capacity. The same applies for thoracic spinal stenosis, which is, however, extremely uncommon. In thoracic disc prolapse, on the contrary, it is not rare for the patient to present with a typical picture of intermittent claudication, particularly when the herniation is located at the lowest thoracic intervertebral discs. Sometimes the clinical picture of intermittent claudication can be seen in association with disorders of the spinal cord or extradural vessels, such as atherosclerosis, vascular malformations (angioma, arterovenous aneurism, extradural cavernous telangiectasia) or neoplasms (haemangioblastoma).

Medullary claudication is clearly differentiated from the lumbo-radicular by the presence of unilateral or bilateral piramidal signs, such as hypereflexia, paraparesis and spastic paraplegia, patellar and ankle cloni, absence of abdominal reflexes, positivity of Babinski's sign, hypoaesthesia or anaesthesia below the level of the cord compression. Sometimes, particularly in the early phases of disease, these neurological signs can become apparent after prolonged walking and may disappear with rest. Furthermore, when the thoracic cord or the conus medullaris are affected, urinary and sexual dysfunctions are often present, while cervical cord involvement causes subjective and objective deficits also in the upper limbs.

Vascular intermittent claudication

It is unusual for claudication due to aorto-iliac or femoral obliterating arteriopathy to be confused with lumbo-radicular claudication, when the vascular deficit is severe enough to cause, together with the typical cramp-like pain, the absence of one or more peripheral pulses and marked trophic disturbances of the extremities. In patients in whom the vascular deficit is relatively mild, however, this type of claudication can be easily confused with lumbo-radicular claudication. The distinguishing features between the two forms are (Table 7.II):

— The different influence of standing on the onset and relief of the claudication symptoms. In lumbo-radicular claudication, the walking induced symptoms often disappear only if the patient sits, whereas in vascular claudication the leg symptoms usually decrease or disappear even simply on standing (Hawkes and Roberts, 1978). In lumbo-radicular claudication, moreover, prolonged standing can often cause lumbar and/or radicular pain (Kavanaugh *et al.*, 1968; Hawkes and Roberts, 1979).

— The higher incidence, in patients with lumbo-radicular claudication, of low back

Table 7.II
MAIN DIFFERENCES BETWEEN LUMBO-RADICULAR CLAUDICATION AND VASCULAR CLAUDICATION

	Lumbo-radicular claudication	**Vascular claudication**
Low back pain	+	—
Walking distance	constant	varying
Time necessary for rest before resumption of walking (in minutes)	10-15	5
Radiation path of the symptoms through the limb	downwards	upwards
Sensory deficits	mono- or biradicular	— (stocking)*
SRLT and Lasègue	(—)+	—
Motor deficits	+ (—)	—
Reflex changes	+ (—)	—
Arterial pulses	normal (foot pulse reduced or absent)	femoral, popliteal and/or foot pulse reduced or absent
Arterial bruit	—	+ (—)

* In brackets alternative less frequent possibilities.

pain at rest and during spinal movements.

— The much greater frequency with which patients affected by vascular claudication show abnormalities of peripheral pulses. Patients with lumbo-radicular claudication may also show absence of a peripheral pulse (Blau and Logue, 1961). Usually, however, it is the foot pulse on only one side, in the presence of normal femoral and popliteal pulses (Hawkes and Roberts, 1978). In patients with vascular disorders, the foot pulse is very often absent on one or both sides and, when it is present, there is often absence of the femoral or popliteal pulses. Quite often, moreover, the vascular patient will have a bruit over the femoral artery or the aorta.

— The higher frequency of sensory disturbances in patients with lumbo-radicular claudication. In these, hypoaestesia usually shows a metameric distribution, whereas in vascular patients it is typically stocking-like (Blau and Logue, 1961; Hawkes and Roberts, 1978).

— The different incidence of muscle deficits and reflex changes in patients with lumbo-radicular, from those with vascular, claudication. In the former, neurological examination often reveals weakness of the quadriceps, extensor hallucis longus, peroneals or calf muscles, and deficit of the knee or ankle jerk. In vascular patients these signs are quite uncommon.

Other differences, of lesser significance, concern: the number of symptoms responsible for claudication, which is usually monosymptomatic (pain) in patients with vascular disorders, and plurisymptomatic (asthenia and pain or paraesthesiae) in those with lumbar stenosis (Kavanaugh *et al.*, 1968; Hawkes and Roberts, 1978); the patient's walking distance, which tends to be constant in vascular claudication and variable from day to day in patients with spinal disorders (Kavanaugh *et al.*, 1968; Silver *et al.*, 1969; Hawks and Roberts, 1978); the radiation path of symptoms, which tend to spread down one or both legs in vascular claudication and up one or both legs in lumbar stenosis.

Despite these differences, it may be extremely difficult to determine the nature of claudication on the basis of clinical data, because none of these can be considered pathognomonic of one of the two types of claudication. In doubtful cases, useful investigations can be electromyography and vascular function tests (oscillography, reography, and doppler). Definite diagnostic information, however, can only be obtained with arteriography, myelography, CT scan or MRI.

Pseudoclaudication due to joint disorders in the lower limb

It is not uncommon that patients with disorders of the knee or, particularly, the hip (avascular necrosis or osteoarthritis) report a history similar to that of patients with intermittent claudication. This pseudoclaudication can easily be mistaken for lumboradicular claudication especially in those patients in whom radicular or pseudoradicular symptoms are also present. In these cases, however, a thorough history would elicit that patients are forced to slow down or stop walking because of progressive worsening of knee or hip pain and not because of lumboradicular symptoms; in addition, clinical examination will reveal the typical clinical and radiological signs of joint disease. In doubtful cases useful diagnostic data can be obtained by neuroelectric investigations (EMG, SEP) as well as bone scanning, which, in patients with joint diseases, may show an increased uptake at the level of the symptomatic joint. When diagnosis remains uncertain, it may be helpful to inject 5-10 ml of local anaesthetic into the joint which is suspected of being the cause of the claudication. This disappears or improves considerably following the injection when it is related to joint disease, while remaining unchanged if it has a spinal origin.

REFERENCES

Blau J.N., Logue V.: Intermittent claudication of the cauda equina. An unusual syndrome resulting from central protrusion of a lumbar intervertebral disc. *Lancet* **1:** 1081, 1961.

Blau J.N., Ruthworth G.: Observations on the blood vessels of the spinal cord and their response to motor activity. *Brain* **81:** 354, 1958.

Breig A.: *Biomechanics of the central nervous system; some basic and pathologic phenomena*. Chicago Year Book Publ., 1960.

Breig A., Marions O.: Biomechanics of the lumbo-sacral nerve roots. *Acta Radiol.* **1:** 1141, 1963.

Ehni G.: Spondylotic cauda equina radiculopathy. *Texas J. Med.* **61:** 746, 1965.

Evans J.G.: Neurogenic intermittent claudication. *Br. Med. J.* **2:** 985, 1984.

Gilliat R.W., Wilson T.G.: Ischemic sensory loss in patients with peripheral nerve lesions. *J. Neurol. Neurosurg. Psych.* **17:** 104, 1954.

Hawkes C.H., Roberts G.M.: Neurogenic and vascular claudication. *J. Neurol. Sciences* **38:** 337, 1978.

Kavanaugh G.J., Svien H.G., Holman C.B., Johnson R.M.: «Pseudoclaudication» syndrome produced by compression of the cauda equina. *J. Am. Med. Assn.* **206:** 2477, 1968.

Lundborg G.: Structure and function of intraneural microvessels as related to trauma, edema formation, and nerve function. *J. Bone and Joint Surg.* **57-A:** 938, 1975.

Nelson M.A.: Lumbar spinal stenosis. *J. Bone and Joint Surg.* **55-B:** 506, 1973.

Parke W.W., Watanabe R.: The intrinsic vasculature of the lumbo-sacral spinal nerve roots. *Spine* **10:** 508, 1985.

Postacchini F.: The diagnosis of lumbar stenosis. Analysis of clinical and radiographic findings in 43 cases. *Italian Journal of Orthopaedics and Traumatology* **11:** 5, 1985.

Rydevik G., Holm S., Brown M.D.: *Nutrition of spinal nerve roots: The role of diffusion from the cerebrospinal fluid*. Transactions of the 30th Annual Meeting of the Orthop. Res. Soc. vol. 9, p. 276, Atlanta G.A., Feb. 7-9, 1984.

Scapinelli R.: Cauda equina compression syndromes from narrowing of the lumbar spinal canal. *Intern. Orthop.* (SICOT) **1:** 267, 1978.

Silver R.A., Schuele H.L., Stack J.K., Conn J. JR., Bergan J.J.: Intermittent claudication of neurospinal origin. *Arch. Surg.* **98:** 523, 1969.

Wilson C.B.: Significance of the small lumbar spinal canal: cauda equina compression syndromes due to spondylosis. Part 3: Intermittent claudication. *J. Neurosurg.* **31:** 506, 1969.

Chapter VIII
Diagnostic investigations

INTRODUCTION

The range of investigations able to demonstrate a stenosis of the lumbar spinal canal, once mainly represented by myelography, has grown over the last twenty years with new techniques, which have contributed to improve the diagnostic definition of the stenotic conditions. Some of these techniques, such as computed tomography, are now employed as a matter of routine, whereas others, such as ultrasonography and epidural phlebography have acquired a secondary role due to technical limitations or poor diagnostic accuracy. All methods available at present may be useful for a correct diagnosis. As a rule, however, the diagnosis of lumbar stenosis is based on plain radiographic studies, water-soluble myelography and computed tomography, with the addition, in the last few years, of magnetic resonance imaging. These investigations are to be considered of primary importance with respect to the others, which are as yet of complementary diagnostic value.

PLAIN RADIOGRAPHY

It is the most simple, but not the least important diagnostic investigation, since patients with lumbar spinal stenosis may show various abnormalities of the plain radiographic picture, some of which are of considerable diagnostic value. Furthermore, measurements of vertebral components and spaces, which may lead to suspect constriction of the spinal canal, can be carried out on plain radiographs. The role of plain radiographic studies is that of confirming the clinical suspicion and justifying the use of investigations of greater diagnostic significance.

None of the radiographic changes which may be observed in patients with lumbar stenosis is pathognomonic of a narrowing of the spinal canal. The diagnostic evaluation should, therefore, derive from the overall analysis of the radiographic abnormalities found in the different projection of the lumbar spine.

ANTEROPOSTERIOR PROJECTION

Length of the laminae and interlaminar angle

In subjects with developmental narrowing of the spinal canal, the laminae generally appear shorter than normal with, consequently, abnormal closeness of the articular processes to the spinous process (Fig. 8.1). Shortness of the laminae, however, may be only apparent and related to their more sagittal orientation. The length of the laminae, in fact, in a bidimensional image, such as that of a radiograph, is strictly related to their orientation in the sagittal plane. Therefore, relatively short laminae which are transversally orientated may seem longer than laminae of normal length sagittally orientated. Due to the shortness of the laminae and/or their sagittal orientation, the interlaminar angle, formed by the lower margins of the laminae of a vertebra, is often very acute (Fig. 8.1b).

Interapophysolaminar space

It is the translucent space seen on the anteroposterior radiograph between the laminae and the articular processes of two adjacent vertebrae. In a normal lumbar spine, this space generally has the shape of an isosceles

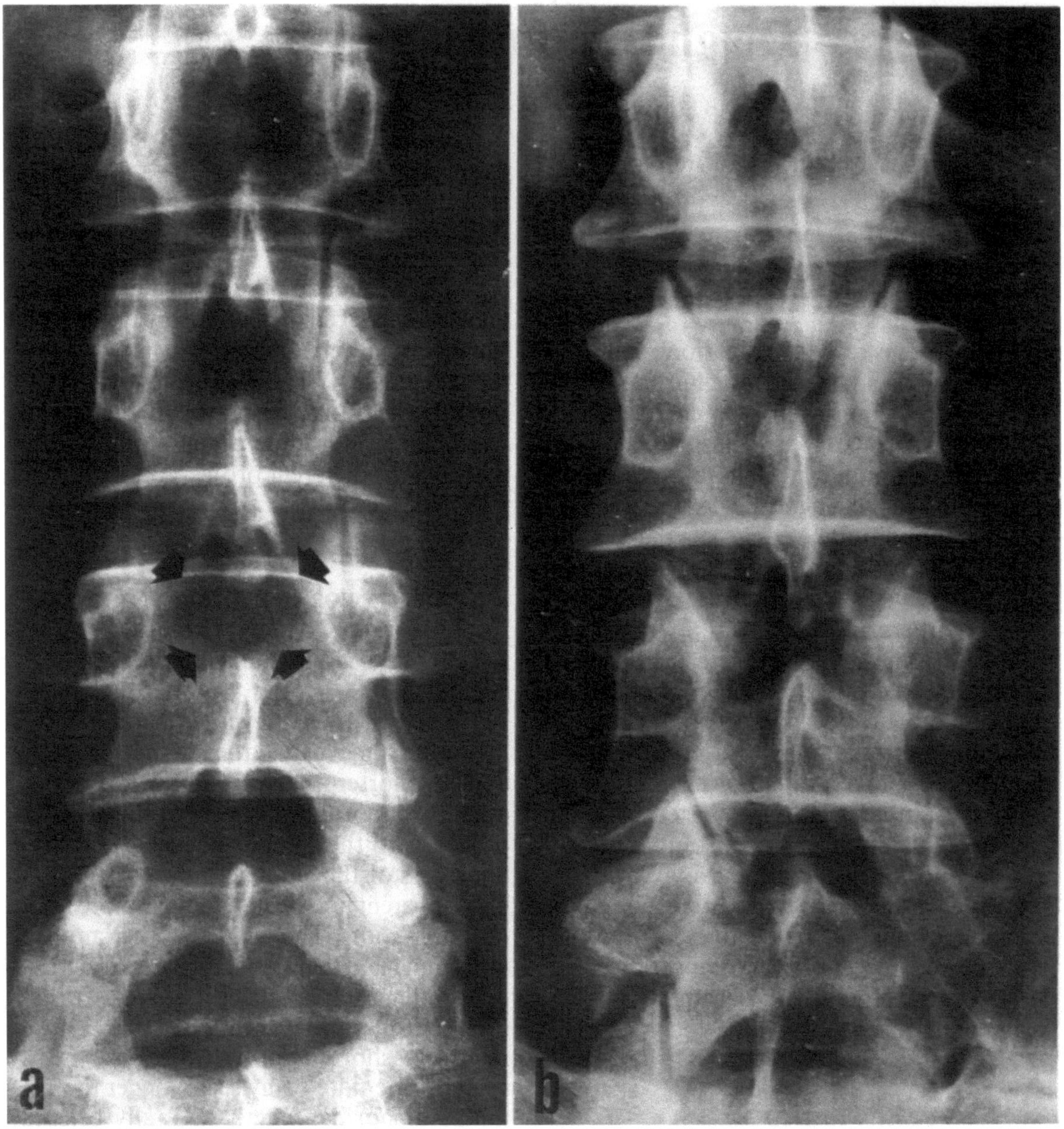

Fig. 8.1- Morphology of the interapophysolaminar space. **a.** In the lumbar spine, this space (arrows) usually has the shape of an isosceles triangle, except for the L_5-S_1 space which is lozenge-shaped. **b.** When the spinal canal is developmentally narrow the interapophysolaminar space is reduced in the transverse direction.

triangle at the upper four intervertebral levels and is lozenge-shaped at the lumbosacral interspace (Fig. 8.1a). In the presence of a developmentally narrow spinal canal, the interapophysolaminar space shows a normal height but it is generally decreased in width (Fig. 8.1b).

Vogue (1980) defined the «width index» as the ratio between the maximum width of the interapophysolaminar space and the width of the vertebral body of L_3. When the spinal canal is normal in size, this index varies from 0.36 ± 5 at L_1 to 0.69 ± 10 at L_5. However, when the canal is developmentally narrow, both the width of the interapophysolaminar space and the width index would be smaller than normal at all intervertebral levels or, in the presence of a single level narrowing, only at the abnormally narrow level. The correlation between the width of the interapophysolaminar space and the narrowing of the spinal canal is certainly valid, but not in such an absolute manner and, however, not only for developmental narrowing. The transverse dimensions of the interapophysolaminar space, in fact, depends upon various factors, such as the length and sagittal orientation of the laminae, and the shape, dimensions and orientation of the articular processes. This space, therefore, may be reduced in subjects with a narrow spinal canal, in whom the laminae are generally short and the articular processes orientated sagittally. However, such a reduction, or an even more marked decrease in width, may be found for a constitutional or degenerative hypertrophy of the inferior articular processes and/or ossification of the ligamenta flava in subjects presenting a normally sized spinal canal or in patients with degenerative lumbar stenosis.

Articular space of facet joints

In subjects with a normally sized spinal canal the interfacetal space is clearly visible at L_2-L_3 level in about two thirds of cases and at L_4-L_5 level in just over half the cases, while at the first and last lumbar level it is rarely seen (De Berail, 1976). In patients with a developmentally narrow canal, the articular space is identifiable, at a given level, with greater frequency, and in a same subject at a larger number of levels than normal. This is probably due to the fact that in subjects with a narrow spinal canal the articular processes (or their posterior portion) frequently show a sagittal or parasagittal direction, which makes the articular interspace visible on a frontal view. Normally, the interfacetal spaces have a vertical direction or are orientated obliquely both latero-medially and cranio-caudally; in the latter instance, the angle that they form with the median line does not exceed 30°. In subjects with a narrow spinal canal, this angle is often greater than normal reaching, in some cases, as much as 60° (De Berail, 1976).

Degenerative changes of the facet joints

In many patients with lumbar stenosis, the articular processes, particularly the inferior ones, appear to be hypertrophic and sclerotic. Hypertrophy of inferior articular processes may be so marked as to obliterate the interapophysolaminar space (Fig. 8.2). At times, the tips of superior articular processes show osteophytic spurs, which prolong the process up to the inferior border

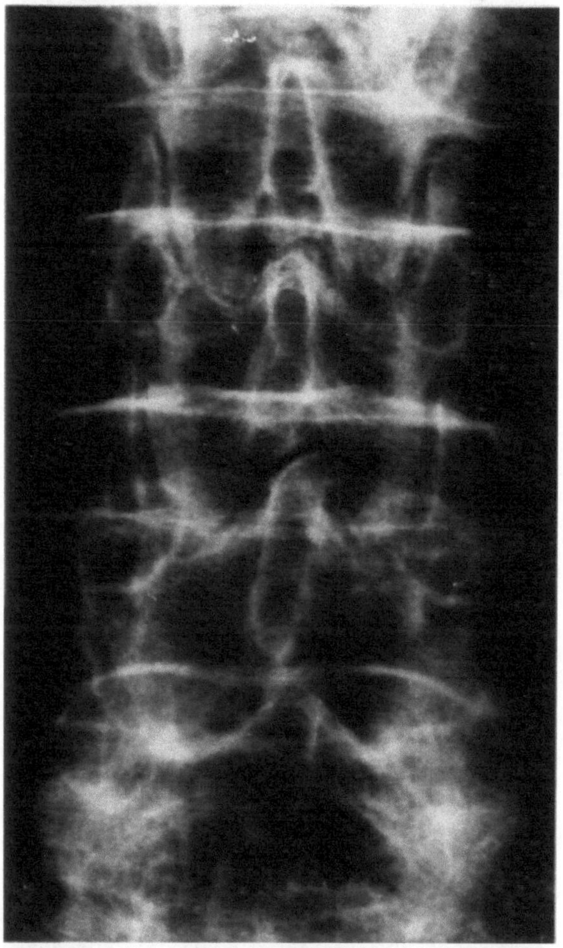

Fig. 8.2 - Considerable degenerative hypertrophy of the inferior articular processes, which almost completely obliterate the interapophysolaminar space at most lumbar levels.

of the pedicle above. The incidence of the degenerative changes is inversely related to the primary dimensions of the spinal canal. The most marked osteoarthrotic changes are found in patients with degenerative stenosis of the spinal canal. The most severe changes are usually observed at the lowest three lumbar levels and, particularly, at L_4-L_5 level.

LATERAL PROJECTION

Length of the pedicles

The length of the pedicles corresponds to the distance between the tangent line to the posterior aspect of the vertebral body and the line, parallel to the former, passing through the junction point between the posterior extremity of the superior vertebral notch and the base of the superior articular process. A precise measurement of the pedicular length may be carried out only in a perfectly lateral radiographic view of the vertebra. If one or more vertebrae are rotated on their vertical axis with respect to the adjacent vertebrae, several projections may be necessary to obtain lateral views of the various lum-

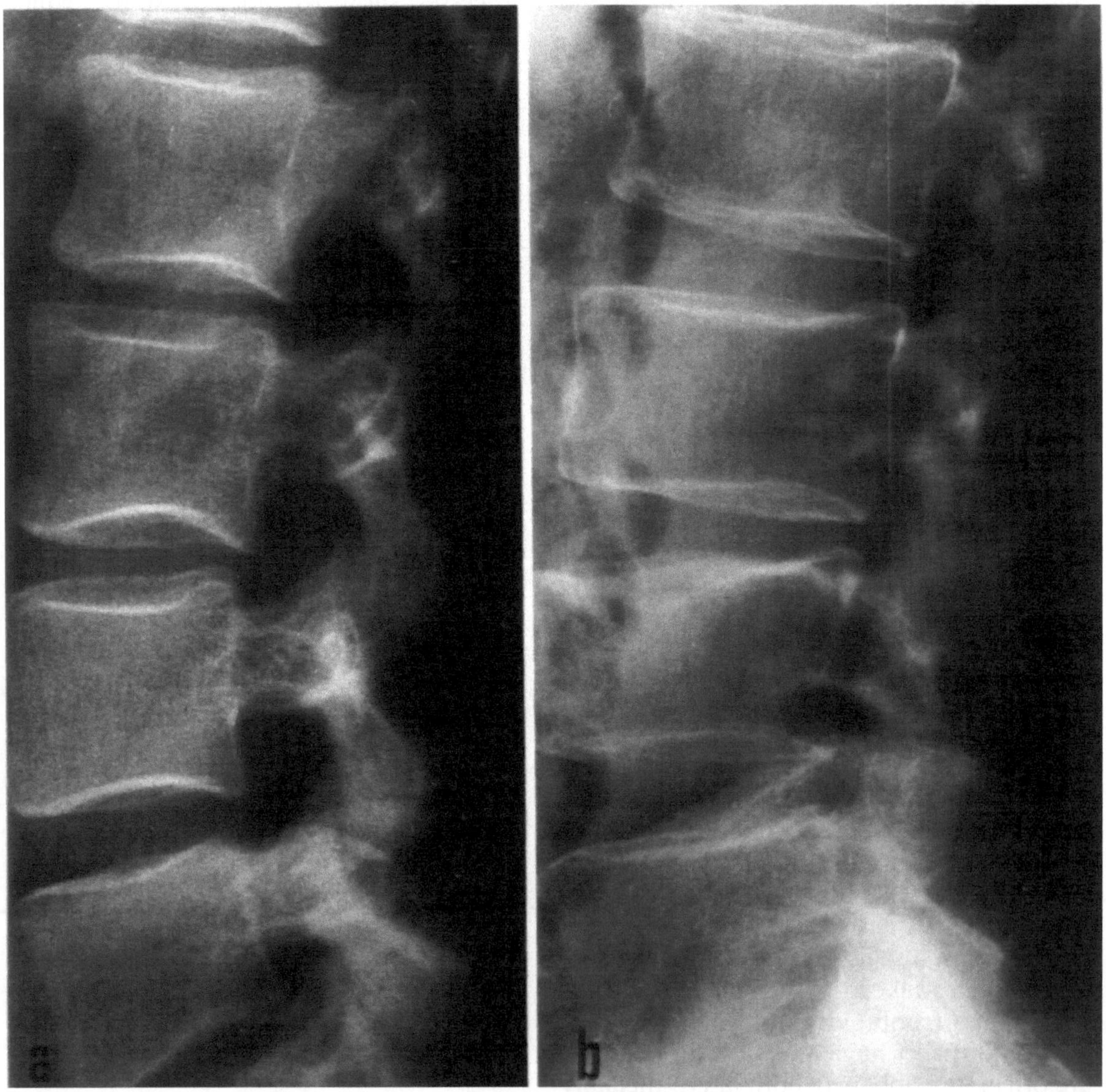

Fig. 8.3 - Comparison of the length of the pedicles in a subject (**a**) with a wide spinal canal and one (**b**) with an abnormally narrow canal.

bar vertebrae.

In normal conditions the length of the pedicles decreases progressively from the first to the fifth lumbar vertebra, so much as that the L_5 pedicles are often very short. The evaluation of the length of the pedicles is an important aspect in the evaluation of plain radiographs since it allows, even at first glance, to establish whether the spinal canal is of normal width, wider than normal or abnormally narrow (Fig. 8.3).

The present author measured the length of the pedicles in 20 asymptomatic subjects and 30 patients presenting acute or chronic low-back pain, but no clinical evidence of nerve root compression, and observed actual mean values (radiographic dimensions reduced by 20%, corresponding to x-ray magnification) varying between 17.1 mm at L_1 to 13.2 mm at L_5.

Furthermore, the length of the pedicles was measured in 35 patients with developmental or combined stenosis of the lumbar spinal canal, in whom primary narrowing of the canal was demonstrated by measurements carried out on CT scans. In 28% of these patients, the length of the pedicles at the stenotic vertebral levels was approximately the same as normal mean values, while in 71% it was lower than mean values. These observations indicate that an increased length of the pedicles with respect to normal values excludes a primary narrowing of the spinal canal, whereas a decreased length represents a sign of developmental narrowing of vertebral canal. This is especially true when the pedicles of all the lumbar vertebrae, and particularly those of the upper three, are exceedingly short.

Vertebral bodies

In patients with a developmentally narrow lumbar spinal canal, the posterior aspect of the vertebral bodies is often markedly concave. This finding, when considered alone, has little diagnostic significance, since scalloping of the dorsal aspect of the vertebral body may also be observed in subjects with a normally sized lumbar spinal canal.

The vertebral body may present a degenerative anterolisthesis or a retrolisthesis. Degenerative spondylolisthesis should always lead one to suspect a stenosis, especially when vertebral slipping exceeds 15%. In these cases, olisthesis is almost constantly associated with a symptomatic or asymptomatic compression of the thecal sac and caudal nerve roots. A retrolisthesis is only very rarely responsible for stenosis of the spinal canal, whereas it often contributes to narrowing of the nerve root canal. On the whole, retrolisthesis is of relatively low diagnostic value, certainly less than anterolisthesis. This is due to the fact that retrolisthesis is rarely associated with marked arthrotic changes of the facet joints, and posterior slipping is usually mild. It is extremely rare, in fact, that it exceeds 15%.

The finding of posterior marginal osteophytes of the vertebral body is relatively uncommon and, in most cases, these are of small dimensions. At times, there may be a posterior prominence of the vertebral end-plate in the form of an osteophytic bar. Such a prominence may only be observed at the level of the lower vertebral end-plate, usually of a single vertebra. Although the pathological effects produced by posterior osteophytes are strictly related to the primary dimensions of the vertebral canal and the lateral recesses, the finding of these osteophytes should lead one to suspect a stenosis, particularly in the presence of other radiographic signs of narrowing, whether developmental or degenerative, of the spinal canal.

Intervertebral foramina

In normal conditions, the sagittal dimensions of the intervertebral foramina, being related to the length of the pedicles, tend to decrease progressively from the first to the fifth neuroforamen. The vertical dimensions on the other hand, are almost constant for the upper four foramina, whereas they decrease at L_5-S_1 level, due to the greater height of the pedicles of the fifth lumbar vertebra (Fig. 8.4a).

In subjects with a developmentally narrow lumbar spinal canal, the intervertebral foramina are usually narrow in a sagittal

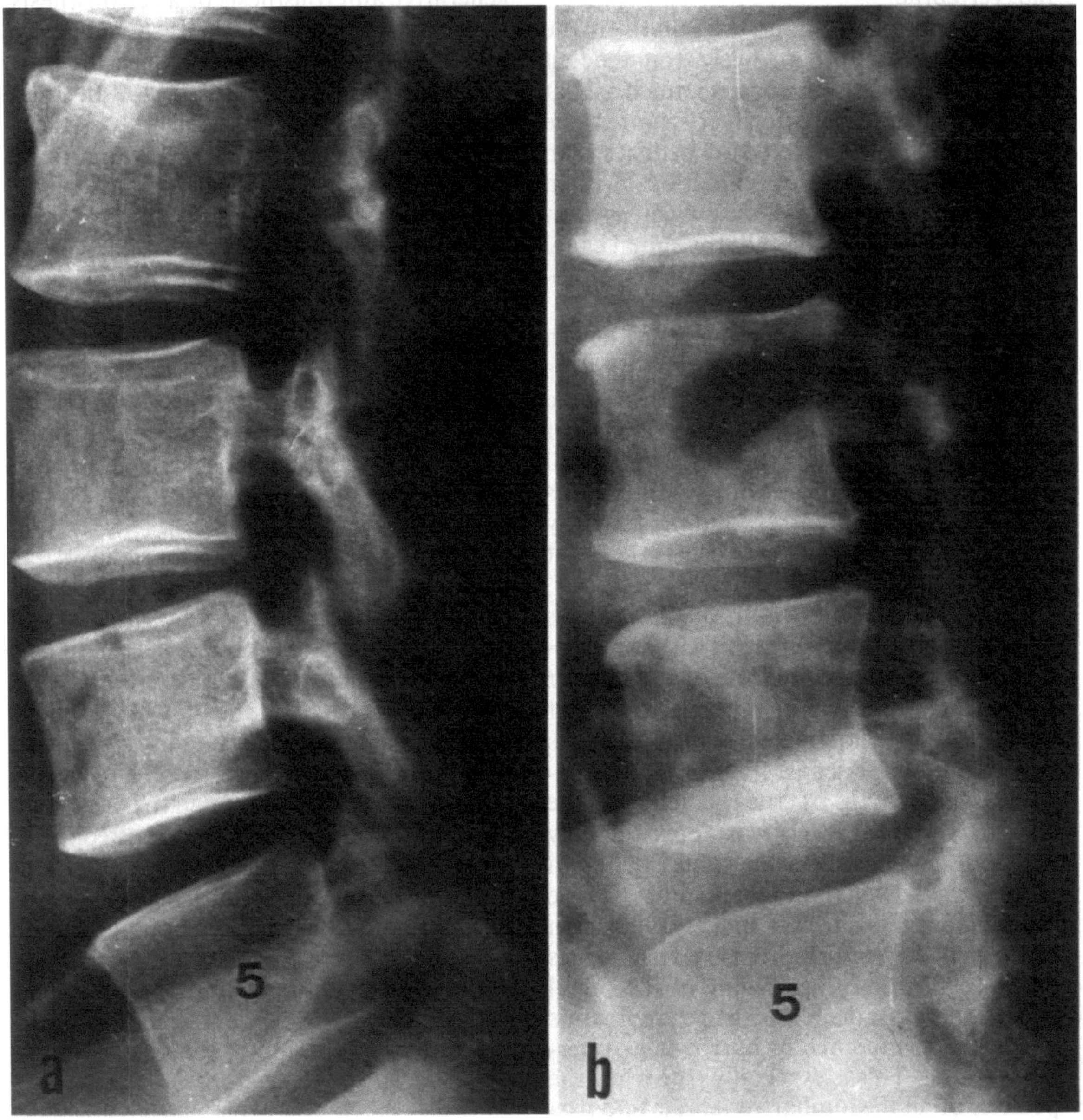

Fig. 8.4 - a. Normal appearance of the lumbar intervertebral foramina, which progressively decrease in size from the first to the fifth lumbar level. **b.** In the presence of a developmentally narrow spinal canal, the intervertebral foramina display short sagittal dimensions and, at times, appear to be divided into two parts due to posterior prominence of the bony end-plate.

direction due to the shortness of the pedicles and, often, to the posterior prominence of the inferior portion of the vertebral body, if the dorsal aspect of the latter shows a marked concavity in the sagittal plane (Fig. 8.4b). Narrowing of the foramina in the vertical diameter is usually due to a decrease in height of the intervertebral disc. In the presence of a marked loss of disc height, the tip of the superior articular process of the distal vertebra may appear to be in contact with the pedicle of the proximal vertebra above. This may occur particularly for the L_5-S_1 neuroforamen, which is the narrowest in the vertical diameter. According to Crock (1976), narrowing of the intervertebral foramen caused by disc resorption may frequently be responsible for compression of the nerve root lying in the foramen. In my experience, this does not occur in the absence of other constrictive conditions — particularly of marked arthrotic changes of the superior articular process — which may narrow the foramen also in the sagittal diameter.

In the presence of posterior marginal osteophytes of the vertebral body, the neuroforamen appears to be invaded by osteophytes. The encroachment, however, may only be apparent and due to the overlapping of the image of the osteophytes on the image of the foramen. The latter, in fact, may be constricted only by posterolateral osteophytic spurs arising at the level of the pedicles. Osteophytes, however, are rarely responsible for compression of the nerve root in the intervertebral foramen, since the root occupies the proximal portion of the neuroforamen, which is not usually invaded by these osteophytes.

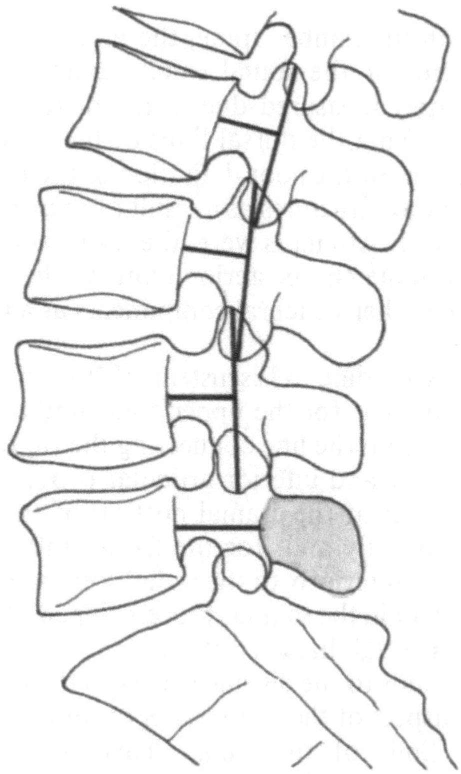

Fig. 8.5 - Eisenstein's method to determine the posterior limit of the vertebral canal and measurement of the midsagittal diameter of the canal in the lateral radiograph.

OBLIQUE PROJECTIONS

In lumbar stenosis, oblique projections do not usually add much to the diagnostic information obtained by means of frontal and lateral view. In most cases, therefore, these projections are of little interest, except in degenerative spondylolisthesis, in which they may be useful to exclude an isthmic defect, or in the presence of abnormalities of orientation and/or shape of the articular processes or the laminae. Oblique views, however, should be used to better analyze the degenerative changes of the articular processes and the relationships (abnormal closeness, neoarthrosis) that the tip of the upper articular process may have with the pedicle of the vertebra above.

MEASUREMENTS OF VERTEBRAL CANAL DIMENSIONS

Interpedicular distance

The interpedicular distance corresponds to the largest transverse diameter of the spinal canal. In a normally sized canal, this diameter is always greater than the midsagittal diameter, whereas in a developmentally narrow canal, the interpedicular distance may be not only below the lower limits of normal, but equal or less than the midsagittal diameter. None the less, measurement of the interpedicular distance, even though useful for the identification of a developmentally narrow canal, is of little diagnostic value in lumbar stenosis, since the compression of the spinal nervous structures is never caused by the pedicles, even if abnormally close.

It should be pointed out, however, that in the measurement of this and other vertebral diameters, the radiographic magnification should be taken into account, which, in standard conditions, is approximately 1.2.

Midsagittal diameter

In the lumbar spine, the midsagittal diameter of the spinal canal cannot be accurately measured due to the difficulty of identifying the dorsal limit of the canal on account of the poor definition of the posterior bony structures as a result of image overlapping. Attempts were, therefore, made to determine the posterior limit of the canal using other vertebral components as a reference.

According to Eisenstein (1976), this limit is situated, for the upper four lumbar vertebrae, on the line connecting the tip of the superior and inferior articular processes at the level of the cranial portion of the vertebral body and, for the fifth lumbar vertebra, anteriorly to the radiolucent area visible within the spinous process (Fig. 8.5). The midsagittal diameter of the spinal canal corresponds to the distance between the posterior aspect of the vertebral body and the dorsal limit of the canal. This method of measurement is not very precise and is not easy to perform, particularly at L_5 level, due to the difficulty in obtaining a precise radiographic definition of the bony structures used as reference. Nevertheless, this may, at times, be useful to approximately determine the spinal canal dimensions, which may lead one to suspect developmental narrowing of the canal.

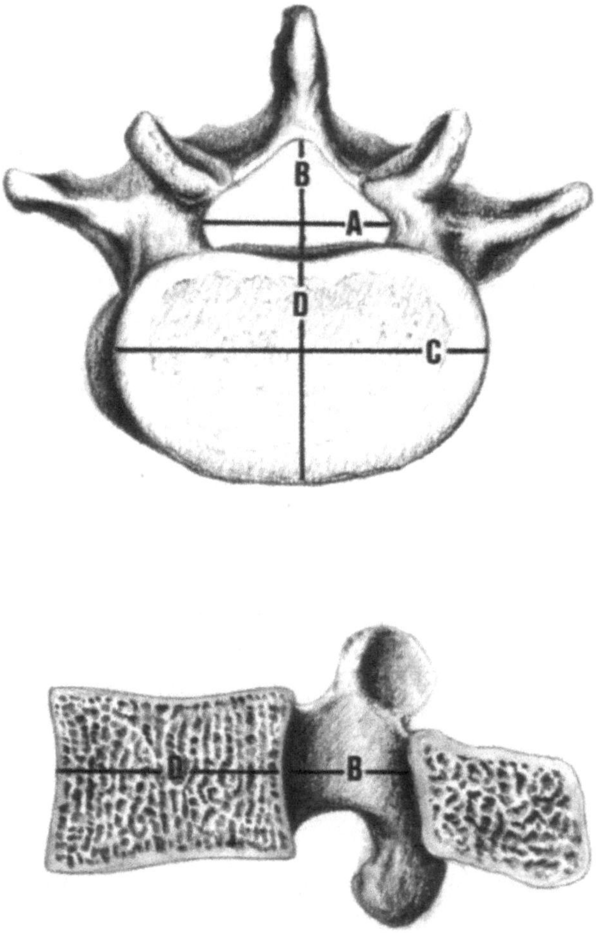

Fig. 8.6 - Jones and Thomson's spinal index. The diameters A (interpedicular distance) and C (width of the vertebral body in its middle portion) are measured in the anteroposterior radiograph. The diameter B (midsagittal diameter of the spinal canal) is measured in the lateral radiograph from the posterior aspect of the vertebral body to the base of the opposite spinous process, which can be recognized by tracing forwards its inferior margin. The diameter D (midsagittal diameter of the vertebral body) is also measured in the lateral radiograph.

Jones and Thomson's spinal index

The Jones and Thomson's index is the ratio of the product of the transverse and midsagittal diameters of the spinal canal to the product of the same diameters of the vertebral body (Fig. 8.6). The transverse diameter of the spinal canal corresponds to the interpedicular distance measured on the anteroposterior radiograph, whereas the sagittal diameter is calculated as the distance between the vertebral body and the base of the spinous process, which would correspond to a line traced anteriorly to the lower margin of the spinous process. The vertebral body is measured at the level of the median portion, corresponding to the narrowest part of it.

According to Jones and Thomson (1968), the ratio between the two products usually varies between 1/4. 5 (0.22), representing the lower limit of normal, and 1/2 (0.50), corresponding to the upper limit of normal. A ratio lower than 0.22 would indicate developmental narrowing of the spinal canal, while a ratio over 0.33 would exclude such a narrowing.

This index, which avoids the need, during measurements, to take the radiographic magnification into account, is, in reality, of little diagnostic value. The dimensions of the spinal canal are, in fact, relatively independent of those of the vertebral body. This implies that a body of large dimensions (in other words, a high denominator) can lower the ratio below the lower limits of normal, even in the presence of a normally sized spinal canal. Moreover, it should be pointed out that measurement of the midsagittal diameter of the spinal canal on plain radiographs is somewhat approximate, and that the ratio accumulates, in itself, a margin of error equal to the sum of the margins of error of the single measurements.

The unreliability of Jones and Thomson's ratio is confirmed by the poor correspondence between the sagittal diameters of the spinal canal and the values of this ratio, as measured in the vertebrae of different skeletal populations (Eisenstein, 1977) and on lumbar CT scans both of normal and stenostic subjects (Postacchini *et al.*, 1980).

CONVENTIONAL TOMOGRAPHY

Tomograms may be useful in evaluating the width of the vertebral canal and the lateral recesses in the sagittal plane. Sagittal tomograms allow precise visualization of the anterior wall of the spinal canal and detection of the posterior limit of the canal, represented by the anterior aspect of the neural arch, which is not visible on plain radiographs. Nevertheless, even on tomograms, the posterior limit of the canal cannot be precisely determined due to overlapping of the images of the laminae, as well as the articular processes, if these are hypertrophied and very close to the midline. For these reasons, and on account of the difficulty in obtaining exactly midsagittal tomographic sections, the width of the spinal canal can be determined approximately and not measured precisely. The same is true for multidirectional tomography, with which is possible to obtain thinner sections, providing a better definition of the bony structures. This technique is, however, still inadequate for exact measurement. Similar considerations are valid for lateral recesses, the width of which can be evaluated, at least visibly, if thin tomographic sections are used. It should be emphasized, however, that, as with other diagnostic investigations, simple assessment of the width of the vertebral canal or the lateral recesses provides little information on the presence of compression of the spinal nervous structures, thus making tomography of little use in the diagnostic evaluation of patients with lumbar stenosis. On the other hand, with the advent of transaxial radiological investigations, conventional tomography has lost even that relative usefulness that it might have enjoyed in the past.

ELECTRODIAGNOSTIC INVESTIGATIONS

The investigations currently employed in the evaluation of patients with lumboradicular syndromes are electromyography (EMG), H reflex analysis and somatosensory evoked potentials (SEPs).

Electromyography

EMG still represents the most important electrodiagnostic study. It is useful to document, and evaluate the severity of, clinically appreciable motor deficits and to demonstrate nerve root compression which does not determine any clinically appreciable sensory or motor deficit.

In patients with suspected lumbar stenosis, electromyography should be carried out bilaterally, analyzing the L_4, L_5 and S_1 nerve roots on each side, and also the L_2 and/or L_3 in the presence of a clinical syndrome suggesting involvement of the upper lumbar roots. In rare instances it may also be worthwhile analyzing the electrical activity of the paraspinal muscles. The electromyographic findings may be normal, may indicate a complete or partial muscle denervation, or may show evidence of a milder radicular motor deficit.

Jacobson (1976) analyzed the electromyographic findings obtained in 49 patients with a herniated disc at a single level or multiple levels and in 53 patients with spondylosis (associated or not with disc herniation), developmental stenosis of the spinal canal or spondylolisthesis. Of the patients in the first group, only 19% had a positive multiradicular or bilateral electromyogram and none showed bilateral pluriradicular involvement. In the series reported by Paine (1972), comprising patients with simple disc herniation and patients with stenotic conditions, associated or not with a herniated disc, EMG showed pluriradicular involvement in 13% of patients in the first group and in 30% to 60% of those in the second group.

In my experience, electromyography is generally positive when root compression occurs in the nerve root canal or the intervertebral foramen. For this reason, in patients with isolated stenosis of the nerve root canal or the neuroforamen, pathological electromyograms are often obtained not only for the root or roots which appear clearly compressed on myelography, but also for those showing slight signs of compression, or even no compression, on myelograms. Conversely, in stenosis of the spinal canal, EMG may, at times, give negative results or show a monoradicular involvement even in the presence of a pluriradicular involvement, such as that occurring in patients with a complete myelographic block. This is probably due to the fact that, in the intradural course, a single nerve root may escape more easily, or more easily adapt to, the compressive agent, which, therefore, only rarely causes functional changes that can be demonstrated by electromyography. In the extradural course, in contrast, the spinal nerve root, having less space and thus less possibility to escape a compressive agent, more easily undergoes significant functional changes. There is no doubt, however, that if negativity or monoradicular positivity of EMG do not exclude stenosis, pluriradicular involvement, particularly when bilateral, is usually indicative of spinal canal stenosis, rather than isolated nerve root canal stenosis or disc herniation.

For the purposes of therapeutic decision, electromyography is particularly useful in two circumstances: in patients presenting nerve root canal or intervertebral foramen stenotic syndromes, in whom myelography is negative and CT scan or magnetic resonance imaging show negative or doubtful findings; and in patients with a severe, clinically symptomatic, stenosis at one vertebral level, and a mild, clinically asymptomatic, stenosis at an adjacent level. In the former, clearly pathological electromyographic findings might tend to suggest surgical treatment when an adequate trial of conservative treatment has been unsuccessful; in the latter, the electromyographic findings may orientate or not toward the extension of surgical decompression even at the asymptomatic level.

H reflex

It is elicited by stimulating the posterior tibial nerve in the popliteal fossa and recording the potentials induced in the soleus muscle. The H reflex may be considered the electric correspondent of the Achilles tendon reflex and, like the latter, it represents an index of functional integrity of the first sacral nerve root. This electrodiagnostic test presents two advantages with respect to electromyography: it becomes positive immediately after the occurrence of a functional deficit of the S_1 nerve root, and may be abnormal in the presence of a purely sensory involvement of this root. The H reflex, however, may be recorded only in the soleus muscle and is, therefore, of value only for the detection of a S_1 radiculopathy.

Study of this reflex is especially helpful in the presence of a S_1 nerve root canal stenosis, which not infrequently causes a functional deficit only of the sensory component of the root. In this instance, there may be an abnormal H reflex in the presence of normal electromyographic findings.

Somatosensory evoked potentials

With monitoring of SEPs, electrophysiological investigations have been endowed with a new technique in the evaluation of neurological pathological conditions, which is able to specifically analyze the function of primary afferent pathways in the spinal nerve roots and the dorsal columns of the spinal cord. However, knowledge of this technique and its diagnostic potentialities is still limited as far as concerns the various aspects of lumbar nerve root pathology and, particularly, the stenotic conditions. In the series described by Keim *et al.* (1985), comprising 20 patients with lumbar spinal stenosis diagnosed by myelography and/or CT scan and confirmed at surgery, somatosensory evoked potentials were found to be abnormal in all cases, including those in which EMG had shown normal findings. In agreement with the results of this study are the findings of Dvonch *et al.* (1984), who recorded dermatomal somatosensory evoked potentials in 70 patients with lumbar radiculopathy and found this technique to have an accuracy of approximately 86% in root-specific diagnosis.

In patients with lumbar stenosis, the posterior tibial and the peroneal are the nerves most frequently showing abnormal SEPs findings. The saphenous nerve is rarely involved, and exclusively when upper lumbar nerve roots are affected. As with electromyography, SEPs are often pathological on both sides even in the presence of a unilateral clinical syndrome. This may be considered a differential diagnostic element with respect to disc herniation, in which SEPs usually show a unilateral monoradicular involvement. The role of SEPs study in the planning of treatment is similar to that of EMG, compared to which somatosensory evoked potentials appear to have a higher diagnostic accuracy.

ULTRASONOGRAPHY

The use of ultrasonography in the study of the spinal canal was first proposed by Meire (1975). However, it was Porter *et al.* (1978 a, b) who introduced echography as a routine clinical

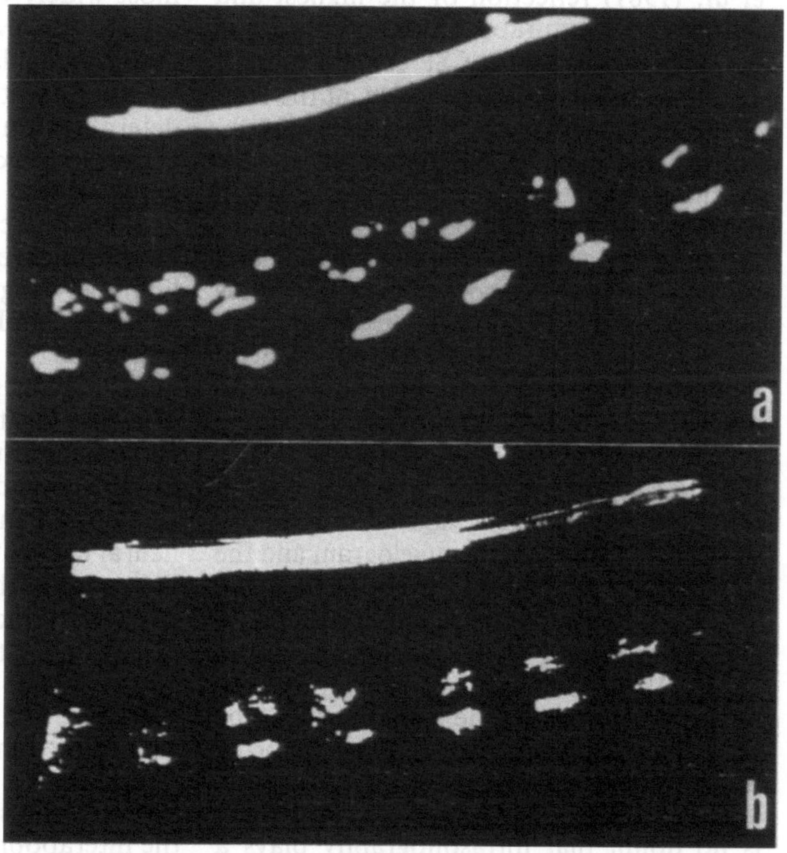

Fig. 8.7 - Type B sonographic scans of a normally-sized (**a**) and a narrow (**b**) spinal canal (sagittal diameter).

investigation to measure the sagittal dimensions of the lumbar spinal canal. According to the technique of these authors, which is that currently employed, the ultrasound beam penetrates into the vertebral canal through the interlaminar spaces, at an angle of 15° to the sagittal plane of the spine. What is measured, therefore, is the oblique sagittal diameter of the lumbar canal, which, although differing from the midsagittal diameter, allows evaluation of the width of the spinal canal at the various vertebral levels and distinction between a normally sized and a narrow spinal canal (Fig. 8.7). Vertebral sonography, however, still presents several obscure aspects as far as concerns both the origin of the echoes recorded by the transducer and the precision of the measurements. According to the original interpretation (Porter *et al.*, 1978a), the echoes originate from the reflection of the ultrasonic energy at the boundaries between the epidural tissue and the laminae, dorsally, and the posterior surface of the vertebral body, ventrally. In contrast, according to Kadziolka *et al.* (1981) reflection of the highest and more easily measurable echoes occurs at the boundaries between the CSF contained in the dural sac and the epidural tissue, at the level of the intervertebral disc. The dimensions obtained, therefore, would reflect the size of the dural sac, rather than that of the vertebral canal. According to Porter *et al.* (1978b), the values of the mean oblique sagittal diameter of the spinal canal recorded by ultrasounds are comparable to those of the mean midsagittal diameter measured on skeletal material, compared to which the oblique diameter is 0.4 to 1.8 mm shorter, depending on the vertebral level. Asztely *et al.* (1983), however, found a very poor correlation coefficient between the sagittal dimensions of the dye column on the myelogram and the size of the spinal canal (or the dural tube, according to the interpretation) measured, in the same subjects, by ultrasounds. Legg and Gibbs (1984), on the other hand, found the mean dimensions of the spinal canal to be some 2 mm less compared to those reported by Porter *et al.* (1978).

Regardless of these discrepancies, there is no doubt that ultrasonography plays a secondary role in the diagnostic evaluation of patients with lumbar stenosis. This is due to the fact that a narrow canal may, or may even not, be a stenotic canal, and a stenotic compression of the neural structures may also occur in a spinal canal of normal size in the midsagittal or oblique sagittal plane. Furthermore, it should be pointed out that ultrasounds, although able to demonstrate the presence of a disc protrusion (Engel *et al.*, 1985), do not provide any information on the width, and thus the presence or not of stenosis, of the nerve root canal. These considerations indicate that ultrasonography, which has the merit of being an innocuous and non invasive technique, is useful in identifying subjects with a narrow spinal canal, but cannot be considered as a reliable diagnostic investigation in lumbar spinal stenosis.

MYELOGRAPHY

Water-soluble myelography, or radiculography, which was until recently the most widely employed investigation in the diagnostic evaluation of patients with lumbo-radicular syndromes, has several disadvantages: it is invasive; it does not allow determination, in some cases, of the precise aetiology of compression of the dural sac or nerve roots; and is unable, at times, to demonstrate compression of the nerve root in the intervertebral foramen. Despite its limits, myelography represents a reliable diagnostic tool with high accuracy and represents the method on which diagnosis of lumbar spinal stenosis is still currently based. This investigation, in fact, by visualizing the nervous structures contained in the vertebral canal, allows direct detection of the presence of a discrepancy between the volume of the neural elements and the capacity of the spinal canal both in static conditions and the dynamic conditions occurring in flexion-extension of the lumbar spine.

TECHNICAL DETAILS

In the presence of marked narrowing of the interapophysolaminar spaces, it may be preferable to perform lumbar puncture with the patient in the sitting position, rather than lying on one side as in the routine technique, in order to obtain a greater opening of the interspinous spaces, which allows easier entry into the spinal canal.

If stenosis is suspected, lumbar puncture should be carried out al L_2-L_3 level, rather than at L_3-L_4 as is routine practice, since the latter intervertebral level is more often stenotic than the interspace above. At a stenotic level, it may, in fact, be difficult to enter the dural sac with the needle or, once having entered, cerebrospinal fluid may not be withdrawn which confirms the correct position of the tip of the needle. In the event puncture at L_2-L_3 level shows no evidence of CSF, puncture should be carried out at the level below, and if again results are negative, an L_5-S_1 lumbar puncture should be performed. The latter, furthermore, may be carried out in addition to high lumbar puncture in the presence of a complete myelographic block extended to more than one lumbar level, in order to confirm or exclude compression of the nervous structures below the area of arrest of the contrast medium.

In addition to myelograms in standard projections (latero-lateral, postero-anterior with the patient in a prone position, and oblique), it is advisable to carry out, if the radiographic equipment permits, a latero-lateral radiograph with the patient in the supine position, using a horizontal beam. The supine position, in fact, bringing the dural sac to lean on the neural arc, makes any dorsal compression on the sac more easily to detect.

Once the investigation in the recumbent position has been carried out, it is useful to perform functional examination in the standing position, to obtain three latero-lateral radiographs: one in an upright position, one in maximum flexion and one in hyperextension of the spine. When carrying out functional radiographs, care should be taken in order that trunk flexion and extension occur also, and particularly, at the level of the lumbar spine and not only of the hips. Functional x-rays in spinal flexion can also be obtained with the patient supine, placed in a squatting position (Urso, 1986). To obtain this position, two cushions are placed under the thoracic spine of the patient, who is invited to bend the knees and hips as much as possible in order to kyphose the lumbar spine. This position, unlike the flexed standing position, enables anteroposterior radiographs to be obtained and, thus, filling defects of the nerve root sheaths, in spinal flexion and extension, to be recognized.

ELEMENTARY SIGNS OF STENOSIS

Uniform narrowing of the dural sac

The dural sac may be narrowed uniformly, for the whole height of a vertebra, in the frontal and/or sagittal plane. Taking radio-

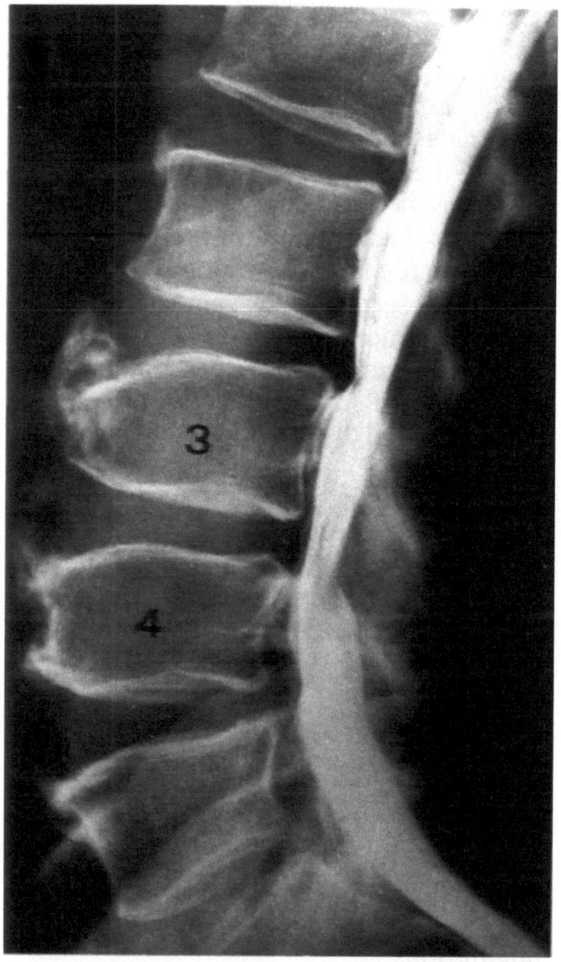

Fig. 8.8 - Segmentary narrowing of the dural sac from the caudal portion of L_2 to the cranial portion of L_4. Note the increase in size of the thecal sac above and below the narrowed area.

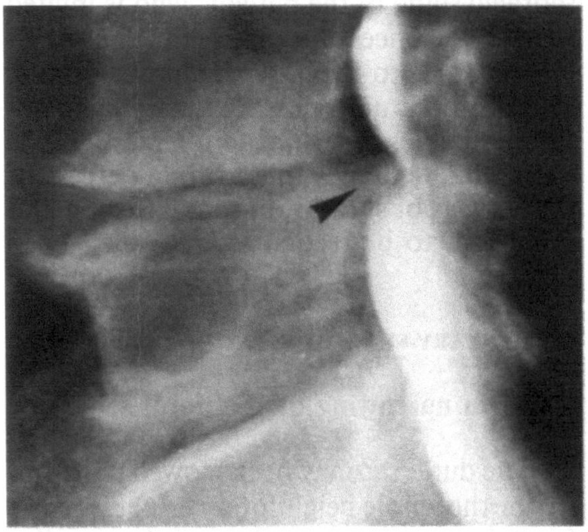

Fig. 8.9 - Ventral indentation of the dural sac caused by a posterior osteophyte of the vertebral body (arrowhead).

graphic magnification into account — which, in standard radiographic conditions, is approximately 1.2 with respect to real dimensions — the dural sac should be consided narrow when the dye column measures less than 18 mm on the anteroposterior, and less than 15 mm on the lateral, myelogram. Narrowing may be segmental or generalized. In the former instance, it usually extends over one or two vertebral levels and is associated with an increase in size of the contrast column proximally and distally to the narrowed area (Fig. 8.8). When generalized, narrowing is extended over the whole lumbar spine and, in some cases, also to the thoracic spine. Of the two forms, only the former is indicative of stenosis. The latter, which is often considered typical of developmental stenosis, is, in fact, the expression of a developmentally narrow spinal canal, but not of stenosis, if there is no evidence of compression of the nervous structures by the osteoligamentous walls of the canal.

Deformations of the dural sac

Indentations

Indentations of the dural sac may be anterior, lateral or posterior.

Anterior indentations may be caused by: posterior osteophytes of the bony end-plate (Fig. 8.9); vertebral retrolisthesis; portions of the vertebral body, if this is deformed as a result of fractures, systemic bone diseases or congenital anomalies; or protrusions of the annulus fibrosus. The latter, which are the conditions most frequently responsible for anterior indentations, are generally mild in entity.

Lateral indentations are caused by hypertrophy and/or osteophytosis of the articular processes, which may or may not be associated with thickening, and in some cases bony metaplasia, of the portion of the ligamentum flavum delimiting anteromedially the facet joint. The indentation usually extends from the pedicle of one vertebra to that of the vertebra below (Fig. 8.10); the greatest deformation of the thecal sac is most frequently observed at the level of the intervertebral space. In some cases, a significant contribution to the formation of lateral indentation is given by a bulging annulus fibrosus which displaces the dural sac dorsally, thus increasing the neural compression by the posterior osteoligamentous structures of the vertebral canal.

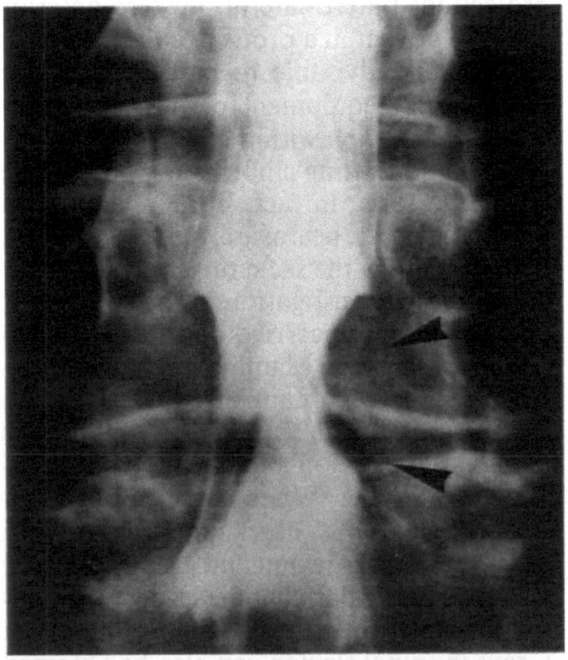

Fig. 8.10 - Lateral indentation of the dural sac (arrowheads) caused by degenerative hypertrophy of the articular processes.

Posterior indentations are caused by the inferior articular processes, with the possible contribution of thickened ligamenta flava. These indentations — which are better demonstrated by a lateral radiograph obtained using a horizontal beam with the patient in the supine position or by functional myelograms — are the most typical myelographic sign of stenosis, whether continous or extended over two or more levels. Generally, two or three vertebral and intervertebral levels, from L_2-L_3 to L_4-L_5, are involved (Fig. 8.11). Frequently, an area of marked stenosis, i.e. a total or subtotal myelographic block at one or two levels, is associated with areas of less severe constriction

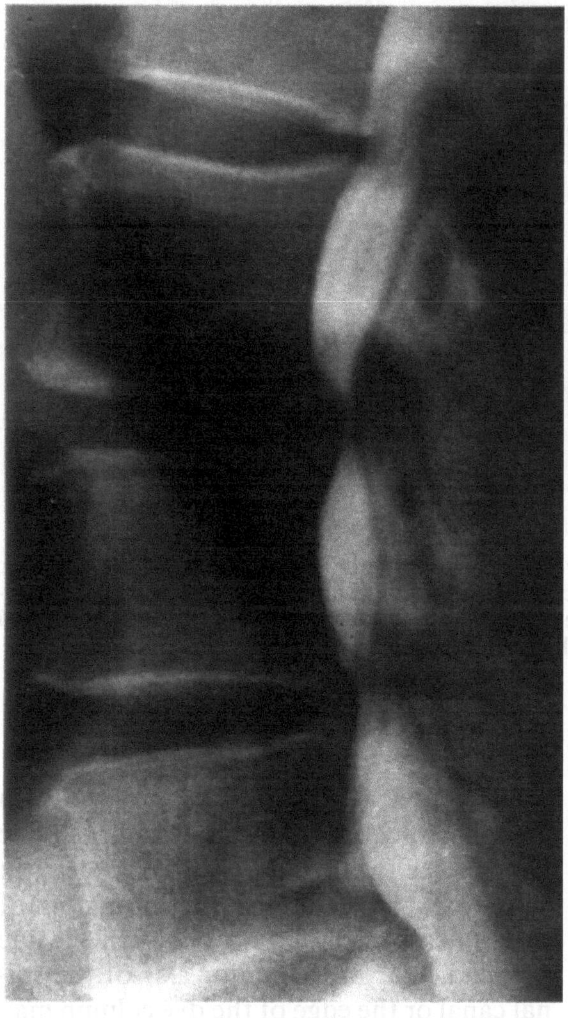

Fig. 8.11 - Posterior indentations of the dural sac at two adjacent intervertebral levels.

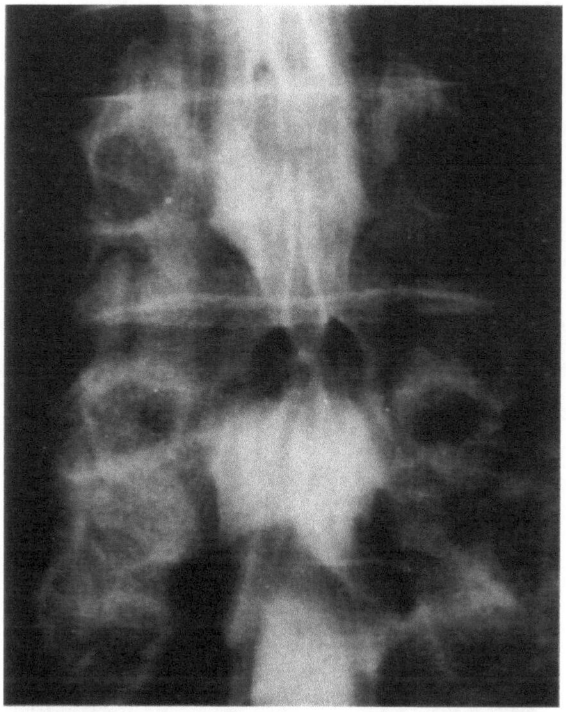

Fig. 8.12 - Hour-glass deformation of the dural sac produced by degenerative changes of the articular processes.

characterized by a posterior indentation of the dural sac, or two lateral indentations facing each other. In these forms, images of redundant nerve roots are more often found than in the other forms of stenosis, probably because the most severe lumbar stenoses are usually those of the combined type.

Hour-glass deformations

The presence of two lateral indentations facing each other determines a characteristic hour-glass deformation of the dural sac in the frontal plane (Fig. 8.12). The same occurs in the sagittal plane, when, at a same level, an anterior indentation produced by the intervertebral disc or marginal osteophytes of the vertebral body is associated with a posterior indentation caused by the osteoligamentous walls of the spinal canal.

Hour-glass deformations on the frontal plane can be distinguished from those caused

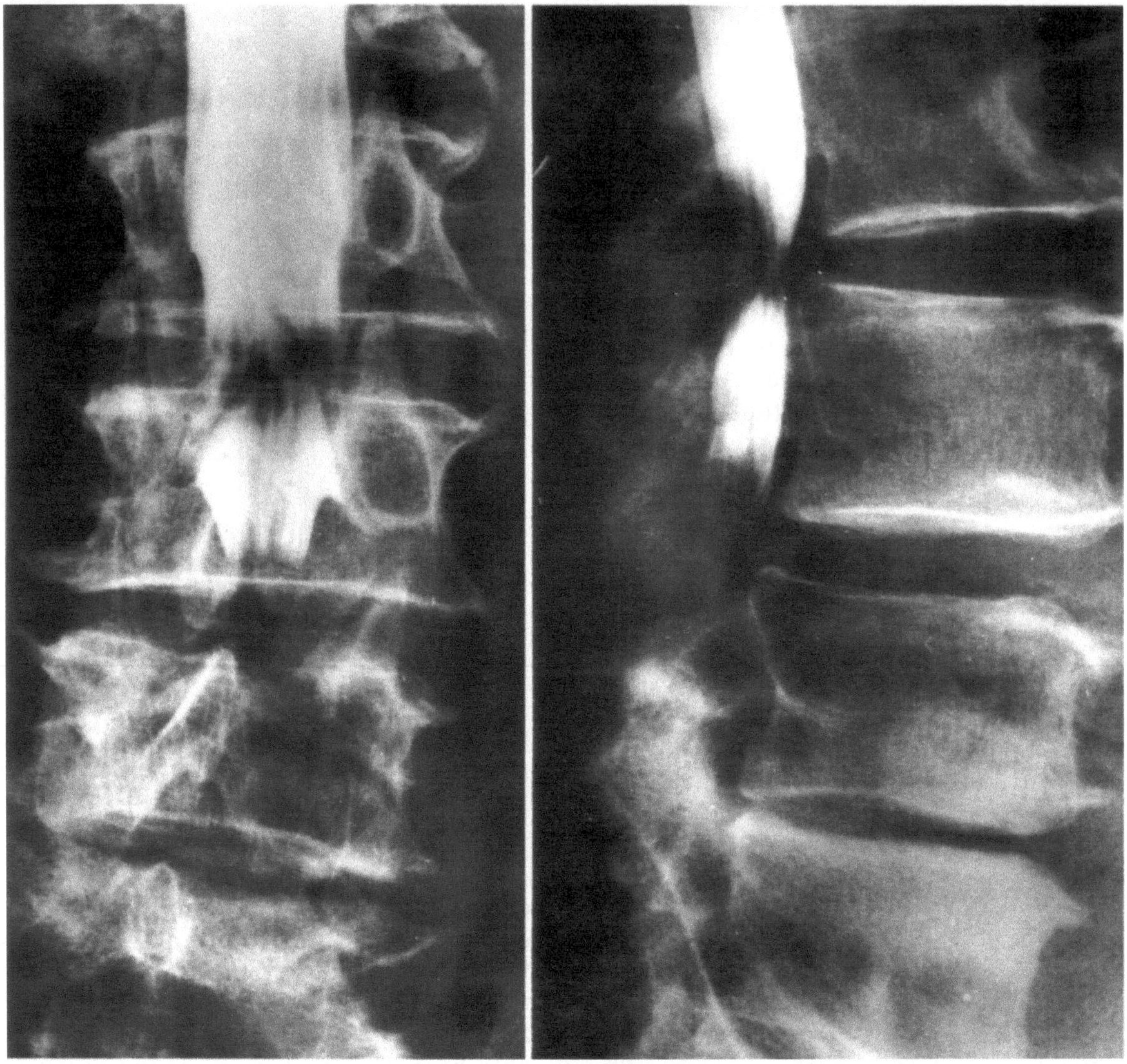

Fig. 8.13 - Complete myelographic block at L_3-L_4 level and marked posterior indentation on the dural sac at the level above. In the anteroposterior view, the block shows a brush-like appearance. In the lateral projection, the margin of arrest of the contrast medium is perpendicular to the vertical axis of the spinal canal and toothed.

by bilateral disc herniations, since in stenosis the lateral indentations usually go beyond the limits of the disc space and the dye column appears as if deviated towards the median line, instead of suddenly interrupted opposite the disc, as in the presence of a bilateral disc herniation. Hour-glass deformation on the sagittal plane is typical of stenosis on account of the characteristic posterior indentation, which may be more or less marked than the anterior.

Block images

The contrast column, at the level of a complete block, usually shows a brush-like appearance in the anteroposterior view; in the lateral projection the inferior margin of the contrast medium may be a straight line perpendicular to the major axis of the spinal canal or the edge of the dye column may be half-conical or typically pointed in shape (Figs. 8.13, 8.14, 8.15). Sometimes, on the

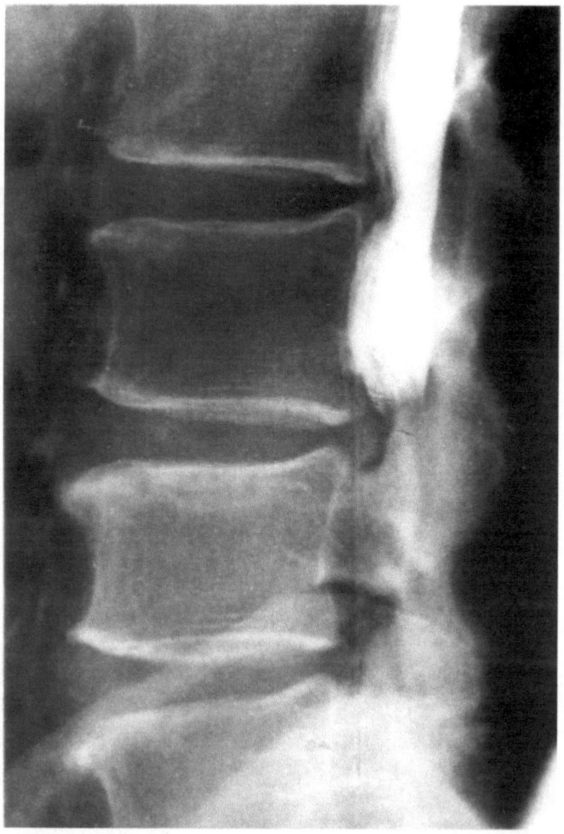

Fig. 8.14 - Complete myelographic block with half-conical appearance of the distal end of the dye column.

other hand, the extremity of the contrast column is half-conical in the frontal plane, whereas in the sagittal view it is slightly concave downwards or dome-shaped and, in both cases, generally toothed.

The block may be located at the level of the superior or inferior border of the laminae or, more often, opposite the intervertebral space. In this instance, the block may be differentiated from that caused by a herniated disc in a normally sized or developmentally narrow spinal canal, since in the block due to a disc herniation the dural sac usually presents a marked ventral indentation or, if the block is subtotal, the posterior margin of the contrast column is straight. In the typical block due to stenosis, on the other hand, the ventral indentation is mild or absent and the posterior margin of the dye column is mostly oblique anteriorly, above and/or below the arrest. When it has a dome-like appearance, the block produced by stenosis may simulate that caused by an intradural neoplasm. In this instance, the stenotic origin of the block is suggested by radiographic abnormalities indicating a primary or secondary narrowing of the spinal canal and, particularly, by myelographic evidence of a neural compression with stenotic features at vertebral levels different from that of the block.

Intrasaccular abnormalities

Translucencies of the caudal nerve roots in the intrathecal course

Normally, the single nerve roots of the cauda equina are not easily identified in the

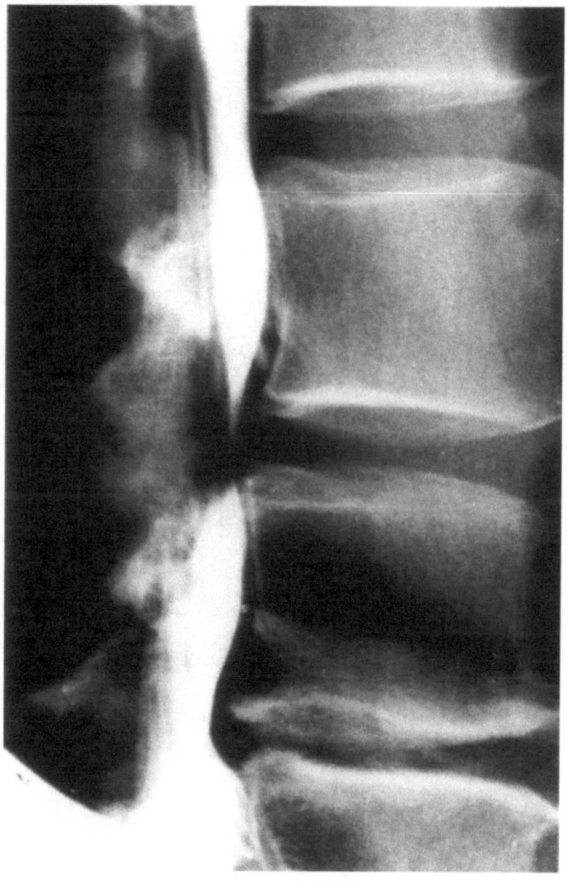

Fig. 8.15 - Complete myelographic block with pointed appearance of the dye column at the level of the block.

intrathecal course, owing to the radiopacity of the surrounding contrast medium. However, in a developmentally narrow or moderately stenotic spinal canal, the radiolucent images of the spinal roots are often more easily identifiable than in normal conditions. This can occur both in the lateral view and, much more frequently, the anteroposterior view. In the anteroposterior myelogram, the radicular translucencies are visible particularly, or only, at the level of the intervertebral spaces, where narrowing of the spinal canal

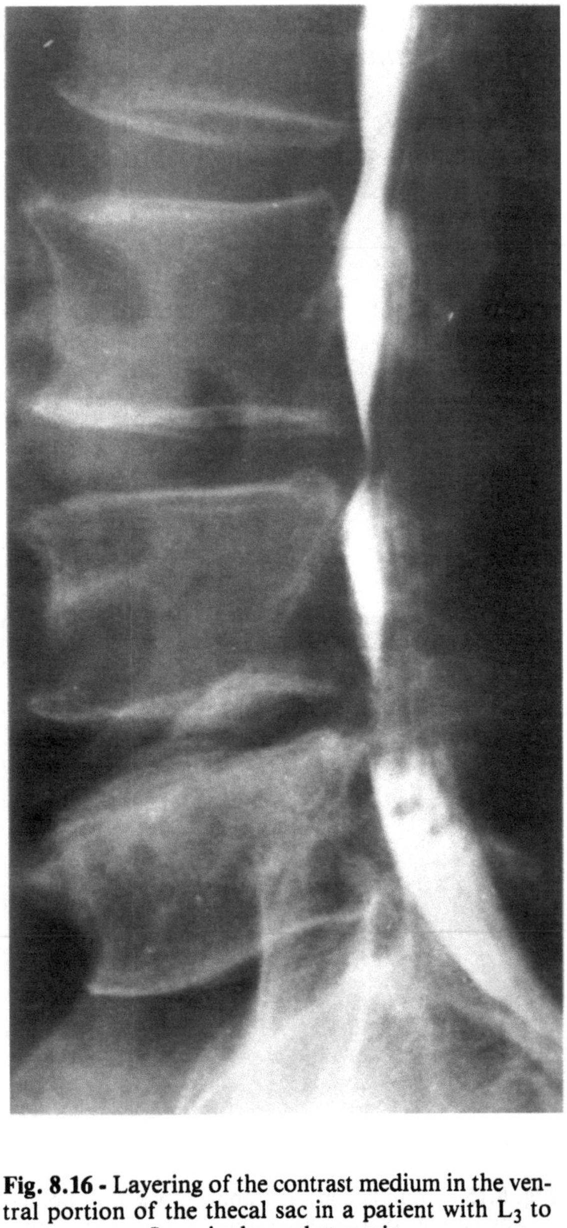

Fig. 8.16 - Layering of the contrast medium in the ventral portion of the thecal sac in a patient with L_3 to L_5 spinal canal stenosis.

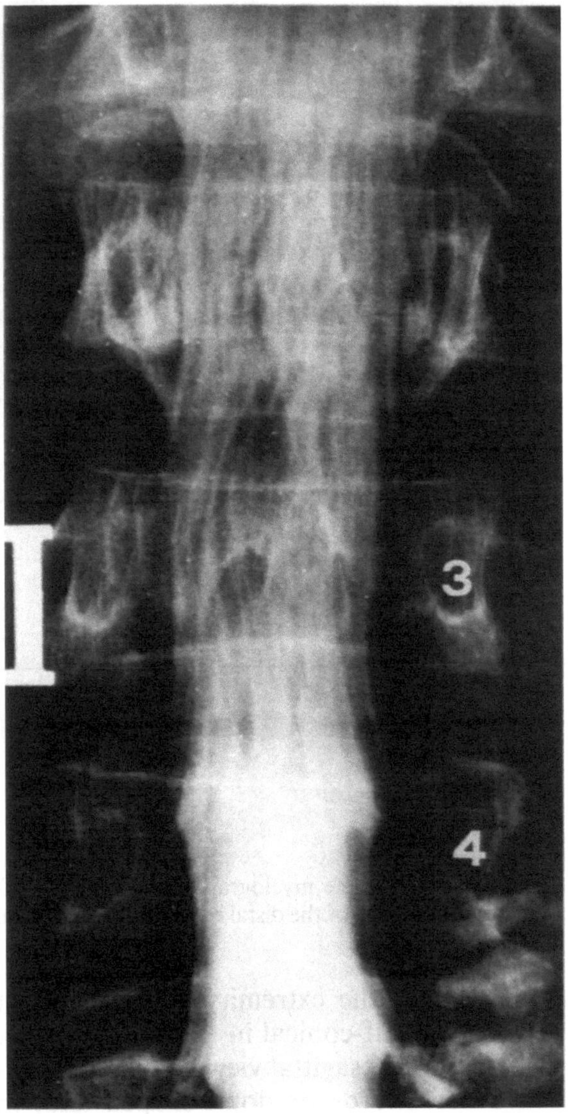

Fig. 8.17 - Mild redundancy of the nerve roots of the cauda equina at L_2-L_3 level. Most nerve roots show an undulated course within the thecal sac.

is generally greater than in the portions facing the vertebral body.

This myelographic sign is due to the fact that, owing to the pressure to which the dural sac is submitted, a smaller amount of contrast medium collects in the narrowed areas, with subsequent better visualization of the individual radicular structures. However, when compression of the dural sac is severe, radicular translucencies are not generally visible because of accumulation and sedimentation of the contrast agent above the stenotic area.

Dyshomogenous distribution of the contrast medium

In a stenotic, or only narrow, vertebral canal, a dyshomogenous distribution of the contrast medium may be seen, due to gravitational layering of the latter in some areas of the dural sac. These are usually located in the ventral half of the sac, at the level of the vertebral bodies (Fig. 8.16). According to Verbiest (1980), layering of the contrast agent occurs when the interpedicular diameter of the vertebral canal is much larger than the transverse diameter of the posterior, i.e. interlaminar, portion of the spinal canal. In my experience, gravitational layering of the contrast agent is observed particularly when the posterior aspect of the vertebral body, regardless of the dimensions of the spinal canal, shows marked concavity, or above an area of canal narrowing which may be stenotic in nature or caused by a disc herniation or a marked bulging of the annulus fibrosus. In both cases, stasis of the contrast medium — which the smaller volume of radioopaque liquid injected, the more likely it is to occur — is due to the tendency of the latter to stagnate and deposit in wider portions of the sac than the immediately adjacent portions. This myelographic sign, therefore, is not so much an expression of stenosis (or however not only of this) but rather of localized dilation of the dural sac.

Redundancy of spinal nerve roots

In spinal canal stenosis the nerve roots of the cauda equina may show a tortuous course inside the dural sac (Figs. 8.17 and 8.18). At times, particularly when stenosis is severe, some spinal roots present a winding course or produce worm-like filling defects of the dural tube (Figs. 8.19 and 8.20). These myelographic abnormalities, which are the expression of redundancy, i.e. a relative increase in diameter and/or length of the caudal spinal roots, can be observed almost exclusively, at least in the typical form, in stenosis of the spinal canal and, as such, they may be considered as pathognomonic of this condition. The tortuosity of the

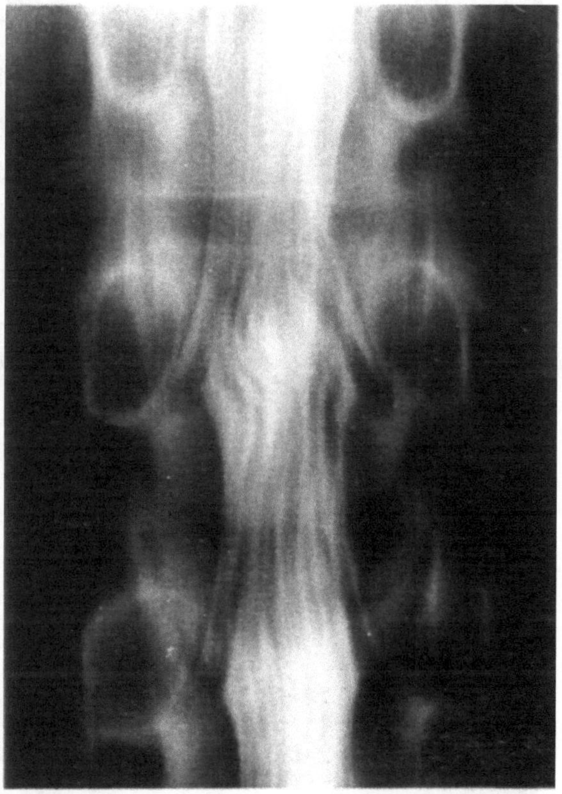

Fig. 8.18 - Winding course of a few caudal nerve roots in a patient with mild developmental stenosis of the spinal canal.

caudal nerve roots, being related to the severity of compression of the dural sac, decreases or disappears in flexion, and increases in extension, of the spine (Tsuji *et al.*, 1985). Occasionally, tortuous filling defects of the dural sac showing a loop-like course may be observed above a stenotic area (Fig. 8.21). These are likely caused by ectasic radicular or medullary veins.

Abnormalities of the nerve root sheaths

Compression of the spinal nerve roots in the extrathecal course caused by a stenotic condition is not characterized by pathognomonic myelographic signs. Often, however, stenotic compression determines different myelographic abnormalities from those usually caused by a herniated disc and such as to allow diagnosis of the origin of the compression to be made.

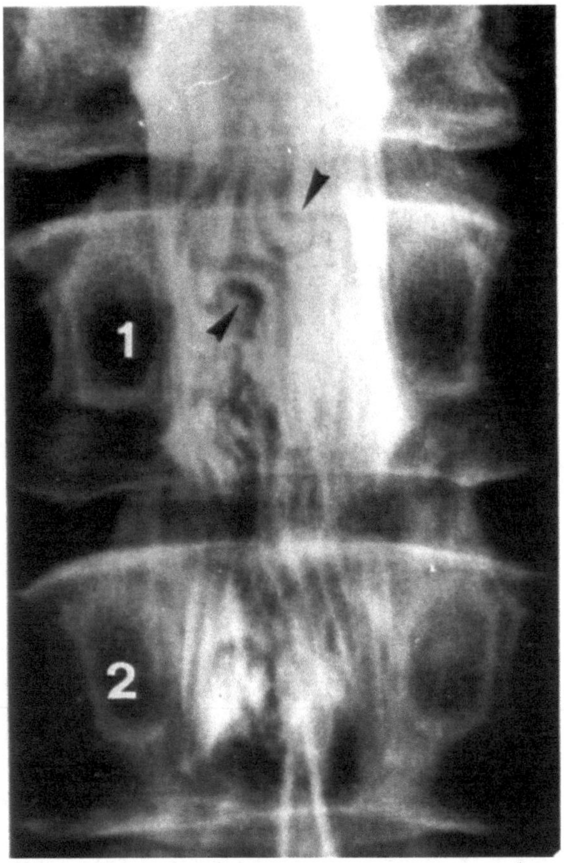

Fig. 8.19 - Winding redundant spinal nerve roots, some of which (arrowheads) show a serpiginous course. Complete myelographic block at L_2-L_3 level.

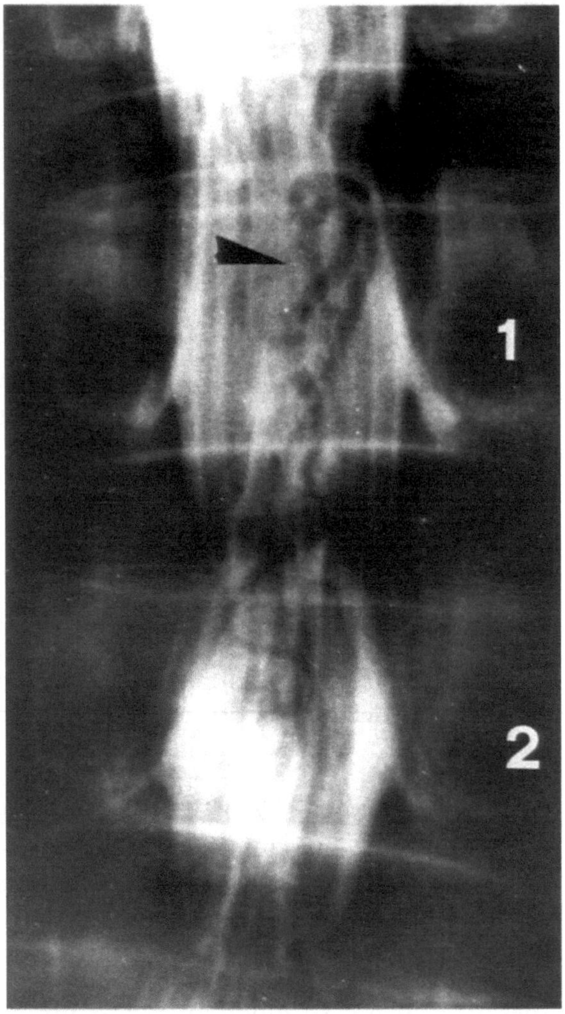

Fig. 8.21 - Loop-like filling defect within the thecal sac (arrowhead), probably due to ectasic radicular or medullary vessels. Complete myelographic block at L_2-L_3.

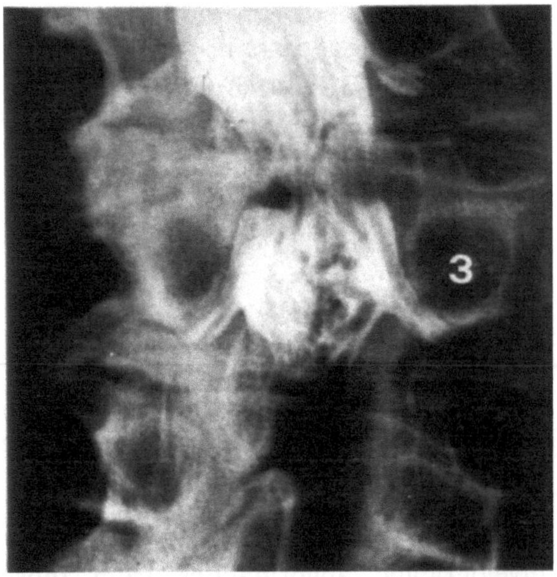

Fig. 8.20 - Worm-like filling defects within the dural sac, which are produced by redundant nerve roots immediately above a complete block of the dye column.

In compression due to stenosis, the nerve root sheath may be deviated medially and/or show a partial filling by contrast medium or may be interrupted at the level of the disc space or the lateral recess (Figs. 8.22 and 8.23). In the latter case, there is usually no nerve root swelling as usually occurs in the presence of a disc herniation. In compression due to stenosis, therefore, the nerve root sheath does not generally show a trumpet-like dilation above the interruption, but is often thinned into a pencil-pointed shape.

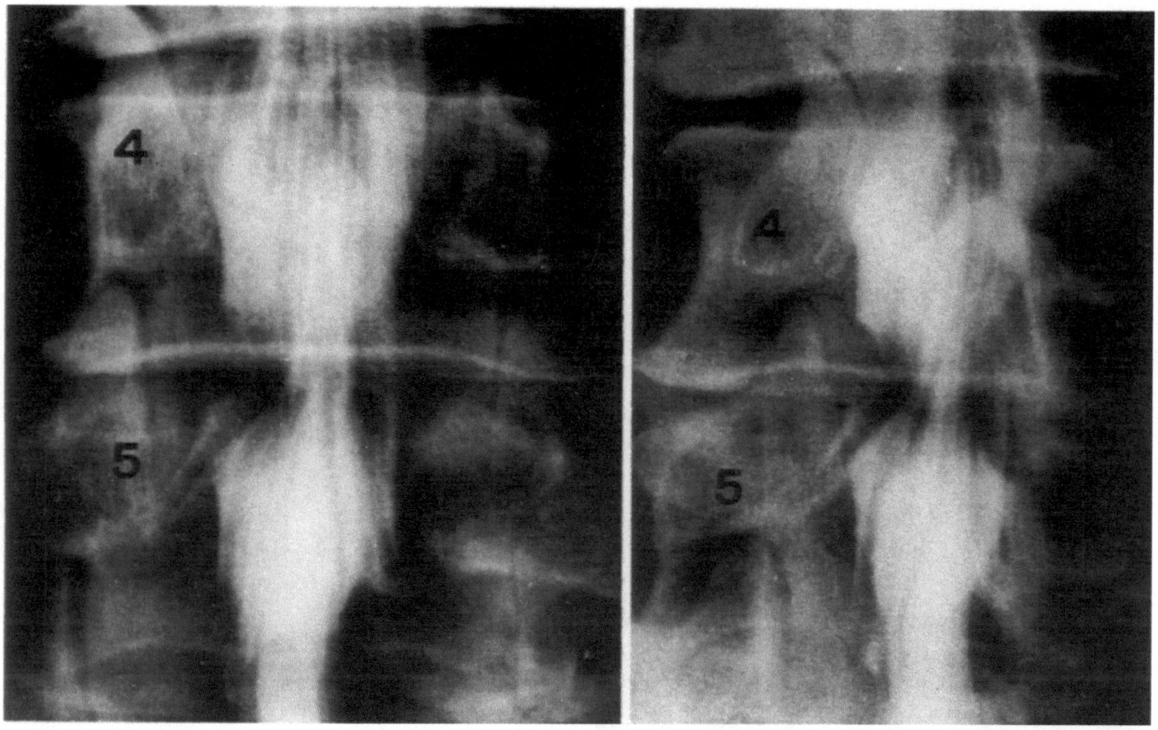

Fig. 8.22 - Medial deviation and partial filling of the right L_5 nerve root sheath due to isolated nerve root canal stenosis.

LONGITUDINAL EXTENSION OF STENOSIS

Single level stenosis

Compression of the nervous structures is limited to a single intervertebral level or a single vertebra (Fig. 8.24). In these cases, an anterior indentation of the dural sac is often visible; the indentation is caused by a bulging annulus fibrosus or, sometimes, a true disc herniation associated with a pathological narrowing of the osteoligamentous spinal canal. Proximally and distally to the stenotic area, the spinal canal may be normal in size or developmentally narrow.

Multilevel stenosis

The nervous structures are compressed at two or more intervertebral levels or over the entire height of two or more vertebrae. Various myelographic patterns may be observed. In most cases, marked compression of the dural sac and caudal nerve roots is present at a single intervertebral level, whereas signs of less severe stenosis, mostly represented by posterior indentations of the dural sac, are visible at adjacent levels. Less frequently, multiple blocks of the dye column are observed, giving the latter a characteristic moniliform appearance (Fig. 8.25). Sometimes, a complete myelographic block extended over two or, very occasionally, more vertebral levels is observed, associated with normal filling of the dural sac above and below the area of block (Fig. 8.26).

The presence of a complete myelographic block with no filling of the thecal sac below the level of arrest of the contrast medium is not, in itself, indicative of multilevel stenosis. Absence of the contrast agent below the block may also be caused, in fact, by such a severe single level compression of the dural sac, as to completely impede the flow of contrast medium. To exactly determine the extent of the stenosis in these cases, it may be useful to inject the contrast agent through

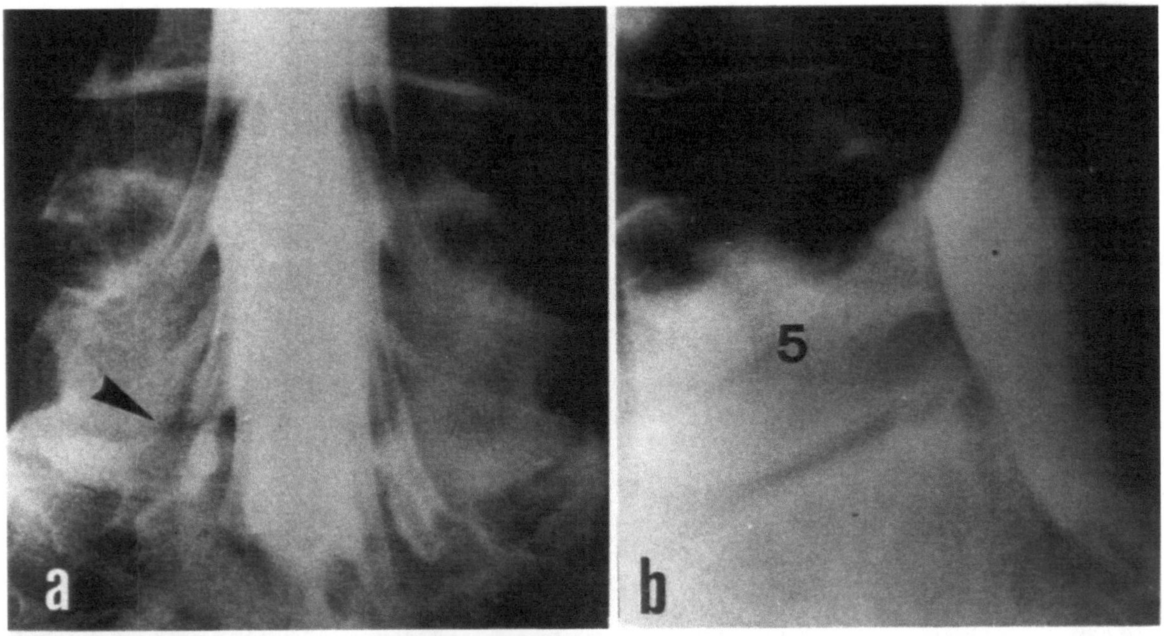

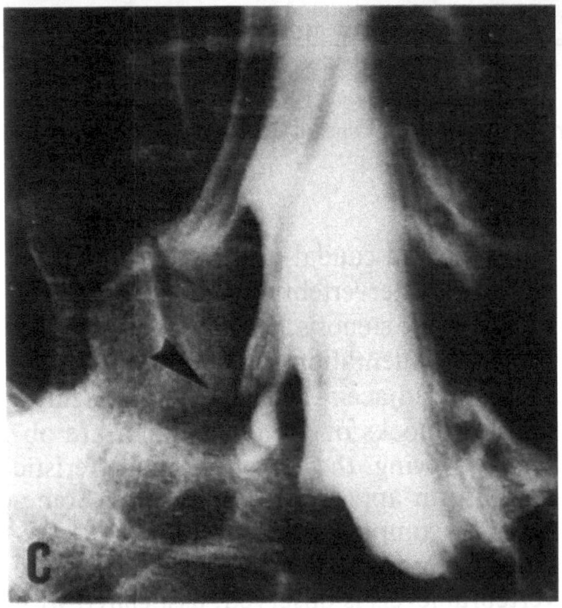

Fig. 8.23 - Nerve root canal stenosis of S_1 on the right. The right S_1 nerve root sheath is interrupted (arrowhead) at the level of the proximal portion of the S_1 lateral recess (**a** and **c**). The L_5-S_1 disc is completely resorbed and the L_5 vertebra shows a mild retrolisthesis (**b**).

a lumbar puncture at L_5-S_1 level, at the same time as or immediately following the high lumbar punture (Fig. 8.27).

FUNCTIONAL MYELOGRAPHY

Functional myelograms may be useful to study the variations in the entity of anterior and, particularly, of posterior compression of the dural sac during flexion and extension of the lumbar spine. Furthermore, lateral myelograms in the standing position may be used to measure the sagittal dimensions of the dural sac. Assessment of the size of the thecal sac may, in fact, be difficult in a recumbent position due to the tendency of the contrast medium to layer ventrally or dorsally in the prone or supine position, respectively, and the consequent difficulty in visualizing the anterior and posterior margin of the dye column in a single myelogram.

In spinal flexion, mild anterior, and especially, posterior compression of the dural sac visible in the standing or recumbent position may decrease or disappear, whereas in extension these tend to increase in entity, sometimes even severely (Fig. 8.28). The functional myelogram in hyperextension, therefore, is able to reveal stenosis of mild severity, which may not be demonstrated by myelograms in the recumbent position. A subtotal myelographic block in the recum-

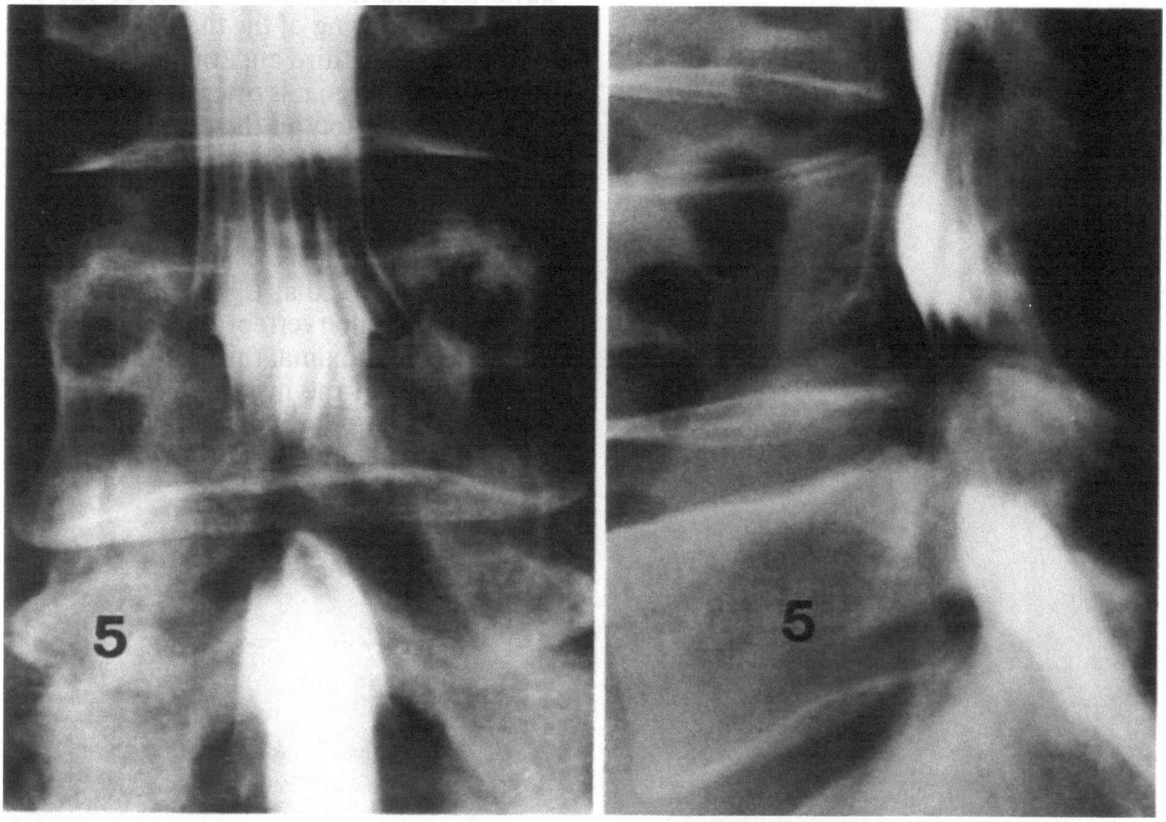

Fig. 8.24 - Single level myelographic block, caused by combined stenosis of the spinal canal at L_4-L_5 level. Upon surgery, a mild posterior bulging of the annulus fibrosus of the fourth lumbar disc was found.

bent position may sometimes disappear in flexion and become total in hyperextension; in contrast, a total block does not usually change on functional myelograms, since marked compression of the thecal sac does not decrease in flexion to such an extent as to allow the contrast medium to flow beyond the block (Fig. 8.29).

The occurrence, or the increase in severity, of posterior compression of the dural sac in hyperlordosis is caused by bulging of the ligamenta flava into the spinal canal. When the latter is wide, buckling of the ligaments has no compressive effect on the neural structures. However, when the spinal canal is narrow or stenotic, even a mild bulge may be sufficient to cause a posterior indentation on the thecal sac or to increase it, if a dural sac compression is already present in the recumbent or standing position. Similarly, the increase in amount, in spinal hyperextension, of an anterior indentation produced by a bulging annulus fibrosus and its decrease in spinal flexion are due to the increase and decrease, respectively, of the annular bulging in the two functional positions.

In nerve root canal stenosis, the anteroposterior myelogram in the squatting position may sometimes show a normal filling, or a better contrast medium filling, of a nerve root sheath presenting no or reduced filling on the myelogram taken in the prone position. These functional changes in opacification of the nerve root sheath, which are better visible on myelotomograms, would be peculiar to nerve root canal stenosis, since they do not occur when the nerve root is compressed by a disc herniation (Ascani *et al.*, 1986).

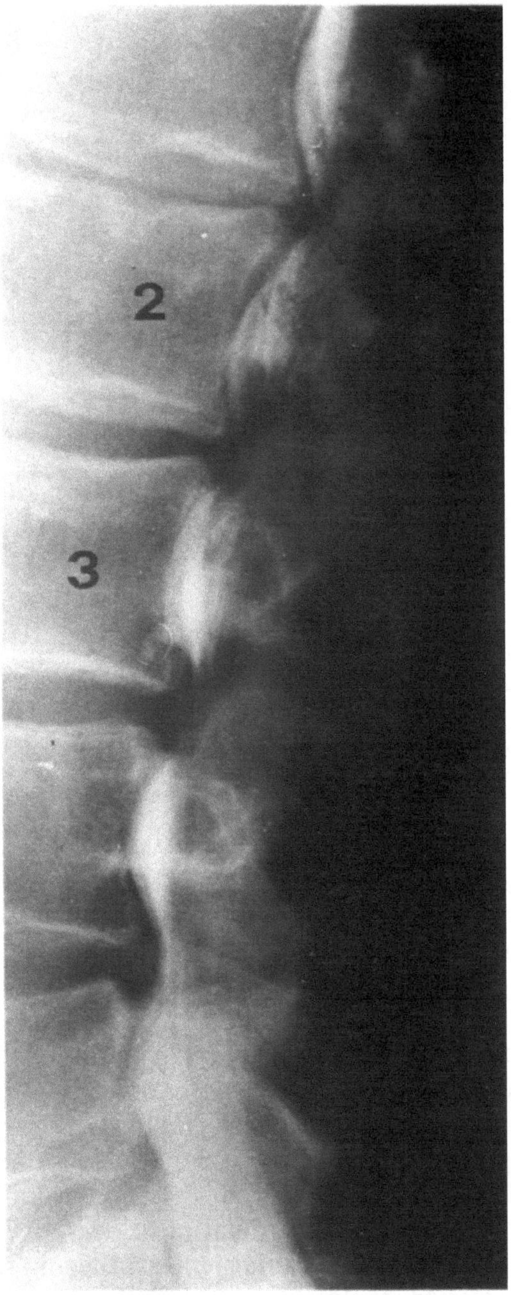

Fig. 8.25 - Typical myelographic pattern of multiple blocks of the dye column.

MYELOGRAPHIC PATTERNS IN THE VARIOUS TYPES OF STENOSIS

Spinal canal stenosis

In primary forms of stenosis the most frequent findings are uniform narrowing of the dural sac and multilevel blocks of the dye column. Narrowing of the thecal sac is mostly located at the third and/or fourth lumbar intervertebral level; it is often associated with ventral indentation on the dural sac caused by mild bulging of the annulus fibrosus and with posterior indentations which appear, or increase in entity, in the functional myelogram in hyperlordosis. The blocks are most frequently observed at L_2 to L_5 levels. They are located at intervertebral level and often extend to the proximal third of the underlying vertebra; in the more typical forms of stenosis, the anterior indentations caused by the disc are relatively mild (Fig. 8.30). A

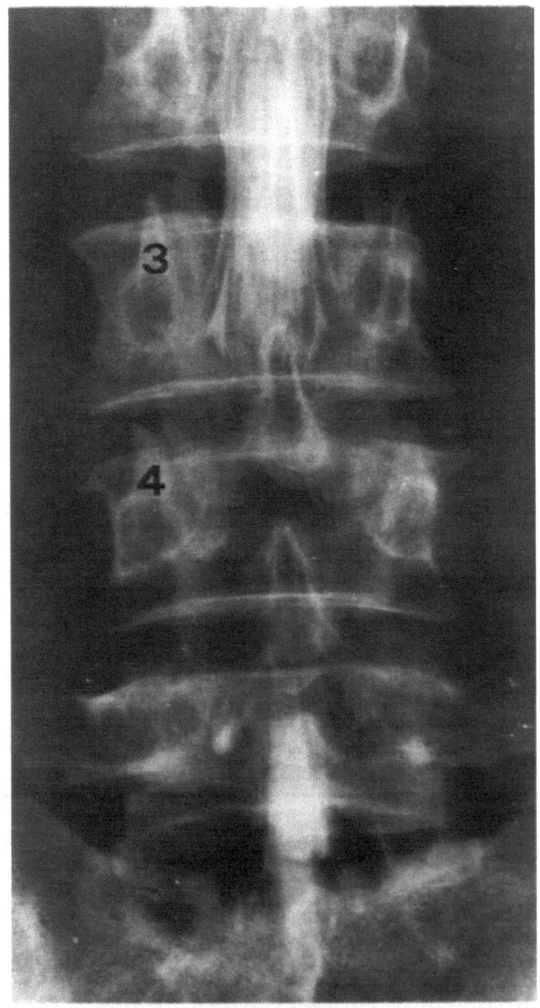

Fig. 8.26 - Complete myelographic block at L_3 level with re-filling of the dural sac at L_5.

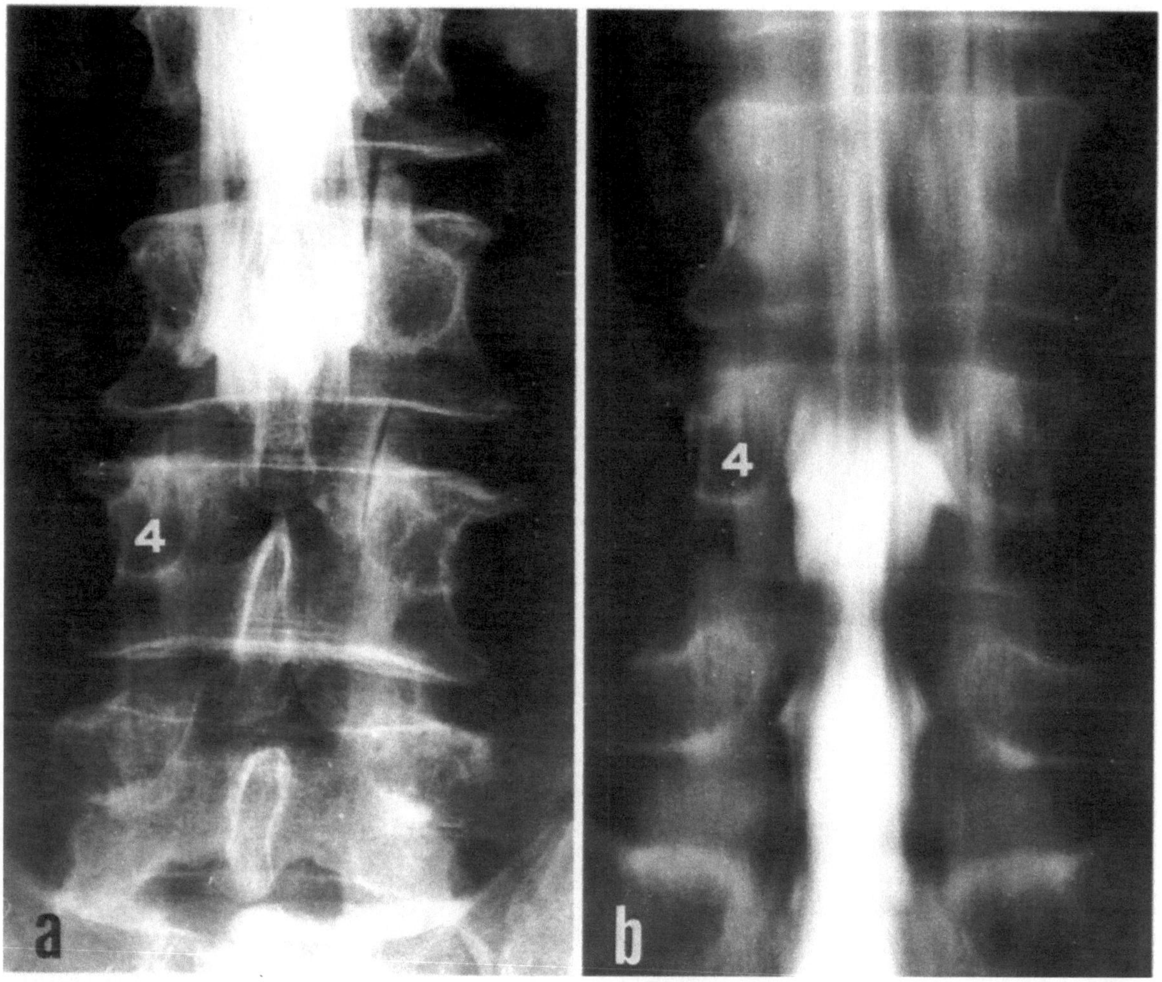

Fig. 8.27 - a. Complete myelographic block at L_3-L_4 level after injection of the contrast medium at L_2-L_3. **b.** The subsequent injection of the contrast agent at L_5-S_1 opacifies the thecal sac below the block and reveals an hour-glass deformation of the sac at L_4-L_5.

single level block of the dye column, which is fairly rare, is usually associated with narrowing of the dye column and, at the level of the block, mild or moderate bulging of the annulus fibrosus. Stasis of the contrast medium is more frequently observed in primary stenoses than in other forms of spinal canal stenosis probably because of the greater frequency with which marked concavity of the posterior aspect of the vertebral body is found in the primary forms.

In degenerative stenosis, the most frequent myelographic findings are the hourglass deformations of the contrast column in the frontal plane and the single level block. The levels most frequently involved are L_4-L_5, followed by L_3-L_4. Rarely are more than two vertebral levels affected. In most cases, marked compression of the neural structures at one level is associated with signs of minor compressions at one of the adjacent levels; these signs are usually represented by posterior indentations on the thecal sac and/or no filling, or filling defects, of the nerve root sheaths due to radicular canal stenosis. At the non stenotic levels, moderate bulging of the annulus fibrosus, as a result of disc degeneration, is frequently observed. In stenosis caused by scoliosis, there may be a partial or complete myelographic

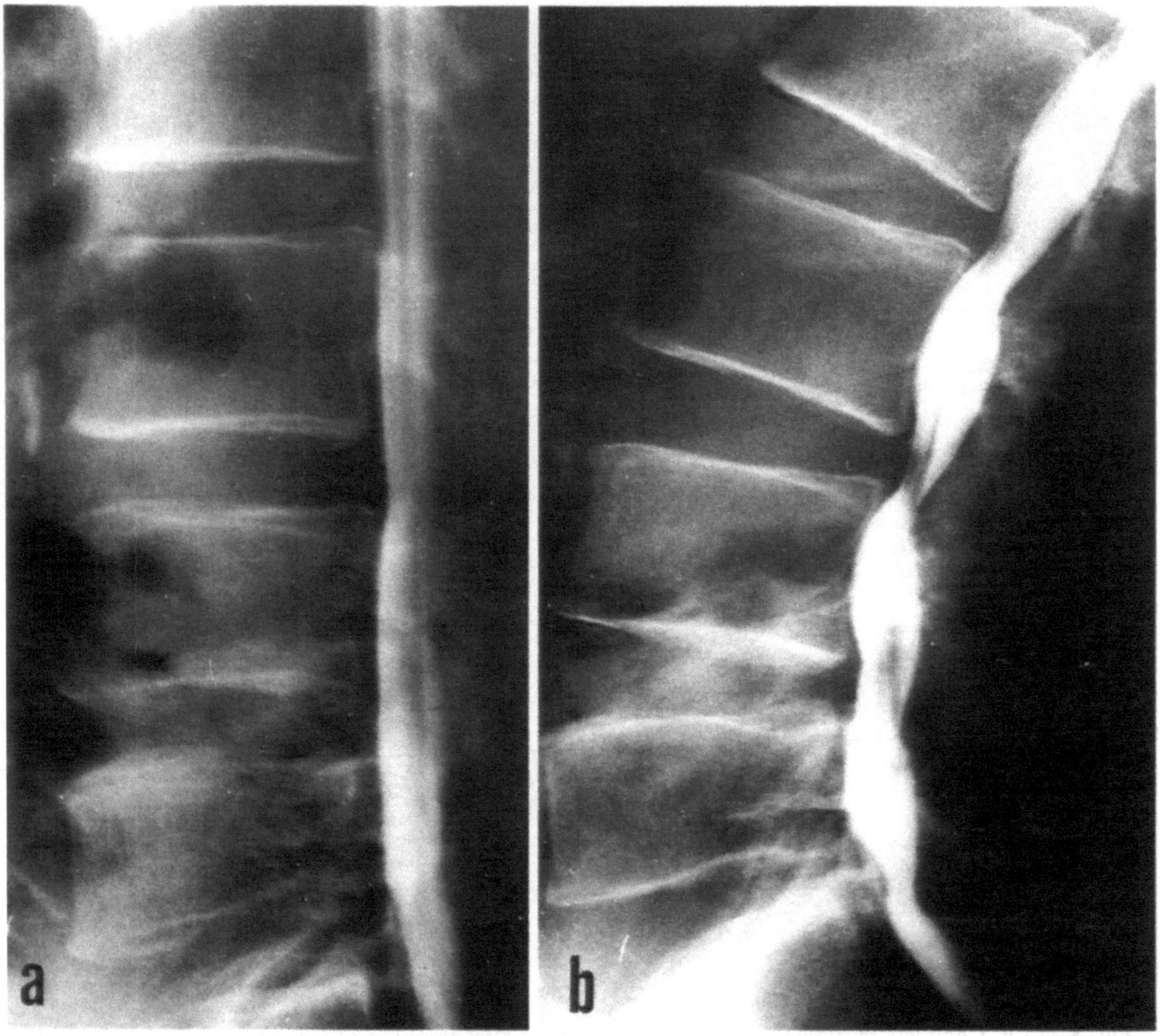

Fig. 8.28 - Functional myelograms in lateral projection. **a.** In spinal flexion, the dye column appears abnormally narrow, but there is no evidence of compression. **b.** In extension, multiple posterior indentations of the dural sac become apparent.

block or a filling defect of the nerve root sheaths and the dural sac only on the side of the concavity of the curve (Fig. 8.31). When scoliosis is associated with kyphosis, the ventral portion of the dural sac may show a filling defect, or a complete myelographic block may be present at the apex of the kyphotic curve.

Combined stenosis is characterized, more often than the degenerative form, by multilevel myelographic blocks (multiple blocks or a continuous block extending over two or three adjacent vertebral levels) or the association of a single level block with signs of lateral and posterior compressions of the dural sac at the other levels (Fig. 8.32). The levels most frequently involved are L_3-L_4 and L_4-L_5, followed by the intervertebral space L_2-L_3.

Stenosis caused by degenerative spondylolisthesis may be characterized by an hour-glass deformation of the dural sac on the frontal plane, associated with a posterior indentation on the sagittal plane or a complete myelographic block. An hour-glass deformation is usually observed when the vertebral canal is primarily wide, and particularly when the olisthetic vertebra is the

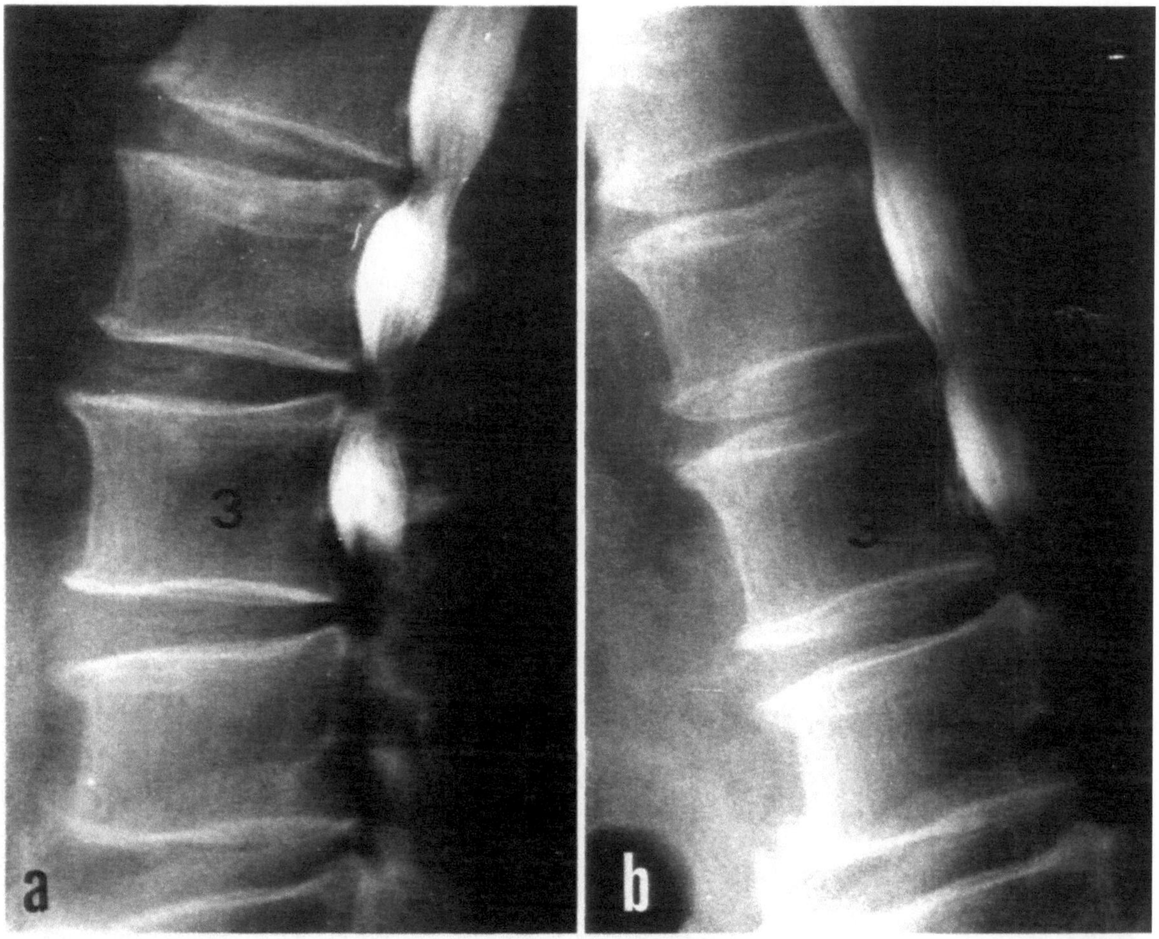

Fig. 8.29 - a. The lateral myelogram in orthostatic position shows a complete block of the dye column at L_3-L_4 level and a subtotal block at L_2-L_3. **b.** In spinal flexion, the subtotal block disappears, whereas the complete block remains unchanged.

L_5, which has a tendentially wider spinal canal than the other lumbar vertebrae (Fig. 8.33). A myelographic block easily occurs when the midsagittal dimensions of the vertebral canal are at, or below, the lower limits of normal, and particularly at L_3 and L_4 levels, where the midsagittal diameters of the spinal canal are shortest (Fig. 8.34).

Nerve root canal stenosis

It may be associated with stenosis of the central portion of the spinal canal, or may occur independently in a spinal canal of normal width. The two conditions are easily distinguished in as much as in the former instance a filling defect of both the nerve root sheaths and the dural sac is seen, whereas in the latter only the nerve root emerging from the dural sac at the stenotic level appears to be compressed (Fig. 8.35).

In the presence of nerve root canal stenosis, the root may be deviated medially and the radicular sheath may show a poor filling or no filling by contrast medium. Medial displacement of the root occurs at the level of the disc space and is often associated with a mild ventral indentation on the dural sac by bulging of the annulus fibrosus. Amputation of the nerve root sheath may be located at the level of the intervertebral space

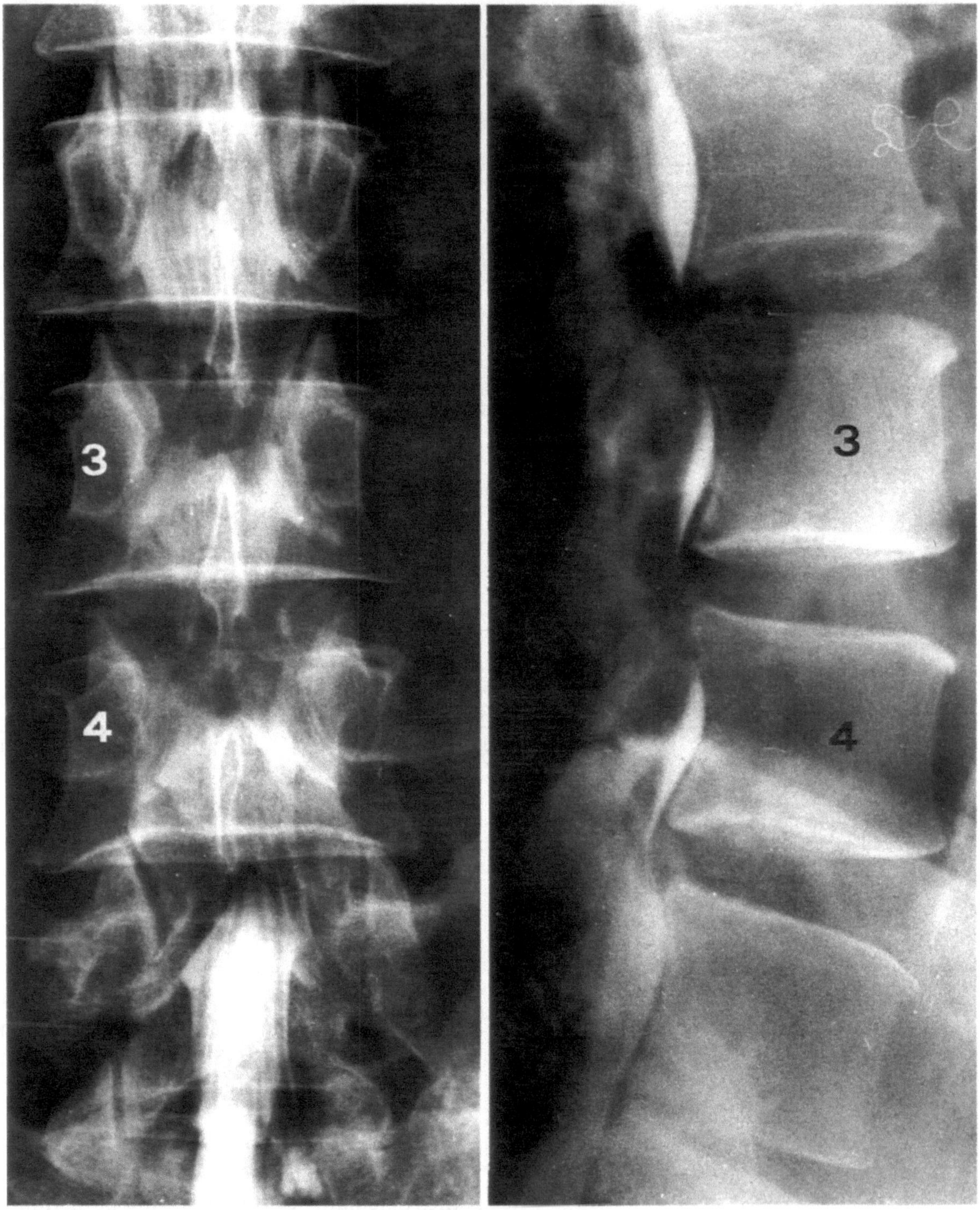

Fig. 8.30 - Myelographic pattern of developmental spinal canal stenosis. In A-P projection, multiple constrictions of the thecal sac are visible, with a complete block at L_2-L_3 and L_3-L_4 level; at both levels, the block extends distally as far as the upper border of the laminae of the vertebra below. In lateral projection, the intervertebral discs show a mild or no posterior bulging in the areas of compression of the nervous structures.

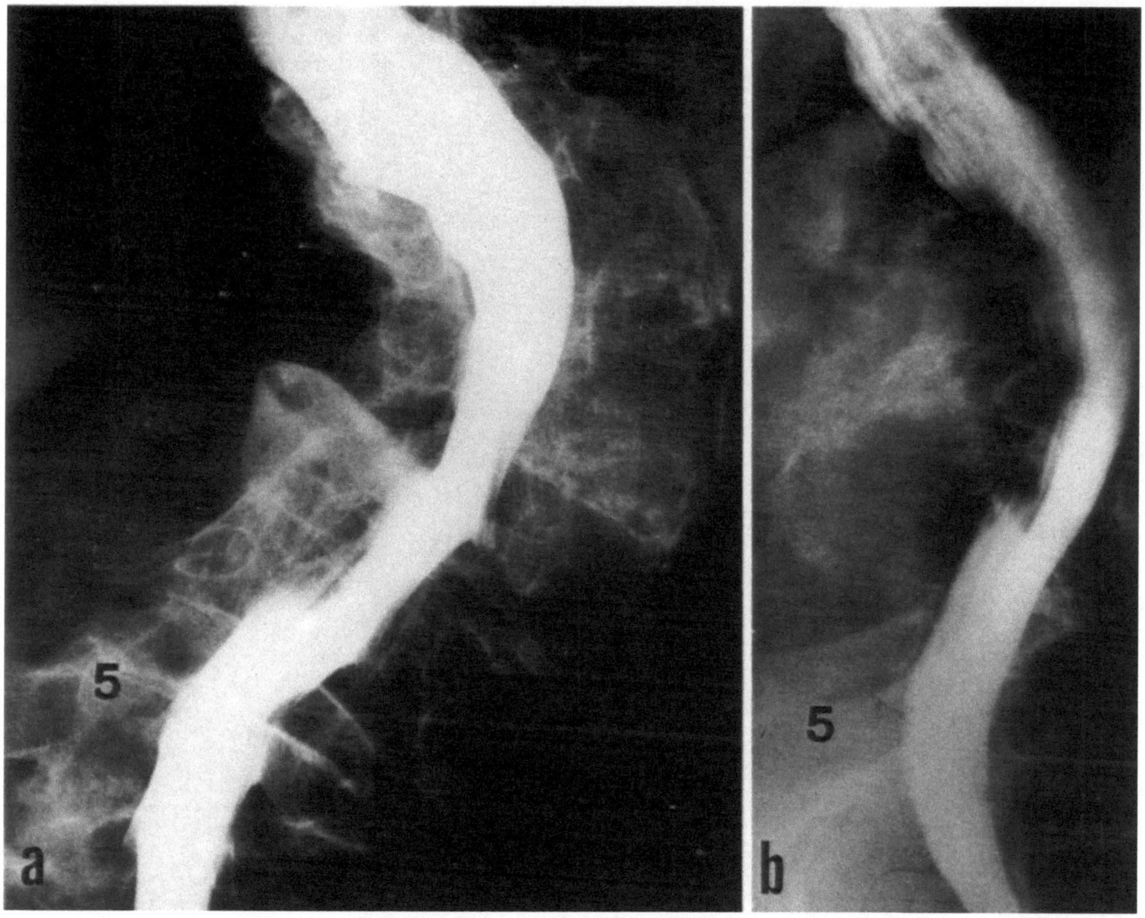

Fig. 8.31 - Severe lumbar kyphoscoliosis responsible for compression of the nervous structures on the side of concavity of the scoliotic curve (**a**). In lateral projection (**b**), the ventral portion of the thecal sac is not filled by contrast medium at the apex of the kyphotic curve.

or, less frequently, of the lateral recess, that is medially to the pedicle.

The fifth lumbar and first sacral roots are those most frequently affected in isolated stenosis of the nerve root canal. The L_5 root may show all the myelographic abnormalities described above, whereas the S_1 usually shows no filling of the sheath at the level of, or immediately below, the intervertebral space. In both cases, however, there may be no abnormality of the myelographic pattern even in the presence of nerve root compression. According to some authors (Getty *et al.*, 1981; Kirkaldy-Willis *et al.*, 1981), this may occur fairly frequently. In my experience, myelography is rarely completely negative, if the examination is carried out carefully and there is significant nerve root compression. The patients in whom myelography will more frequently display false negative results or findings of uncertain interpretation are those presenting a short dural sac, in whom the L_5 and S_1 nerve roots emerge proximally to the intervertebral space and the root sheaths end at the level of the disc or the initial portion of the lateral recess. In these cases nerve root compression in the radicular canal may produce a mild or even no filling defect of the nerve root sheath.

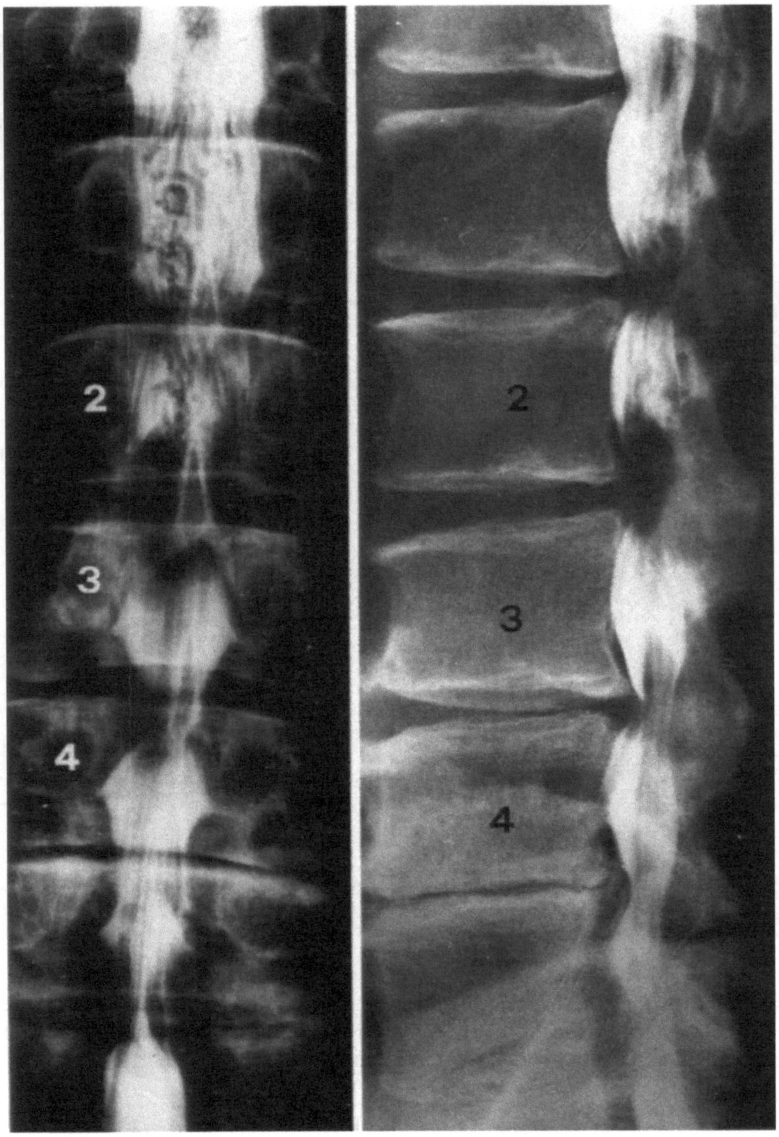

Fig. 8.32 - Combined stenosis of the spinal canal, with marked compression of the nervous structures at all lumbar levels. The dye column shows a subtotal block at L_1-L_2 and a complete block at L_2-L_3. At the levels below, hourglass deformations and/or anterior compressions of the dural sac are visible.

Stenosis of the intervertebral foramen

When the root is compressed in a stenotic intervertebral foramen, the myelographic pattern may be normal or show non-filling of the nerve root sheath at the level of the infero-medial portion of the pedicle. This finding, however, should be interpreted as pathological only when the nerve root shows signs of swelling or the radicular sheaths at the adjacent vertebral level, or the contralateral nerve root sheath in the presence of a unilateral root compression, appear to arrive more distally than the radicular sheath affected. In these cases, however, myelographic diagnosis of stenosis of the neuroforamen is generally presumptive. Furthermore, it should be confirmed — unless the intervertebral disc is completely or almost completely resorbed — by surgical findings excluding foraminal disc herniation, which is more frequent than a pure stenosis of the neuroforamen.

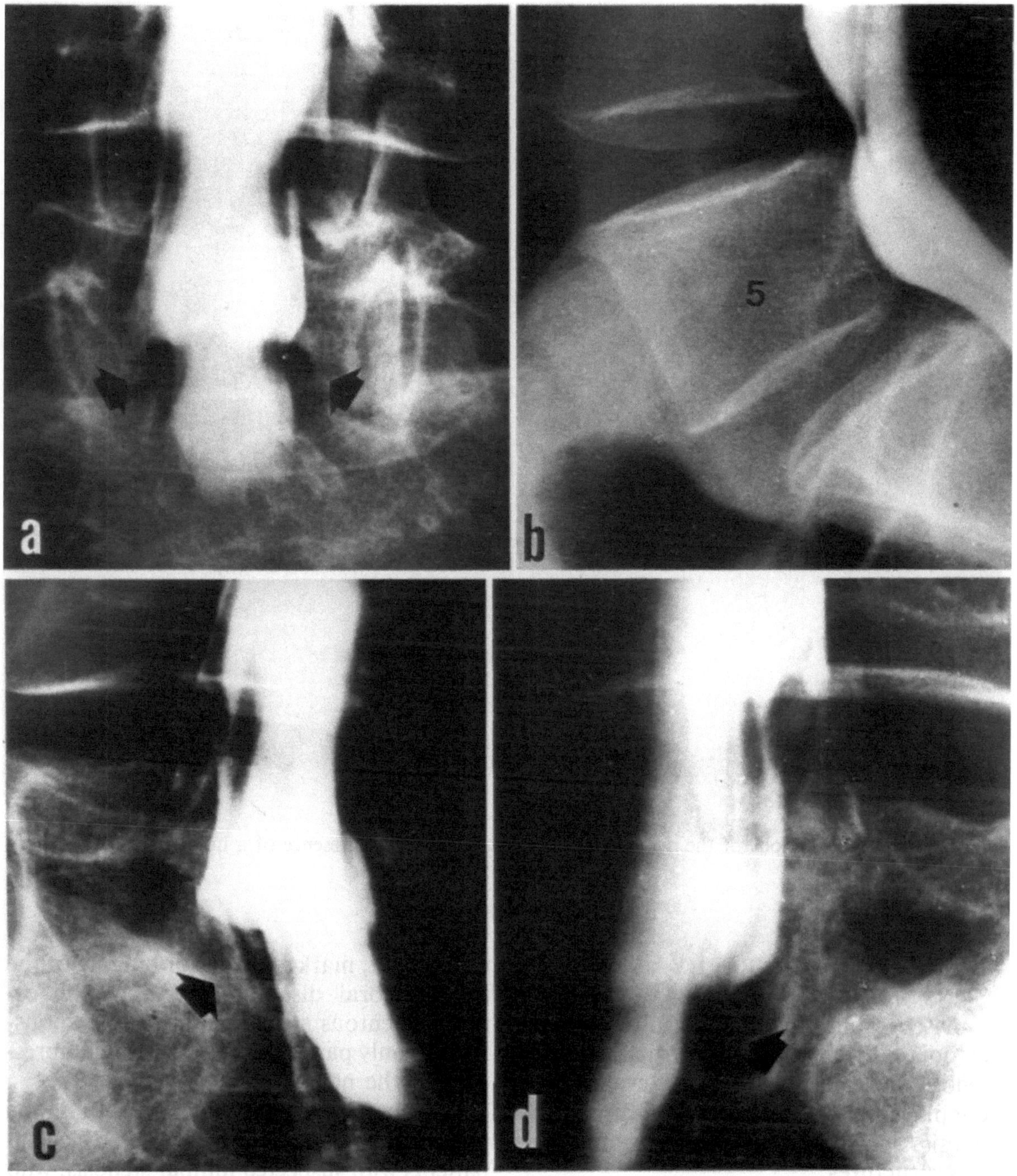

Fig. 8.33 - Degenerative spondylolisthesis of L_5. Non-filling of both S_1 nerve roots (arrows) and bilateral indentation of the dural sac (**a, c** and **d**). The wide sagittal diameter of the dye column at the level of L_4 and L_5 vertebrae (**b**) indicates a normal anteroposterior diameter of the spinal canal.

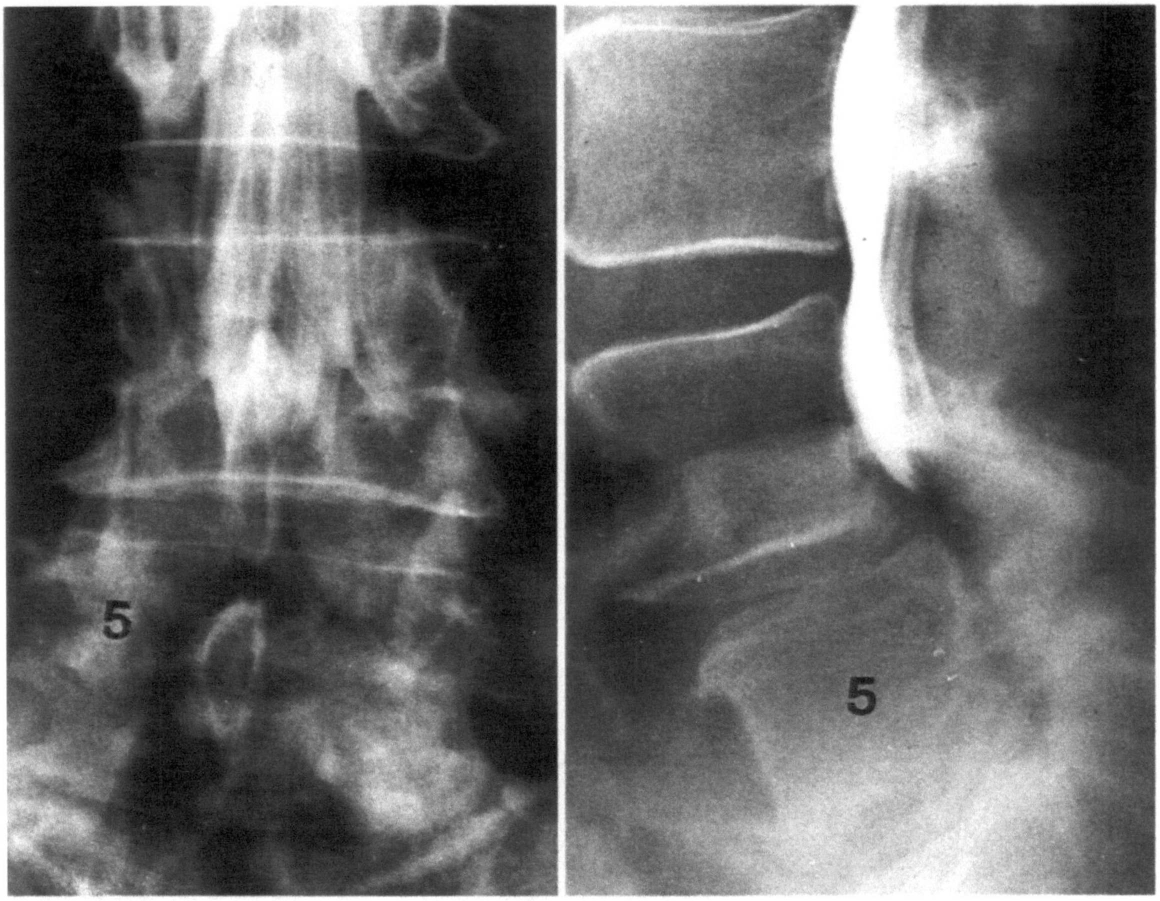

Fig. 8.34 - Complete block of the dye column at L_4-L_5 level, in the presence of a mild degenerative spondylolisthesis of L_4.

DISCOGRAPHY

Discography represents a usuful diagnostic tool to differentiate disc herniation from stenosis and, more in general, to evaluate the role played by the intervertebral disc in the genesis of a compression of the spinal nervous structures.

In patients with lumbar spinal stenosis, the intervertebral discs are often degenerated, but do not usually protrude, or protrude only slightly, into the vertebral canal (Fig. 8.36). The absence of significant disc bulging at an intervertebral level at which the nervous structures of the spinal canal appear to be compressed, indicates that compression is caused exclusively or essentially by the osteoligamentous walls of the canal. On the other hand, marked posterior bulging of the intervertebral disc indicates that the osteoligamentous structures are not responsible, or only partly responsible, for compression of the neural elements (Fig. 8.37).

Discography is particularly useful in the presence of a complete myelographic block in patients with suspected lumbar stenosis, who show no significant spondylotic changes at the level of the block. In these cases, in fact, it may be difficult to determine, on the basis of myelography or computed tomography, whether the block is produced by disc herniation or mild posterior bulging of the annulus fibrosus in a pathologically narrow lumbar spinal canal. The precise assessment of the role played by the intervertebral disc in the genesis of compression of the neural

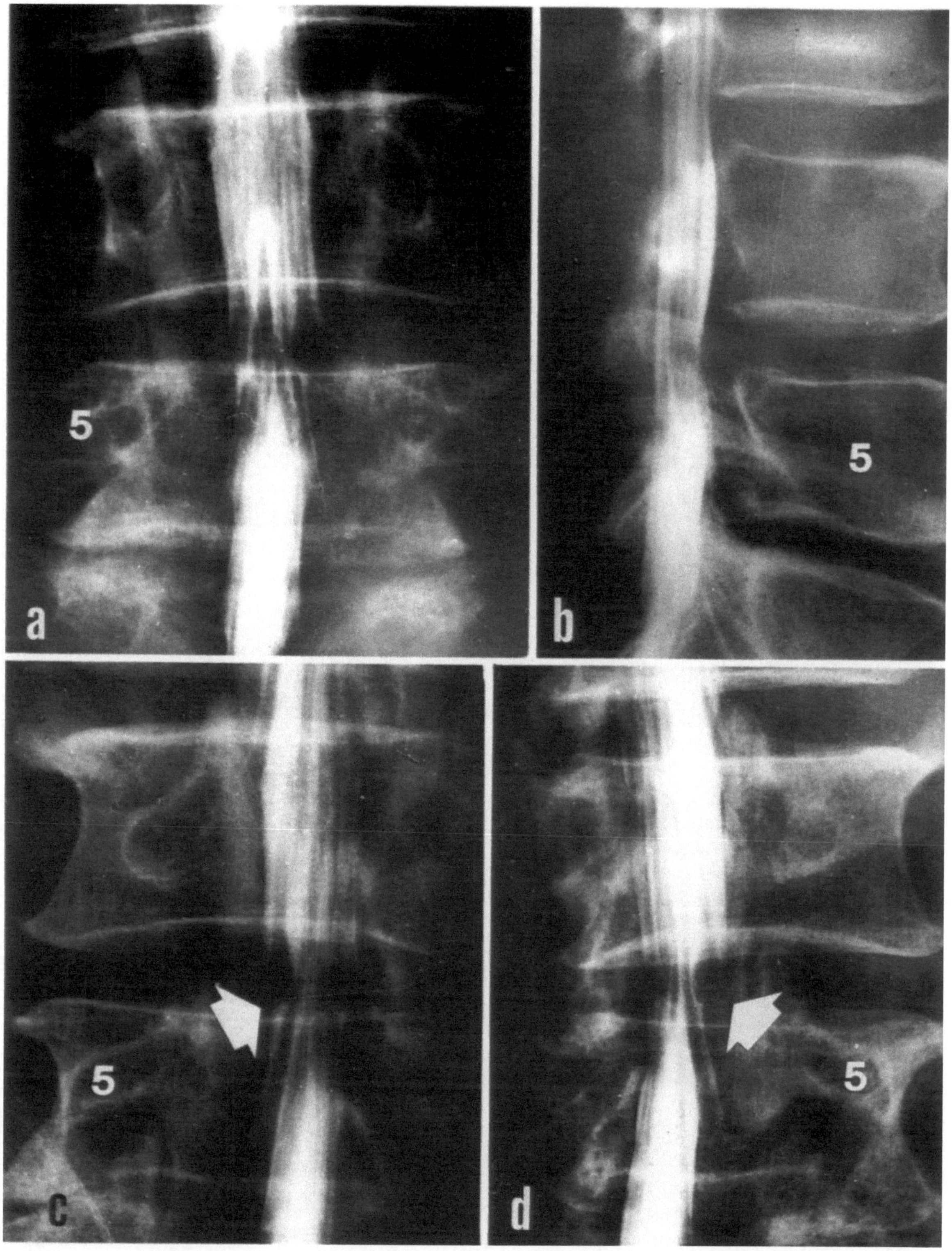

Fig. 8.35 - Bilateral isolated stenosis of the L_5 nerve root canal in a patient with a developmentally narrow spinal canal. The anteroposterior and oblique projections (**a, c** and **d**) show non-filling of the L_5 nerve root sheaths; on the left, the root sheath appears enlarged also above the site of compression. The lateral view displays short sagittal dimensions of the dye column and mild posterior bulging of the L_4-L_5 disc. At surgery, this disc bulged into the spinal canal but did not appear to be herniated.

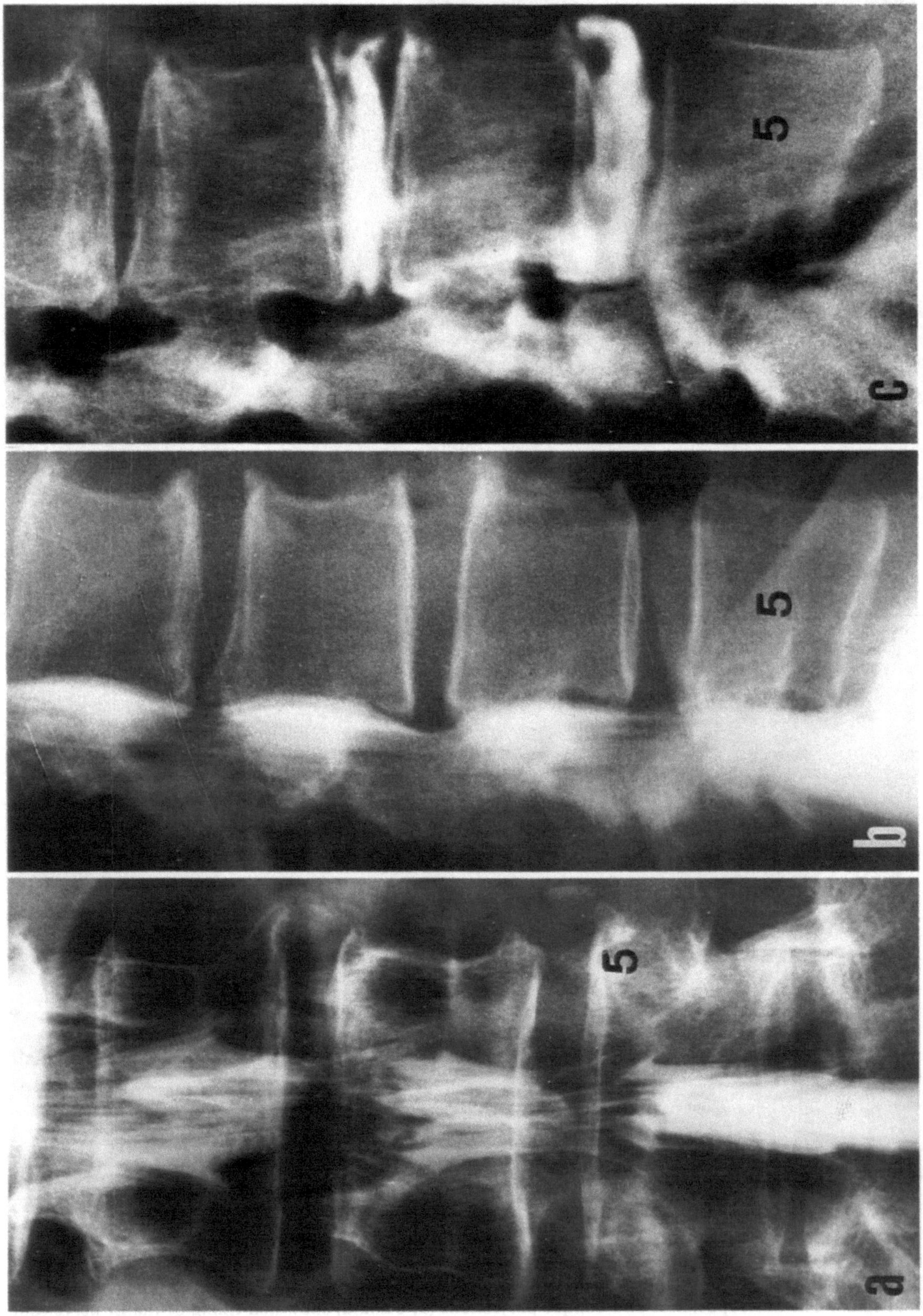

Fig. 8.36 - Spinal canal stenosis at L_4-L_5 level (**a** and **b**). Discography (**c**) shows degenerative changes, but no significant posterior protrusion, of the L_3-L_4 and L_4-L_5 discs.

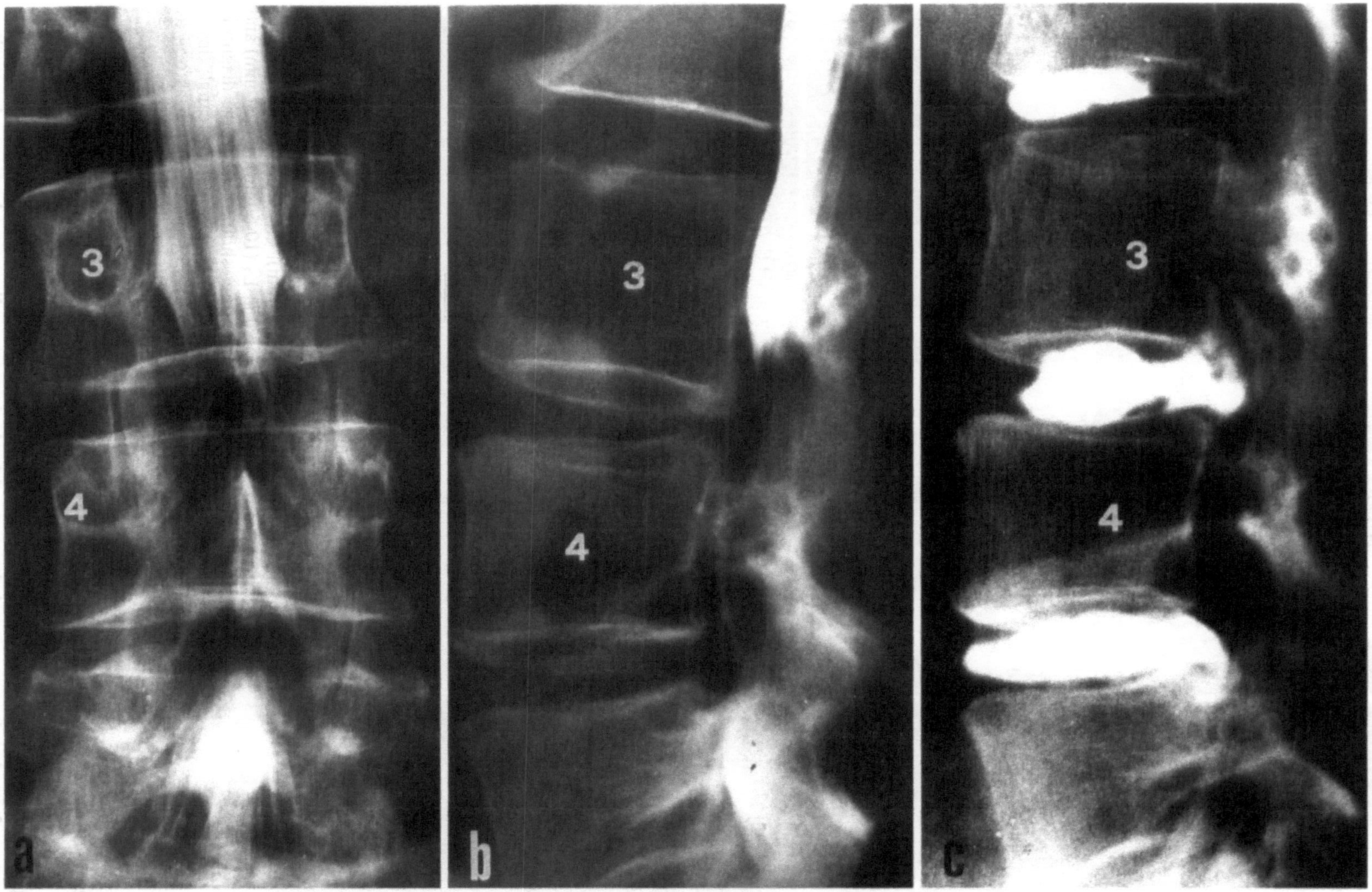

Fig. 8.37 - Complete block of the dye column at L_3-L_4 with almost complete block of the contrast column at L_4-L_5 level (**a** and **b**). The myelographic pattern is compatible with a diagnosis of spinal canal stenosis. However, discography (**c**), showing a marked posterior protrusion of the L_3-L_4 disc and a milder protrusion of the L_4-L_5 disc, leads to the diagnosis of disc herniation in a relatively narrow spinal canal. This diagnosis was confirmed by surgical findings.

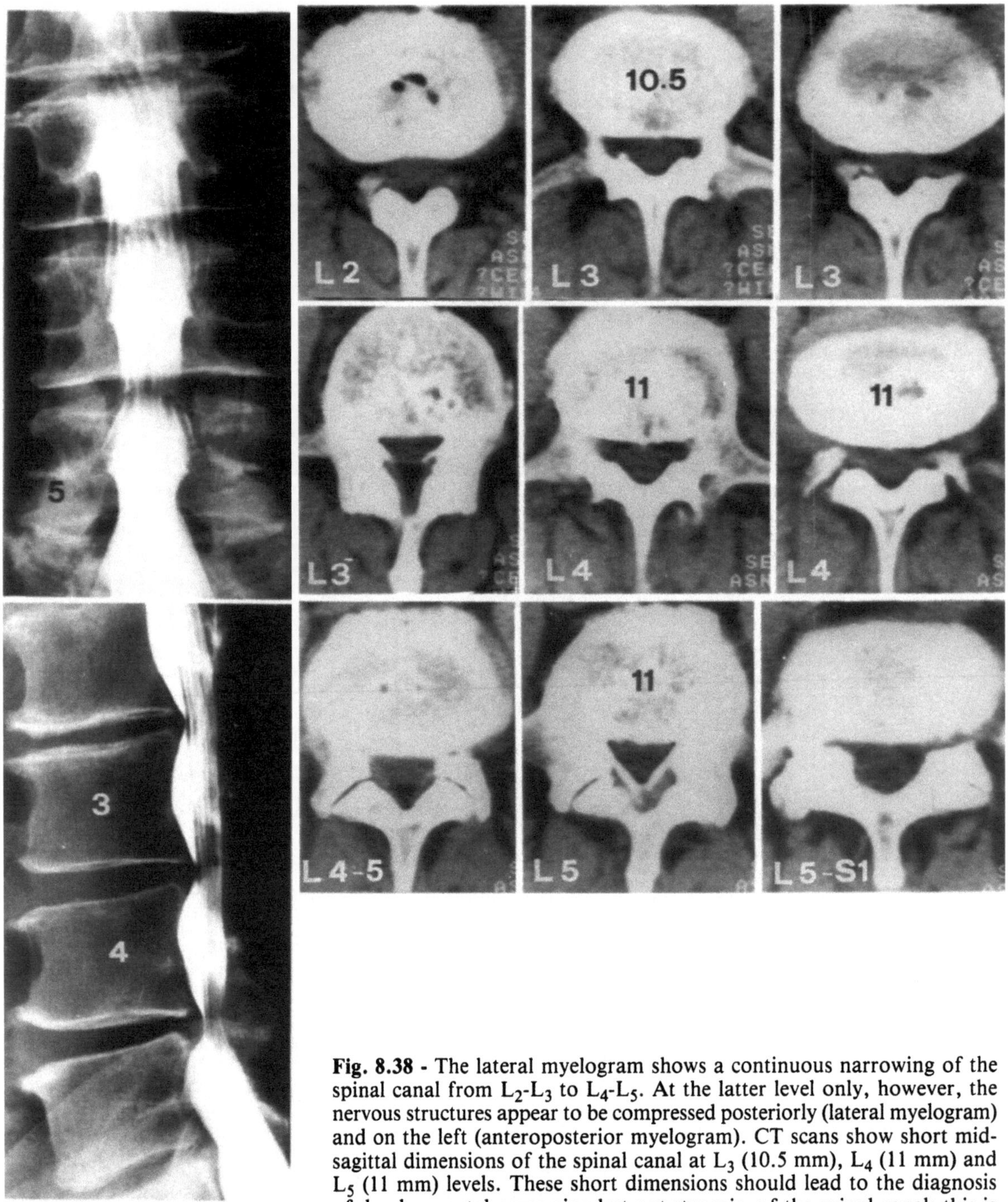

Fig. 8.38 - The lateral myelogram shows a continuous narrowing of the spinal canal from L_2-L_3 to L_4-L_5. At the latter level only, however, the nervous structures appear to be compressed posteriorly (lateral myelogram) and on the left (anteroposterior myelogram). CT scans show short mid-sagittal dimensions of the spinal canal at L_3 (10.5 mm), L_4 (11 mm) and L_5 (11 mm) levels. These short dimensions should lead to the diagnosis of developmental narrowing but not stenosis, of the spinal canal; this is confirmed by the absence of deformations of the dural sac, as well as myelographic findings.

structures is extremely important in planning surgical treatment, since the presence of a marked posterior protrusion of the disc may lead one to perform laminotomy and, in any case, a discectomy, whereas the absence of a significant disc pathology tends to suggest that bilateral laminectomy not associated with disc excision would be preferable. Even in the absence of a complete myelographic block, however, discography may play an important role in determining preoperatively the opportunity or not of carrying out a disc excision at a given stenotic level. Discography should certainly not be performed in all patients with lumbar stenosis. However, this investigation (or MRI) should be carried out in all those cases of uncertainty concerning the cause of compression of the nervous structures, particularly when a better knowledge of the pathology may influence the surgical procedure.

Discography should be performed by a lateral approach with the patient in left or right lateral decubitus (McCulloch and Waddel, 1978). However, the prone position may also be used. The risks of infective discitis may be minimized using an 18 gauge 10 cm long guide needle, and a 22 gauge 18 cm long needle (straight for the upper four lumbar discs and curved for the fifth) which is inserted into the intervertebral disc. The tip of the needle should be positioned exactly in the centre of the disc to avoid injection of the contrast medium into the annulus fibrosus, rather than into the nucleus pulposus. Discography should be performed at all the intervertebral levels in the stenotic area or at all the levels at which it is necessary to assess the cause of compression of the nervous structures. Into each disc an adequate volume of contrast agent should be injected, in order to demonstrate the presence and entity of a possible posterior protrusion of the intervertebral disc. When injection is made into a disc at the level of which there is a complete myelographic block, the contrast me-

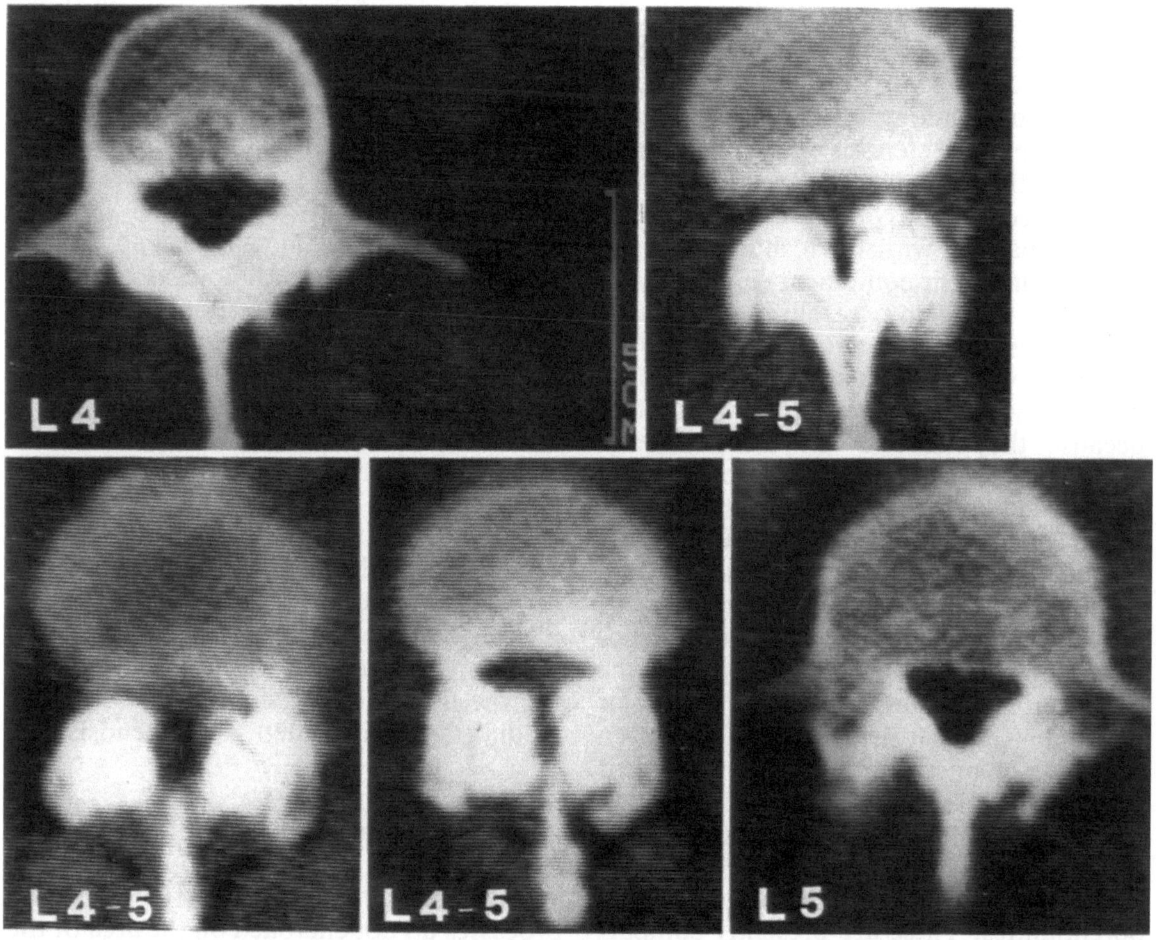

Fig. 8.39 - Marked narrowing of the spinal canal at L_4-L_5 level due to degenerative changes of the facet joints. Narrowing of such severity necessarily leads to compression of the neural structures and in itself leads to diagnosis of stenosis.

dium must be introduced very slowly to avoid that a sudden rise in intradiscal pressure in a possibly herniated disc may increase the compression of the neural elements. For this reason, during injection of the contrast medium, the patient should frequently be asked whether a marked increase in severity of the radicular symptoms is felt. Assessment of the effects on radicular symptoms is in any case useful to determine the role played by the disc in compression of the neural elements and, thus, to decide at surgery whether or not to carry out a disc excision.

COMPUTERIZED TOMOGRAPHY

The advent of computerized tomography has opened new perspectives in the diagnosis, and significantly contributed to the knowledge of pathomorphology, of the various forms of lumbar spinal stenosis. The contribution made by this technique, as well as its diagnostic accuracy, have progressed considerably, in parallel with the technological improvements of the equipment employed. Indeed, the first, low resolution, scanners allowed visualization, almost exclusively, of the bony vertebral canal. Their diagnostic precision was, therefore, somewhat limited, because they allowed the morphometric characteristics of the container, but not (or not adequately) those of the content of the spinal canal, to be analyzed (Postacchini and Pezzeri, 1981). Since in many cases it was not possible by means of the morphometry of only the container to ascertain the existence of a dimensional disproportion between the calibre of the container and the volume of the content, diagnosis of stenosis was often inductive or uncertain. With the advent of high resolution scanners, which allow visualization of the intervertebral disc and the nervous structures in the spinal canal, computerized tomography enjoyed its full diagnostic potentialities. These are presently comparable to, although not the same as, those of myelography, CT having the advantage of not being invasive.

SPINAL CANAL STENOSIS

CT diagnosis of spinal canal stenosis, which is often less easy and immediate than that based on myelographic findings, stems from the analysis of a series of morphometric characteristics of the vertebral canal and the dural sac.

Vertebral canal

Midsagittal diameter

The midsagittal diameter of the spinal canal can be measured on the pedicular and subpedicular sections, in which the posterior wall of the canal is formed by bony structures. The lowest values of this diameter are mostly found in the sections through the upper border of the laminae, since the latter are usually orientated obliquely downward and posteriorly.

As a general rule, midsagittal dimensions greater than 12 mm should be considered normal, whereas lower values indicate a developmental narrowing of the vertebral canal. Such narrowing may be a physiological condition, or a pathological condition, that is a stenosis, if it is responsible for compression of the nervous structures contained in the spinal canal. In itself, therefore, the value of the midsagittal diameter of the vertebral canal cannot be considered a reliable parameter for the diagnosis of stenosis, at least when this value is greater than 10 mm (Fig. 8.38). Values of less than 10 mm indicate a probable stenosis, whereas values lower than 8 mm are unequivocally pathological. Assessment of the sagittal dimensions of the spinal canal, however, is determinant for the definition of the type — primary, secondary or combined — of stenosis.

Articular processes

In normal conditions the articular processes do not encroach on the area of the spinal canal, which is approximately triangular at intervertebral level. Transverse narrowing, associated or not with deformation, of this area as a result of congenital malformations, hypertrophy or osteophytosis of the articular processes, particularly of the inferior, is a sign of stenosis of the spinal canal. This is particularly true when distortion and/or narrowing of the central portion of the vertebral canal are severe (Fig. 8.39). When these are mild, it is difficult or impossible to determine, regardless of other morphometric characteristics, whether the nervous structures of the spinal canal are compressed.

Intervertebral disc and vertebral body osteophytes

Posterior bulging of the annulus fibrosus in the presence of developmental narrowing of the spinal canal at the adjacent vertebral levels, or a significant hypertrophy of the articular processes, should lead to suspect stenosis. Similarly, posterior osteophytosis of the vertebral end-plates represents an important diagnostic element, particularly in subjects showing a developmentally narrow spinal canal.

Ligamenta flava

Thickening of the ligamenta flava, particularly in the presence of bony metaplasia, may contribute to critical narrowing of the spinal canal, if the latter is narrow on a developmental basis or due to degenerative changes of the facet joints.

Dural sac

Midsagittal and transverse dimensions

The sagittal dimensions of the dural sac, in normal conditions, are proportional to the corresponding dimensions of the vertebral canal, compared to which they are slightly inferior. A very wide spinal canal, therefore, generally contains a dural sac of greater dimensions than normal, whereas the dimensions of the thecal sac in a narrow vertebral canal are tendentially situated at the lower limits of normal. The midsagittal dimensions of the dural sac are to be considered normal when they are greater than 11.5 mm, whereas lower values are indicative of thecal sac narrowing, which may be physiological or pathological. In the latter instance, the midsagittal diameter of the dural tube usually increases above and/or below the narrowed area. Similar considerations may be made for the transverse dimensions of the sac, which, in the absence of deformations of the latter, are similar to, or only slightly different from, the midsagittal.

Area

Bolender *et al.* (1985) measured the transverse area of the dural sac in 30 asymptomatic subjects (as far as concerns the lumbar spine) and 24 individuals with spinal canal stenosis diagnosed from myelograms and confirmed by surgical findings. In the former, the area of the dural sac ranged from 130 to 230 mm^2, whereas in the latter it was less than 130 mm^2 at the stenotic levels. According to these authors, values of less than 100 mm^2 indicate spinal canal stenosis, while values of 100 to 130 mm^2 suggest mild stenosis. The same authors (Schonstrom *et al.*, 1985) found a close relationship between the transverse area and the midsagittal diameter of the dural sac.

Certainly, the finding of values of the transverse area of the dural sac below the lower limits of normal is of considerable diagnostic significance. However, diagnosis of stenosis on CT scans cannot be based only on these values. The area of the thecal sac, in fact, may be below the limits of normal both in subjects with a developmentally narrow spinal canal and in individuals showing a short dural sac, ending, for example, at the level of the lumbosacral interspace. In the latter instance, the dural sac, at the level of its caudal tapering portion, may show a subnormal area, even in the absence of compression. On the other hand, an osteoligamentous compression of the dural sac and caudal nerve roots may often be observed in the presence of normal values of the transverse area of the dural sac. This is especially true for degenerative stenosis in which the sac, primarily large, is compressed by hypertrophic articular processes or posterior osteophytes of the vertebral body. The finding of subnormal values of the dural sac area — as observed for the finding of uniform narrowing of the dural sac on myelograms and the midsagittal narrowing of the sac or CT scans — leads to suspect or diagnose stenosis, particularly when the area of the sac increases significantly above and/or below the narrowed area.

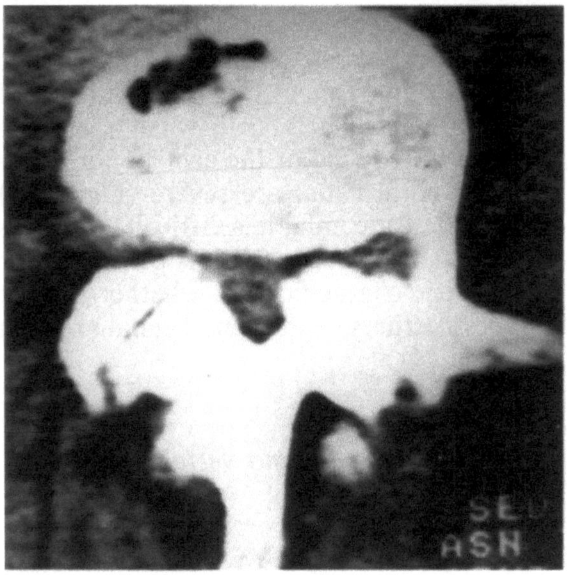

Fig. 8.41 - CT scan at L_4-L_5 level. The thecal sac appears narrow in the transverse diameter and constricted by hypertrophied articular processes.

Morphology

In normal conditions, the shape of the dural sac is round or slightly oval, the widest diameter being the transverse or sagittal.

Deformation of the profile of the dural sac, and particularly the presence of indentations produced by osteophytes of the vertebral end-plates and/or the osteoligamentous structures of the posterior arch, is the most indicative tomographic sign of spinal canal stenosis (Fig. 8.40). Deformations of the dural sac are generally observed in the areas where stenosis is severe, in which also the shape of the spinal canal is altered. The indentations are usually located in the lateral or posterolateral portion of the thecal sac, since they are produced by hypertrophy or degenerative changes of the articular processes and/or hypertrophy, associated or not with bone metaplasia, of the ligamenta flava (Fig. 8.41). For these reasons, deformations are generally seen in the intervertebral portions of the spinal canal. In the pedicular or subpedicular portions, the dural sac regains its normal shape or shows mild symmetric deformations caused by hypertrophic ligamenta flava.

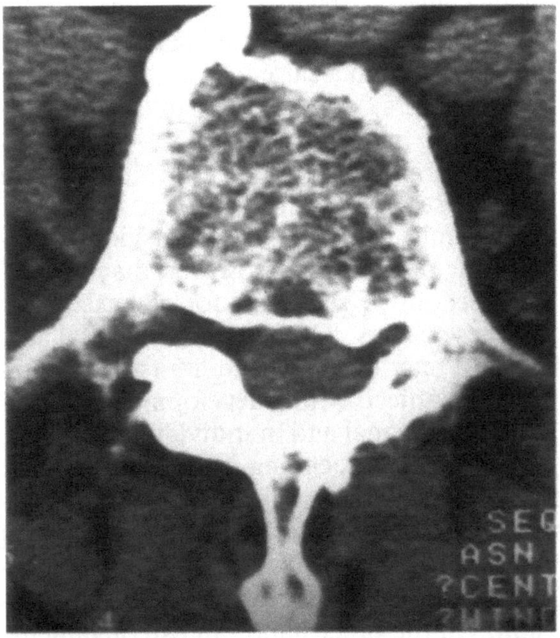

Fig. 8.40 - The thecal sac is deformed and constricted by the anterior and posterior bony components of the spinal canal. This finding enables diagnosis of spinal canal stenosis to be made with certainty.

NERVE ROOT CANAL STENOSIS

On CT scans, the entire length of the nerve root canal can be visualized and narrowing at the level of the intervertebral portion or the lateral recess is easily appreciated. Isolated stenosis of the intervertebral portion of the radicular canal is characterized by abnormalities of the superior articular

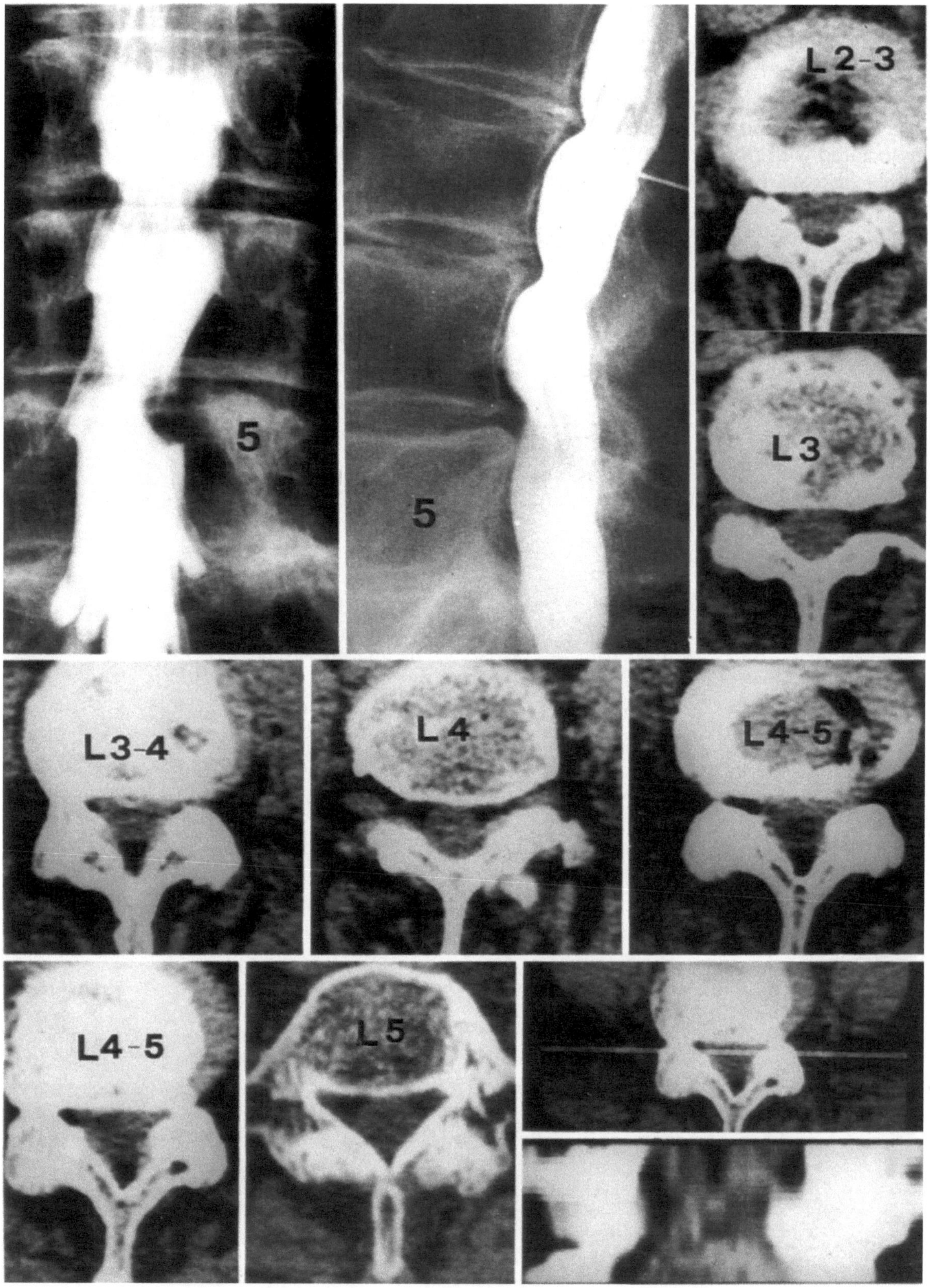

Fig. 8.42 - Bilateral nerve root canal stenosis at L_3-L_4 on both sides and, to a greater extent, at L_4-L_5 on the left. CT scans show at L_3-L_4, narrowing of the intervertebral portion of both nerve root canals due to hypertrophy of the superior articular processes of L_4; at L_4-L_5 level, in addition to hyertrophied inferior articular processes, there is evidence of posterior bulging of the intervertebral disc (which is almost completely resorbed, as shown by the lateral myelogram), which is more marked on the left. Diagnosis of L_5 nerve root canal stenosis on the left was confirmed at surgery.

process — abnormally transverse orientation, osteophytosis and/or hypertrophy — often associated with posterior bulging of the annulus fibrosus (Fig. 8.42). The inferior articular process may show degenerative changes, but not so severe as to produce significant constriction of the spinal canal or cause distortion of the image of the dural sac.

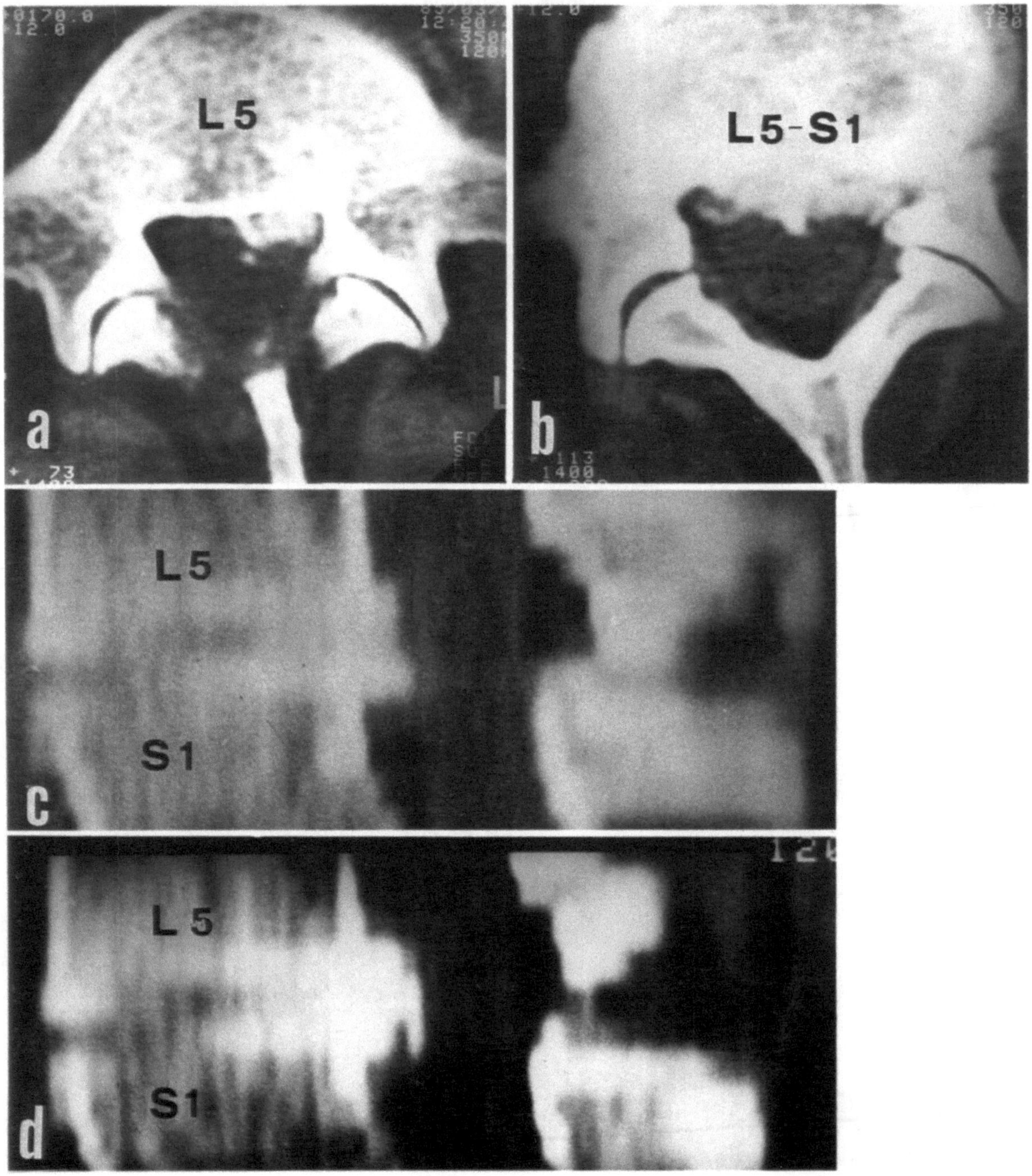

Fig. 8.43 - Axial CT scans (**a** and **b**) and median (**c**) and left lateral (**d**) sagittal reconstructions in a subject with posterior osteophytosis of the vertebral end-plates at L_5-S_1. Osteophytic spurs appear to encroach on the central spinal canal and, even more, the left nerve root canal (**a** and **d**). However, since the nervous structures are not visualized by CT scans, it is impossible to determine whether they are compressed. This patient had no clinical symptoms or signs of S_1 nerve root involvement.

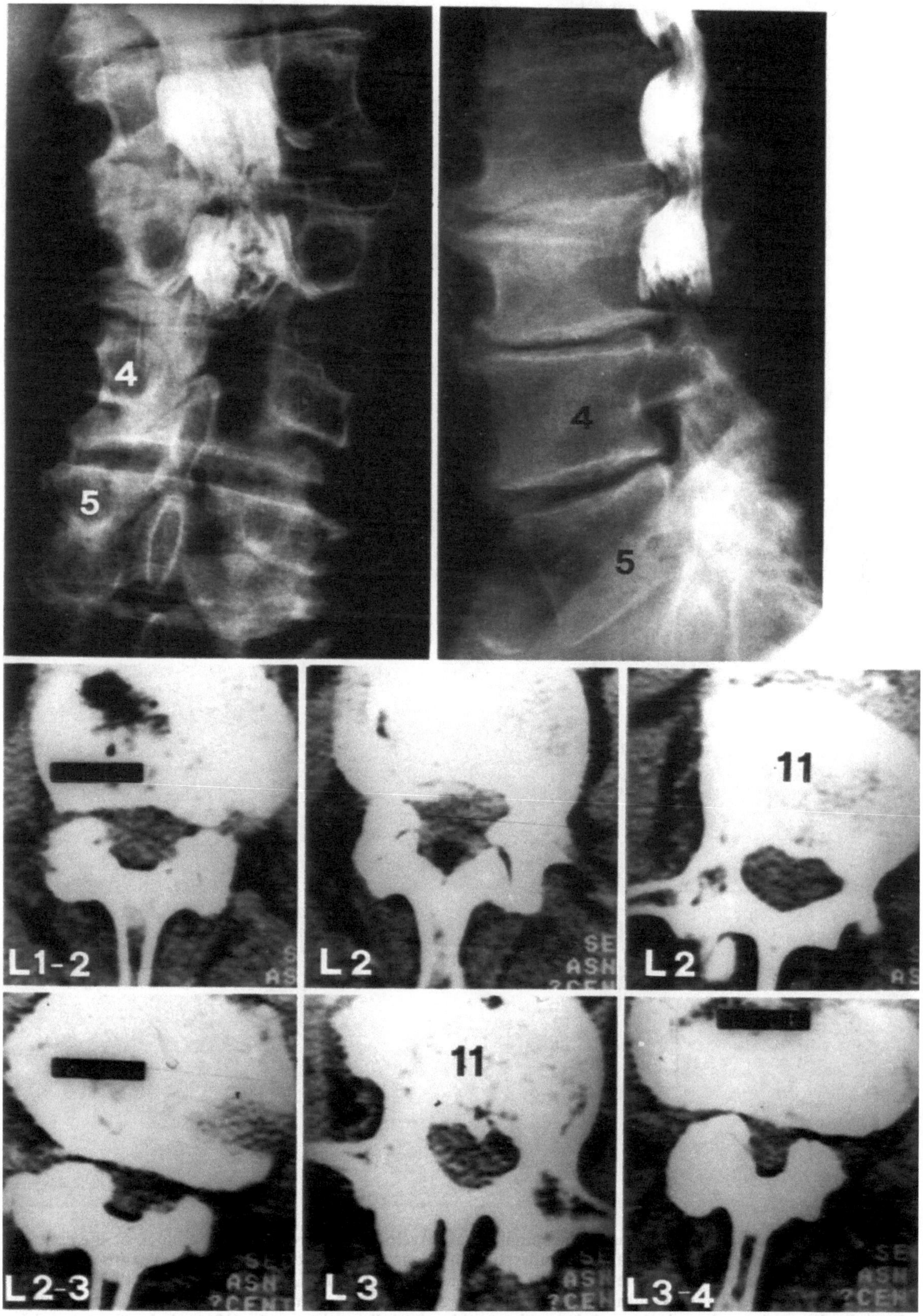

Fig. 8.44 (legend on the following page).

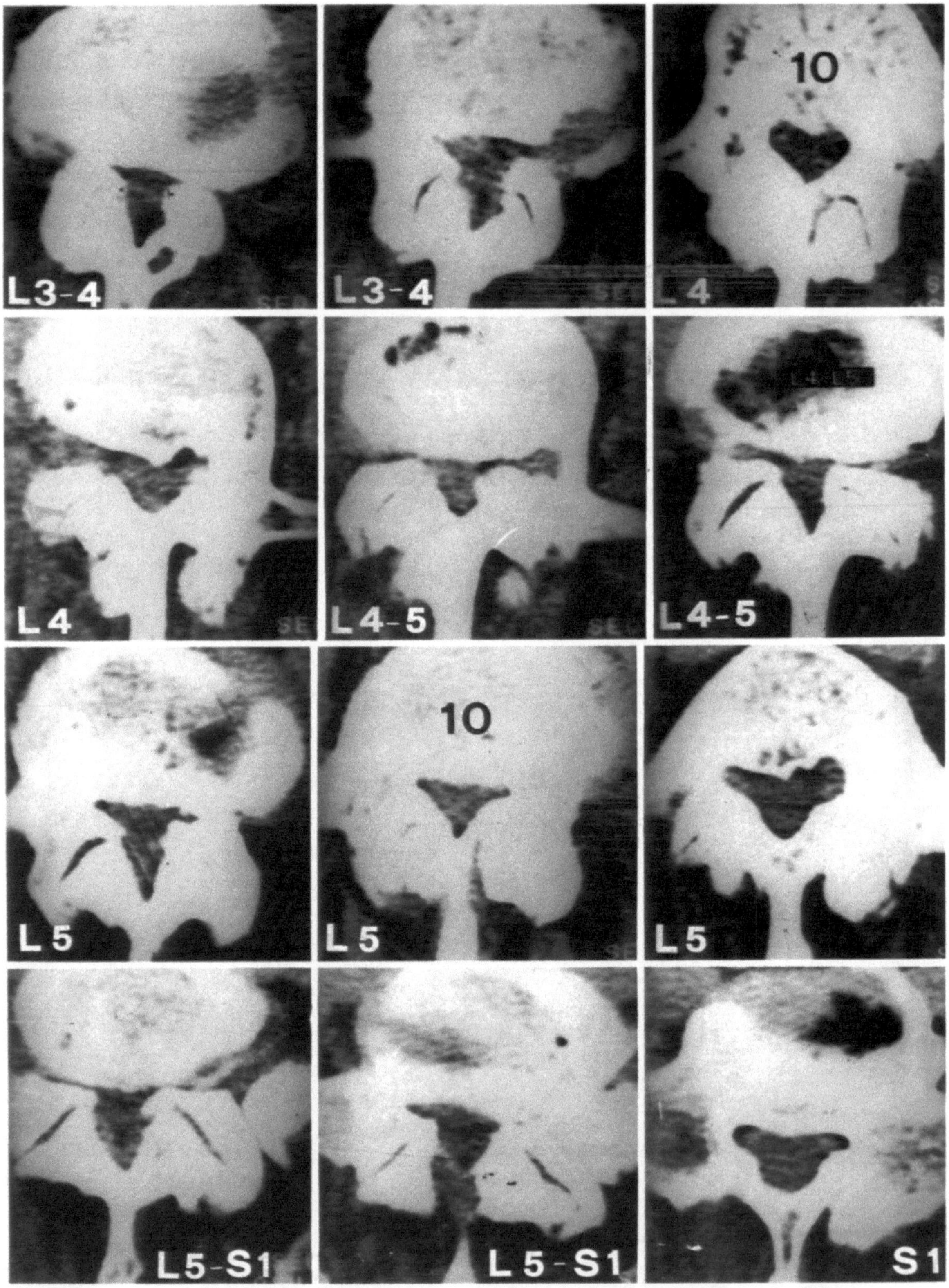

Fig. 8.44 - Severe combined stenosis of the spinal canal. Myelograms show a complete block of the contrast medium at L_3-L_4 level and a less marked compression of the nervous structures at L_2-L_3. CT scans show compression of the dural sac at L_2-L_3 level and, to a greater extent, at L_3-L_4,L_4-L_5 and L_5-S_1. At these levels the dural sac is narrowed in the sagittal and/or transverse direction and, in many scans, appears deformed. In the pedicular sections, the spinal canal shows short midsagittal dimensions at L_2 (12 mm), L_3 (9 mm) and L_4 (10 mm). CT scan is more diagnostic than myelography, since it is able to demonstrate the presence of stenosis also below the block of the contrast column.

The midsagittal dimensions of the spinal canal may be within or below the limits of normal. In stenosis of the distal portion of the nerve root canal, the lateral recess appears to be abnormally narrow and the vertebral canal is often trefoil shaped. In stenosis of both portions, sagittal and coronal reconstructions may contribute to reveal the degenerative changes of the facet joints and vertebral body, and the narrowing of the nerve root canal.

It should be emphasized, however, that narrowing of the radicular canal does not necessarily involve nerve root compression and, therefore, cannot always be identified as stenosis. Very often, CT scan does not visualize the nerve roots in the extradural course — with the exception, generally, of the first sacral root — and does not allow one to determine whether, and to what extent, these are compressed (Fig. 8.43). Therefore, the diagnosis of nerve root canal stenosis on CT scans is frequently presumptive and is based on the evaluation of severity of canal narrowing, rather than on evidence of nerve root compression.

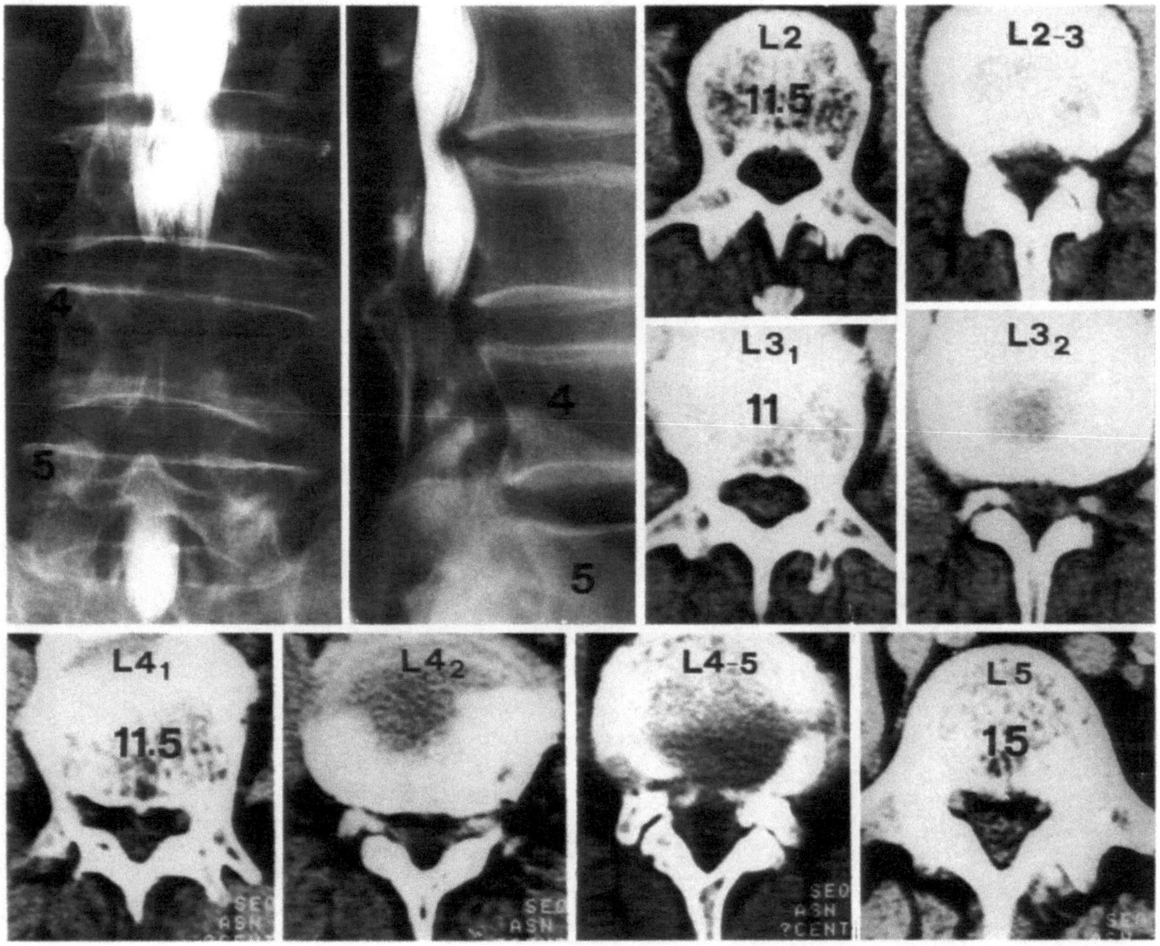

Fig. 8.45 - Combined spinal canal stenosis from L_3 to L_5. Myelograms show a complete block of the contrast medium at L_3-L_4 level and a discal indentation at L_2-L_3. CT scans display developmental narrowing of the spinal canal in the midsagittal dimensions, which are reported in millimetres at a few vertebral levels. The CT scan findings at L_2-L_3 may be interpreted as central disc herniation or narrowing of the thecal sac. CT scan at L_3 shows a reduced transverse area of the dural sac. Similar findings are observed in CT scans at L_4 level. In this patient the CT scans, although indicating a stenosis, does not allow definite diagnosis.

STENOSIS OF THE INTERVERTEBRAL FORAMEN

The presence, in transaxial sections, of narrowing of one or more intervertebral foramina is a fairly frequent finding, which, in most cases, is of no pathological significance. The apparent narrowing is generally due to obliquity of the tomographic section on the transverse plane due to incorrect positioning of the patient during examination, or to a lumbar scoliosis. Narrowing of the foramen can be considered pathological if it is also detectable in the sagittal reconstructions. However, computed tomography, which does not usually visualize the spinal nerve root, cannot demonstrate whether narrowing of the foramen is responsible for nerve root compression. This assessment, as emphasized for nerve root canal stenosis, is inductive and results from the analysis of the severity of narrowing and deformation of the neuroforamen.

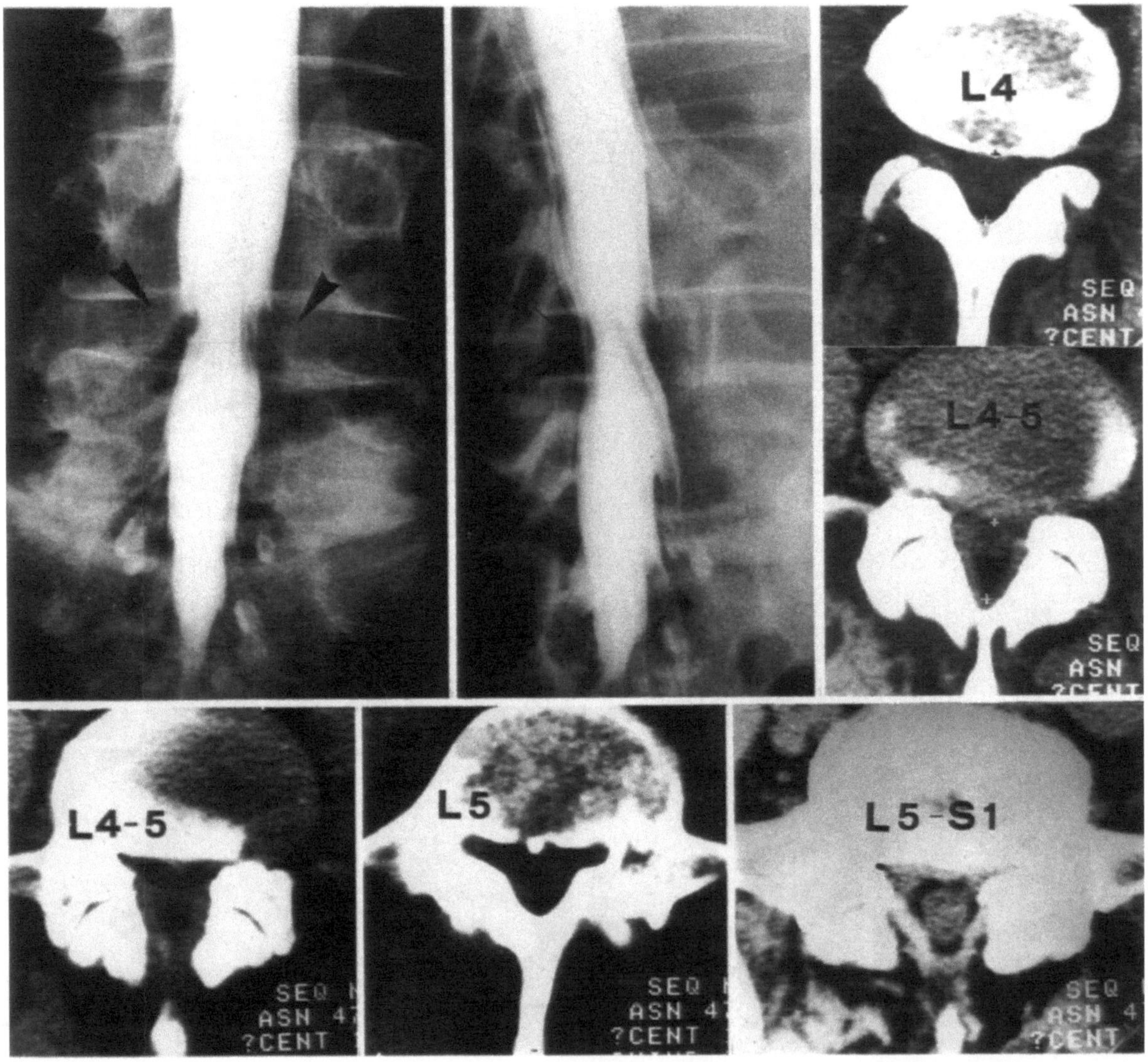

Fig. 8.46 - Bilateral nerve root canal stenosis at L_4-L_5 level in a patient with L_5 radiculopathy on the right side. Myelograms show non-filling of the L_5 nerve root sheaths (arrowheads). CT scan reveals hypertrophied superior articular processes at L_4-L_5 level: these findings lead to suspect, but do not demonstrate, nerve root canal stenosis. A severe S_1 nerve root canal stenosis is detected on the left side at L_5-S_1 level to which, however, compression of the S_1 root does not appear to correspond as shown by the oblique myelogram.

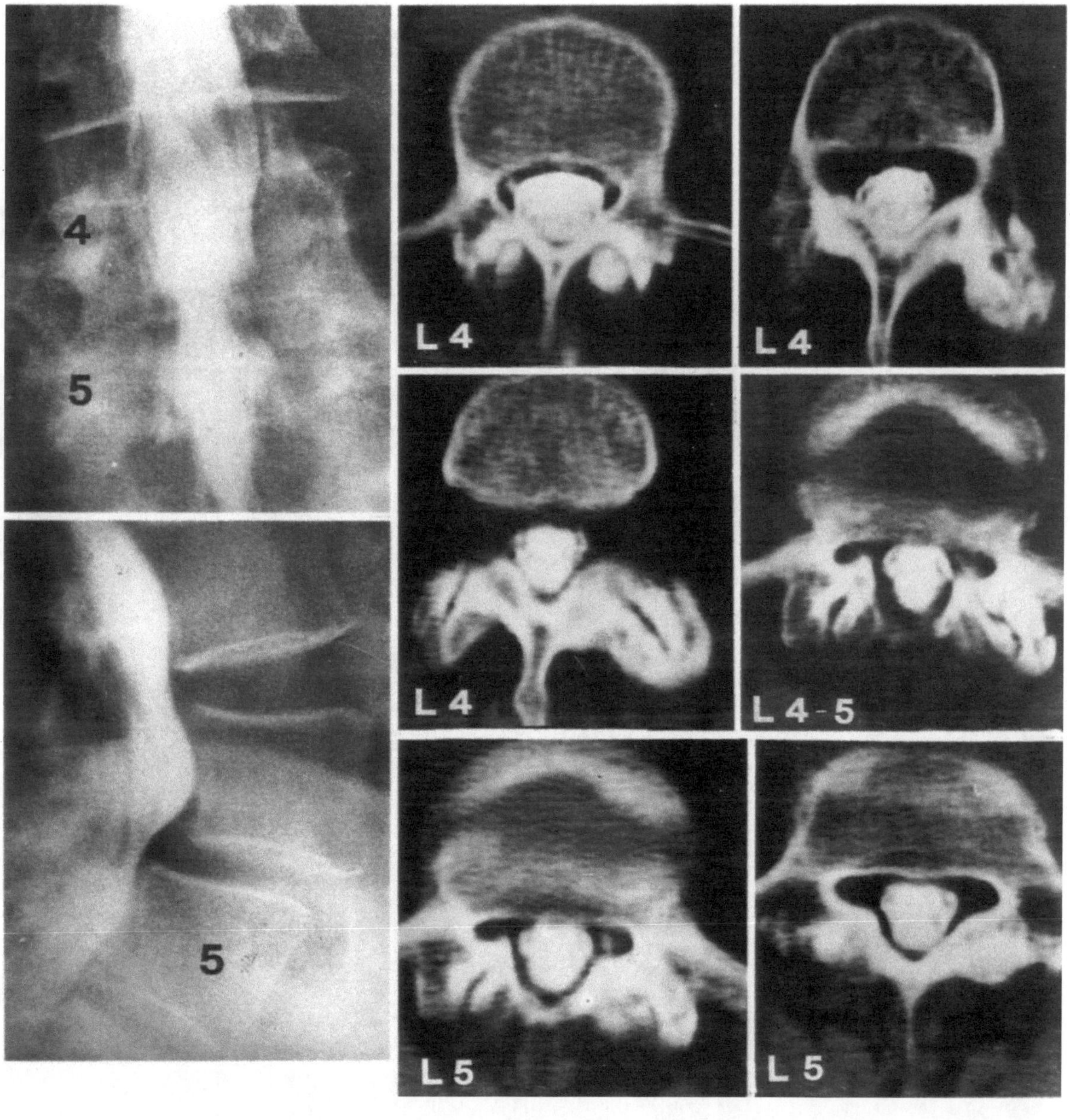

Fig. 8.47 - Myelograms and myelo-CT scans of a patient with L_4-L_5 lumbar stenosis and degenerative spondylolisthesis of L_4. Myelo-CT scans show normal midsagittal dimensions of the spinal canal and severe degenerative changes of the facet joints at L_4-L_5. At this level, the thecal sac presents a reduced transverse area compared with the L_4, and L_5 levels: these findings indicate compression of the dural sac at L_4-L_5 level. The L_5 nerve root canal shows bilateral narrowing and the right L_5 nerve root shows non-filling, whereas that on the left displays a reduced transverse area; this indicates compression of the L_5 nerve root in the radicular canal.

DIAGNOSTIC ACCURACY OF CT SCAN

Bell *et al.* (1984) analyzed the diagnostic accuracy of myelography and CT scanning with respect to surgical findings in 122 patients with either herniated lumbar disc or spinal stenosis or both. They detected three degrees of correlation — strong, firm and weak — between the diagnostic CT scan and myelogram and the surgical findings. There was considered to be a strong correlation if the interpretation of the diagnostic test pre-

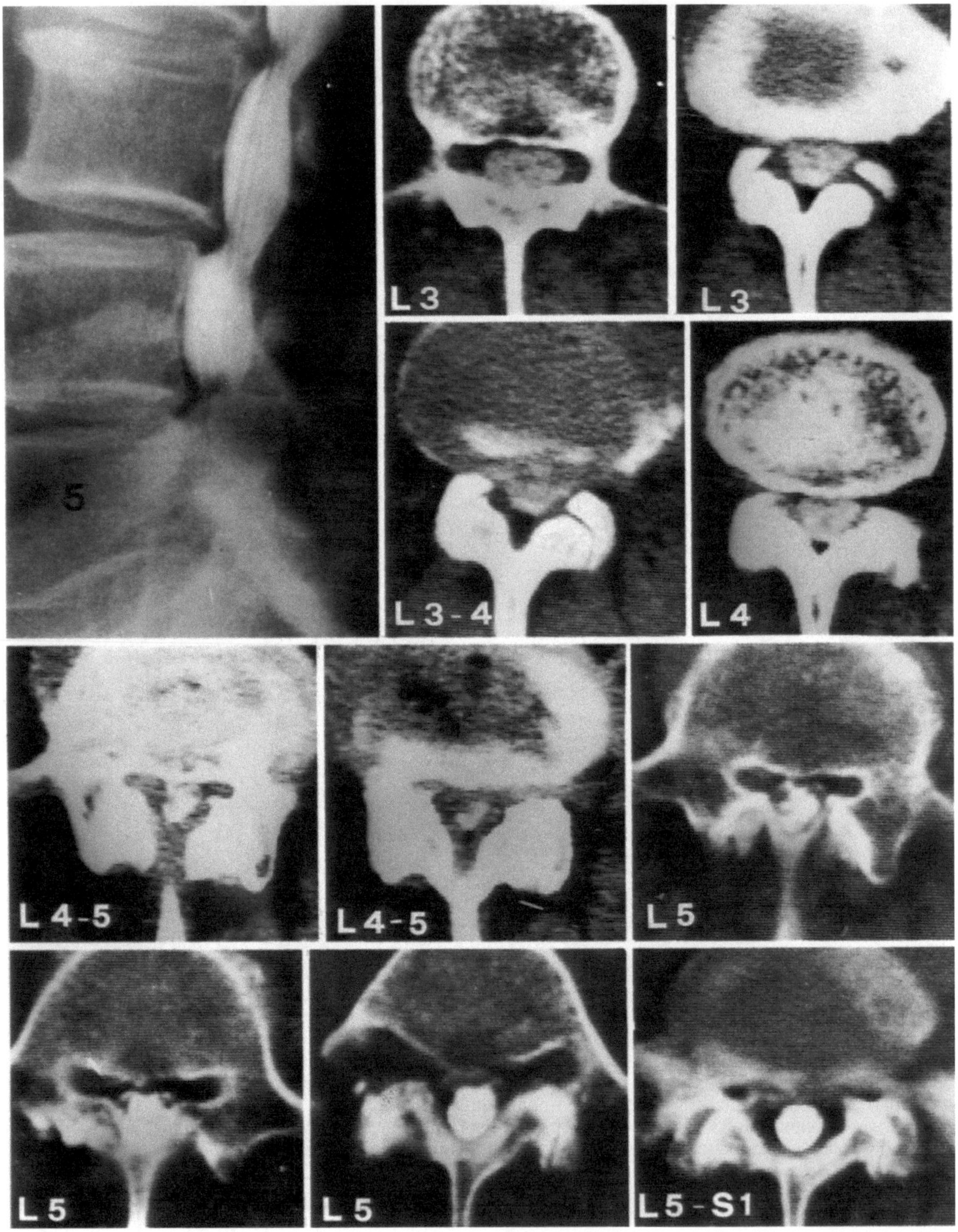

Fig. 8.48 - Lateral myelogram and myelo-CT scans of a patient with degenerative spinal canal stenosis. Myelo-CT scans show a reduced transverse area and partial filling of the dural sac at L_3-L_4 level. The area of the thecal sac decreases considerably at L_4-L_5 level, increasing again in the scans below. At L_4-L_5 level, the dural sac is irregular in shape due to lateral and posterior constrictions. These findings are in complete agreement with the myelographic findings.

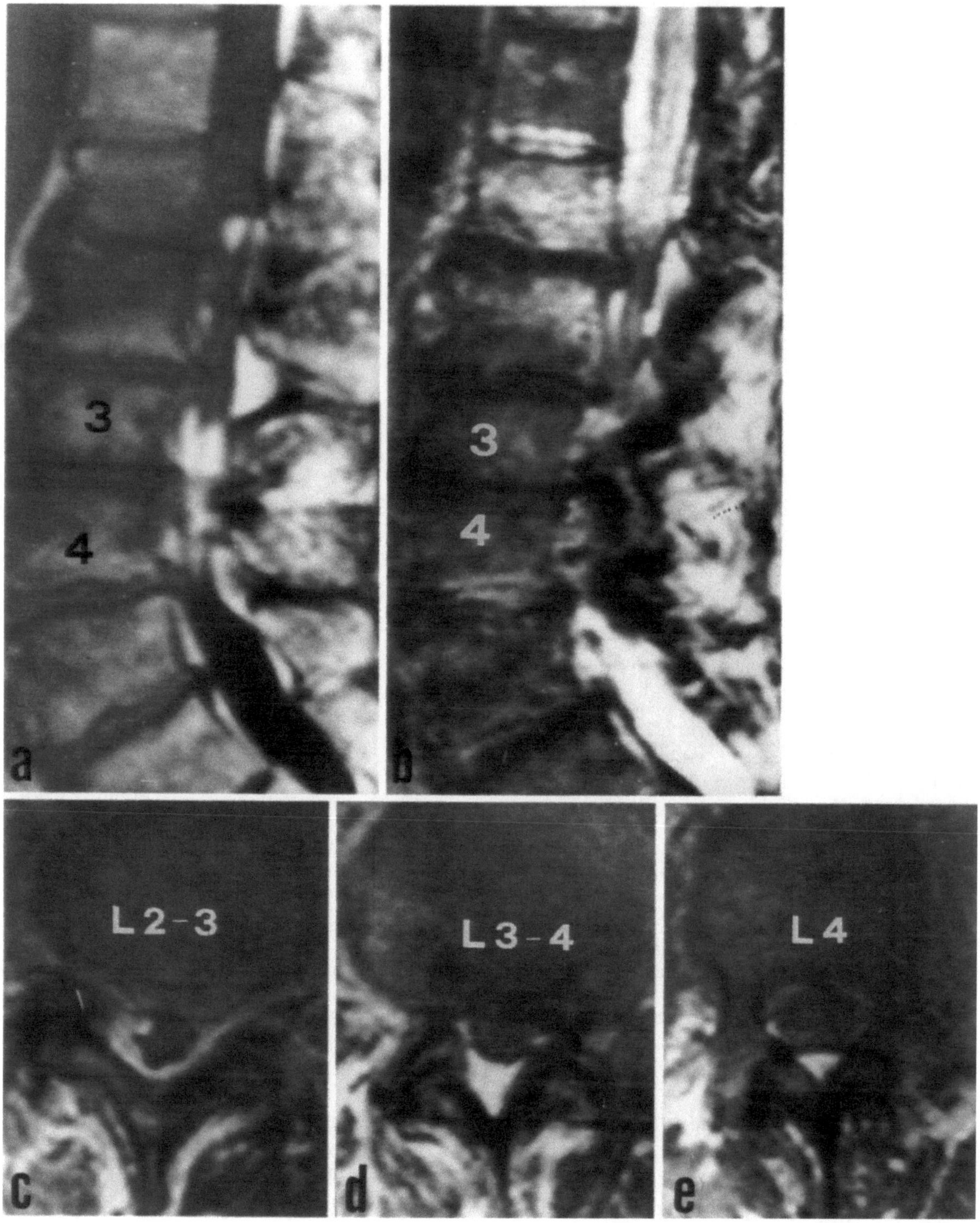

Fig. 8.49 - Spinal canal stenosis from L_1-L_2 to L_4-L_5. **a** and **b**. Midsagittal T_1-weighted (**a**) and lateral sagittal T_2-weighted (**b**) images showing a complete or almost complete interruption of the image of the neural structures in the stenotic area; compression of the neural elements is clearly caused by the osteoligamentous walls of the spinal canal. **c**, **d** and **e**. The cross-sectional area of the dural sac is reduced at L_2-L_3 and L_3-L_4 intervertebral levels, while it is normal in size at the level of the pedicles, that is behind the vertebral body, of L_4.

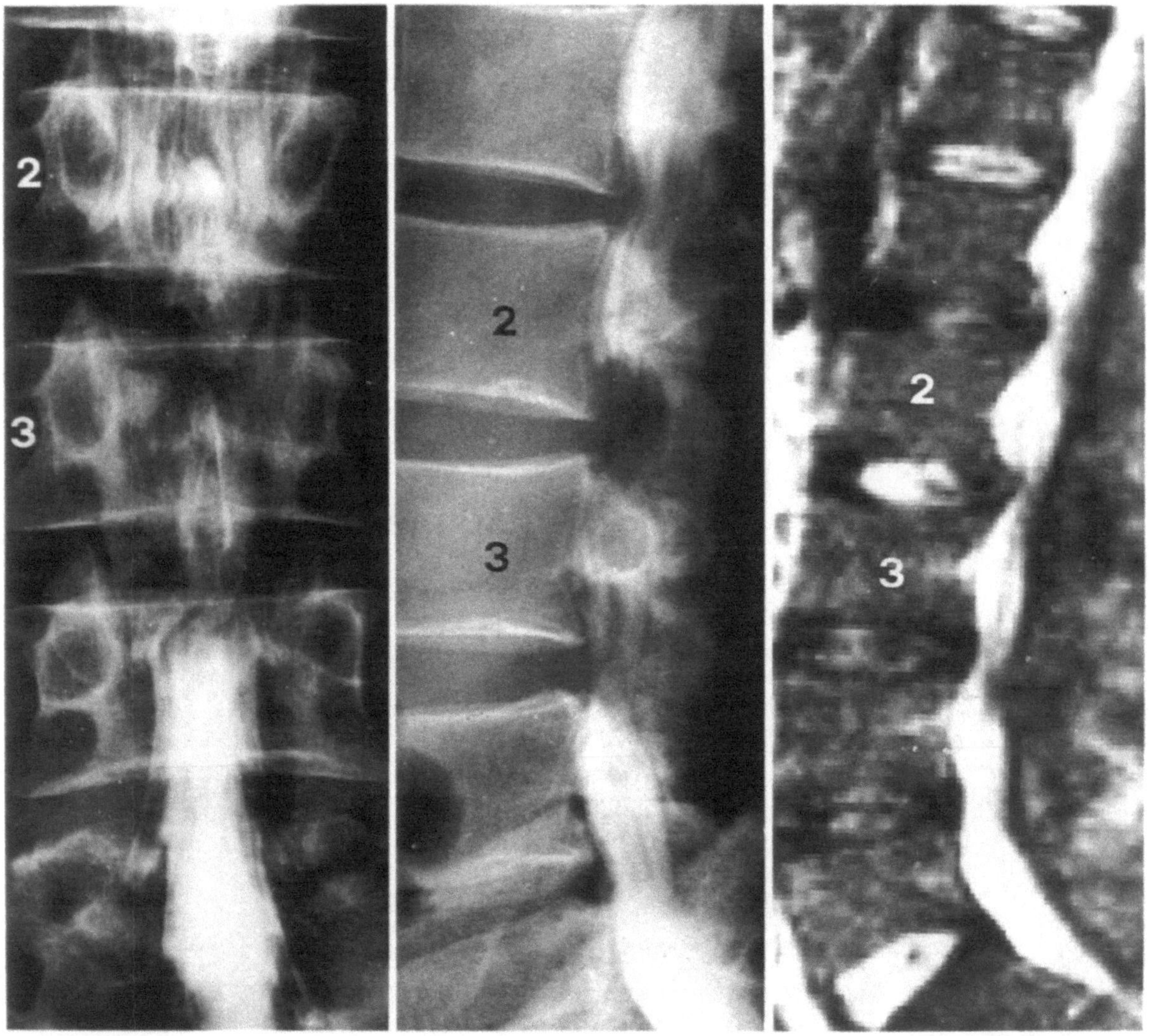

Fig. 8.50 - Spinal canal stenosis at L_2-L_3 and L_3-L_4 levels. Myelograms show a complete block of the contrast medium at L_2-L_3 and a partial block at L_3-L_4. MRI-T_2 weighted midsagittal scan displays narrowing of the thecal sac in the stenotic area and posterior compression of the sac at L_2-L_3 and L_3-L_4 levels. At L_2-L_3 level, anterior compression of the dural sac is also present; compression is due to bulging of the annulus fibrosus rather than true disc herniation, as also suggested by the high signal intensity of the nucleus pulposus.

cisely matched the surgical findings as far as concerns both level and type of pathology; correlation was firm, if the test diagnosed, at least in part, the pathology identified at surgery; finally, correlation was graded as weak, if the test diagnosed some form of pathology at the level noted at surgery, albeit a different type of pathology. In patients with lumbar stenosis, the percentages of diagnostic accuracy of myelography, for the three degrees of correlation, were 67%, 87% and 93%, whereas the diagnostic accuracy of computerized tomography were, respectively, 50%, 74% and 89%. Postacchini and Massobrio (1985) compared the diagnostic accuracy of computerized tomography and myelography in 48 patients with surgically proven stenosis of the spinal canal or nerve root canal. Results of this study, in agreement with those of Bell *et al.* (1984), indicate that the diagnostic accuracy of high resolution computerized tomography is high

Fig. 8.51 - Spinal canal stenosis at L_3 to L_5. **a.** and **b.** Myelograms show a complete block of the dye column at L_3-L_4 level and a filling defect of the lateral portions of the dural sac at L_4-L_5 (**a**). In this case, compression of the nerve structures occurs in the lateral portions of the spinal canal. **c.** MRI. T_1-weighted spin-echo scan (low TE); midsagittal section. The dural sac is abnormally narrow at L_3 to L_5, but appears to be uninterrupted. **d.** MRI. Image obtained with a higher TE than in **c**; lateral sagittal section. The dural sac is severely compressed at L_3-L_4 and L_4-L_5. **e.** MRI. T_2-weighted image (high TE); lateral sagittal section as in **d**. Compression of the thecal sac, occurring in the lateral portions of the spinal canal, is even more evident.

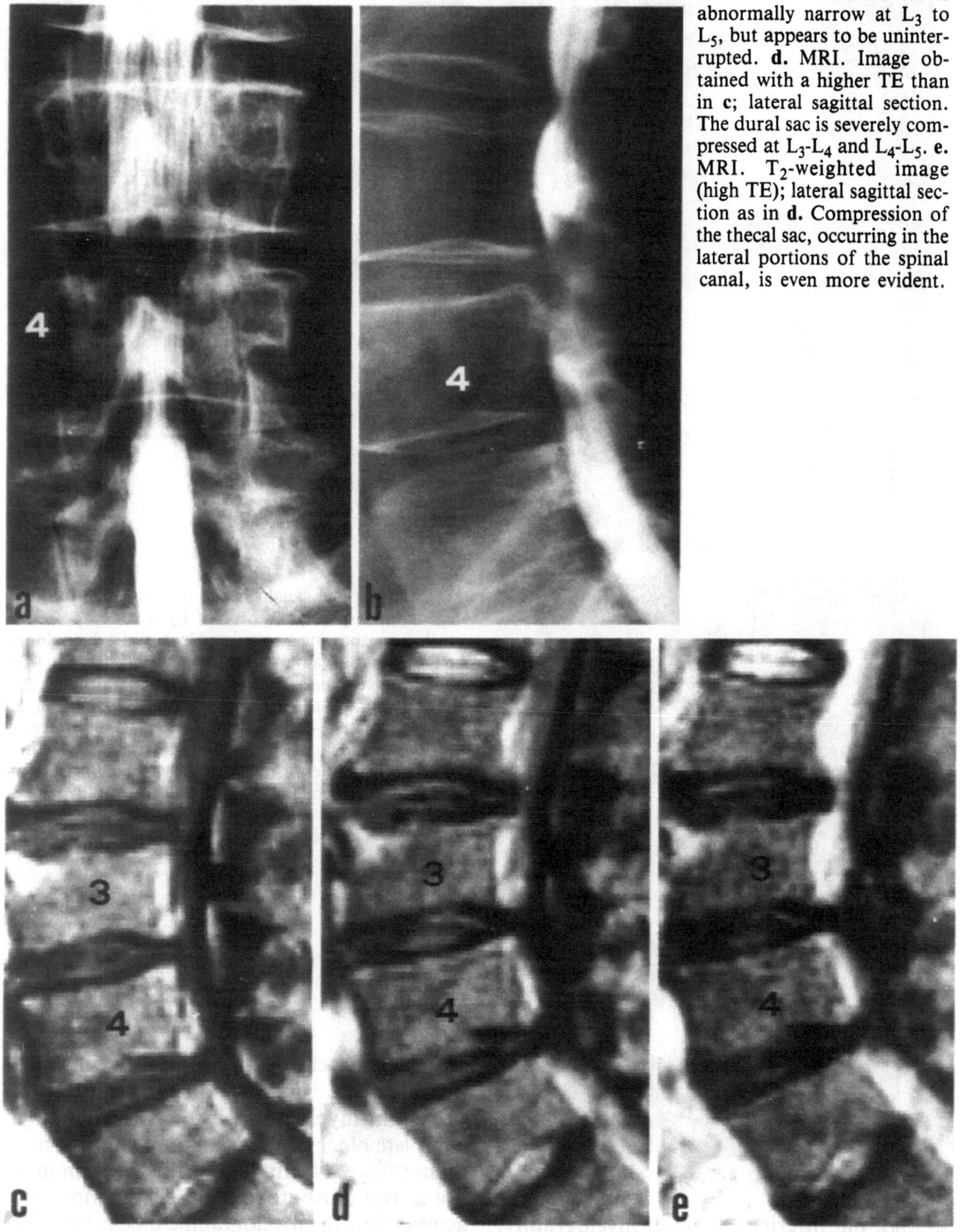

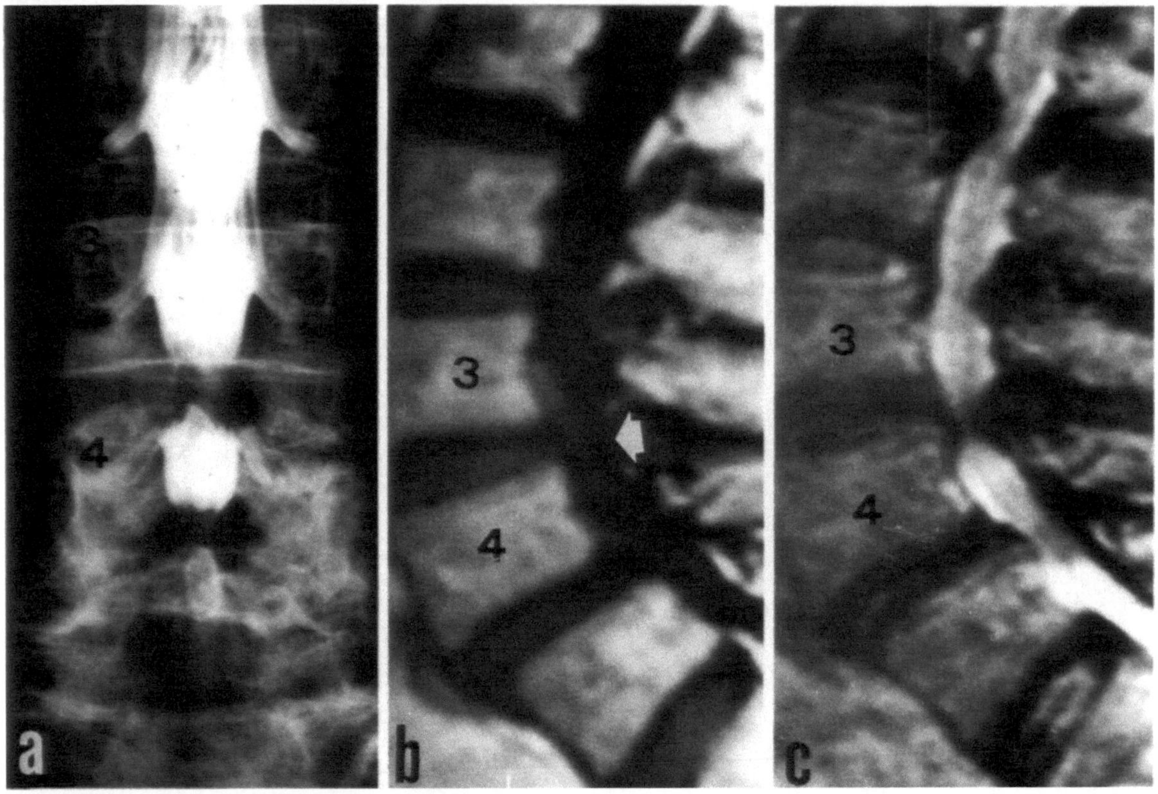

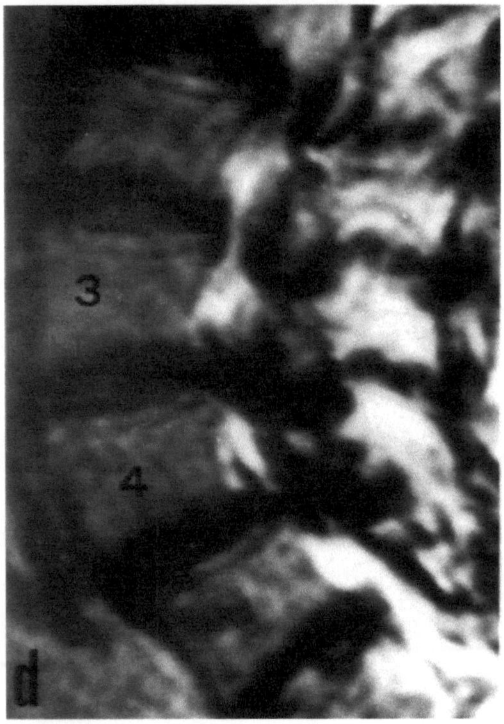

Fig. 8.52 - Spinal canal stenosis in a patient with mild degenerative spondylolisthesis of L_4. **a** Anteroposterior myelogram showing a complete block of the dye column at L_4-L_5 and an almost complete block at L_3-L_4. **b, c** and **d**. MRI scans: T_1-weighted midsagittal image **(a)** shows a mild posterior compression of the dural sac at L_3-L_4 (arrow); T_2-weighted midsagittal scan **(c)** reveals a posterior indentation of the thecal sac at L_3-L_4 and L_2-L_3 and an anterior indentation by a bulging disc at L_1-L_2; on the lateral sagittal T_2-weighted scan **(d)** a complete interruption of the image of the neural structures is visible at L_3-L_4 and L_4-L_5.

(77%), but inferior to that of myelography.

Computerized tomography enables a precise diagnosis to be made in most patients with severe stenosis, in whom CT scans may provide more exhaustive diagnostic information than myelograms in the presence of a complete block of the column of contrast medium (Fig. 8.44). In these cases, CT scan may not only contribute to precisely diagnose the aetiology of the myelographic block, but also to determine the presence of a stenosis below the area of arrest of the column of contrast medium. It should be noted, however, that CT scan, although able to demonstrate the presence of a stenotic pathology, may sometimes provide false positive or false negative results or, more often, results of uncertain interpretation (Figs. 8.45 and 8.46). This occurs particularly in mild spinal stenosis, which is not characterized by marked morphometric changes of the vertebral canal or the dural sac.

MYELO-CT

This investigation consists in CT scanning after injection of contrast medium in the dural sac. The volume of the contrast agent may be the same as, or less than, that used for conventional myelography (10 to 13 ml). In the former instance, the usual myelograms are obtained and then CT scanning is carried out, placing the patient in the supine position with the head and the upper part of the trunk slightly higher than the lumbar spine to avoid rise of the contrast medium. In the second instance, only 5 to 8 ml of contrast medium are injected, which are inadequate for excellent myelographic images, but sufficient to allow adequate visualization of the dural sac on CT scans. Of the two methods, the former is to be preferred, since it adds the diagnostic information provided by myelography to that obtained from CT scans. The disadvantage of computerized tomography with contrast medium in the dural sac is that, like myelography, this diagnostic method is invasive, with necessarily the same complications as the latter.

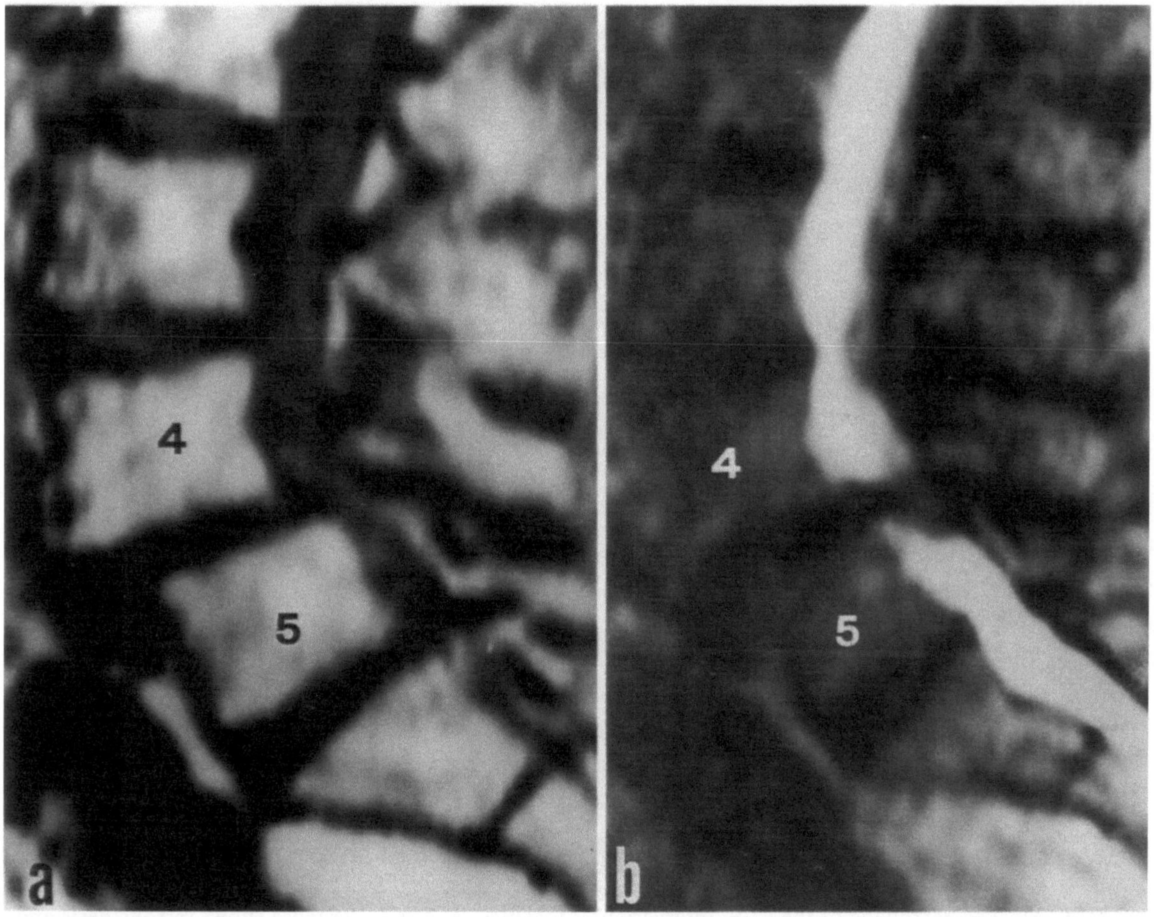

Fig. 8.53 - Degenerative spondylolisthesis of L_4. **a.** T_1-weighted midsagittal scan. The thecal sac appears buckling and severely constricted at L_4-L_5 level. **b.** T_2-weighted image near the midline. Complete interruption of the dural sac at L_4-L_5 level.

Myelo-CT allows more accurate diagnosis of spinal canal stenosis than with CT scanning alone, since, compared to the latter, it permits better visualization of the dural sac and spinal nerve roots. Diagnosis is based on the findings of narrowing and/or deformation of the profile of the dural sac. As already pointed out for myelography, narrowing of the dural sac may be considered pathological only when associated with an increase in size of the sac above and/or below the stenotic area (Fig. 8.47). Much more significant, from the diagnostic point of view, is the finding of deformations of the dural sac caused by hypertrophic or arthrotic articular processes and, even more, the association, in the same tomographic section, or the presence in adjacent sections, of a segmentary narrowing of the dural sac and deformations of the profile of the sac (Fig. 8.48). These changes may be associated with anterior indentations of the thecal sac produced by disc protrusions and filling defects of the nerve root sheaths (Fig. 8.47).

In nerve root canal stenosis, myelo-CT may show a filling defect or a reduced transverse area of the sheath of the nerve root lying in the stenotic radicular canal. Also in these forms of stenosis, therefore, the diagnostic value of myelo-CT is greater than that of plain CT scans, but less than that displayed in stenosis of the spinal canal. In transaxial section, in fact, it may be difficult to appreciate slight filling defects of the nerve root sheaths. Furthermore, as occurs also for myelography, results may sometimes be

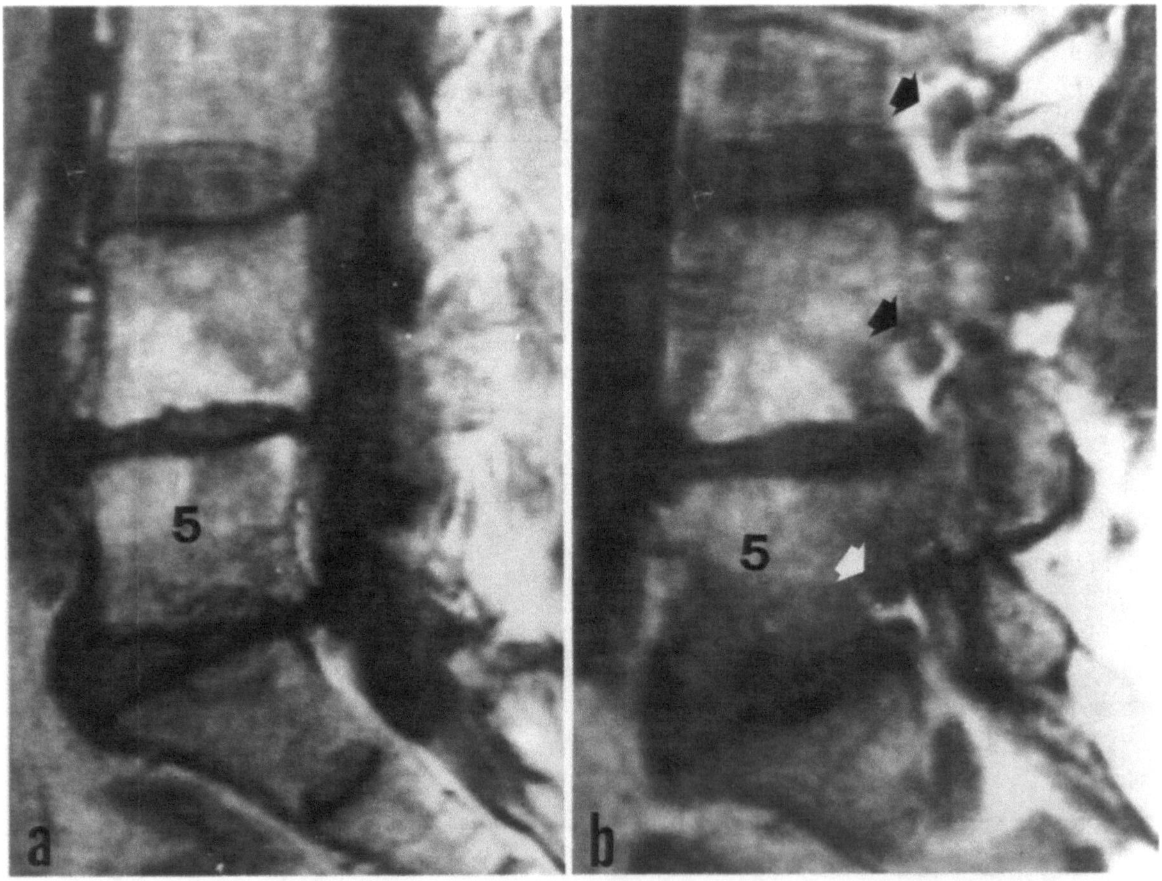

Fig. 8.54 - Marked narrowing of the L_5-S_1 intervertebral foramen. **a.** The L_5 vertebra shows retrolisthesis and the L_5-S_1 disc protrudes slightly into the spinal canal. **b.** The intervertebral foramina at L_3-L_4 and L_4-L_5 are of normal width and the spinal nerve roots (arrows) do not appear to be compressed. The L_5-S_1 neuroforamen is narrowed; the spinal nerve root is reduced in calibre and appears compressed by the pedicle of L_5 and the superior articular process of S_1.

negative even in the presence of nerve root compression.

In stenosis of the intervertebral foramen, the diagnostic accuracy of myelo-CT is similar to that of plain computerized tomography, since the nerve root sheath terminates before the nerve root enters the intervertebral foramen.

MAGNETIC RESONANCE IMAGING

The advent of magnetic resonance imaging revolutionized the diagnostic approach to vertebral diseases, particularly to intradural conditions. In the evaluation of intervertebral disc disease and lumbar stenosis, MRI represents the investigation with the highest accuracy among non-invasive diagnostic studies. Compared with computerized tomography, MRI has the advantage not only of not utilizing ionizing radiations, but also of allowing better visualization of the contents of the spinal canal, an easier and more precise evaluation of the anatomical structures in tridimensional planes and a more detailed evaluation of the degenerative changes of the intervertebral disc. As far as myelography is concerned, no studies have as yet been carried out to compare the diagnostic accuracy of the two methods in patients with lumbar stenosis. However, it is increasingly evident that the diagnostic value of MRI, at least in stenosis of the spinal canal or the neuroforamen, is similar or greater than that of myelography. Considering that, at present, the clinical use of MRI and the technical aspects of this diagnostic tool are still in evolution, it is likely that in the near future this method will by itself be able to concentrate the diagnostic capacity of the two investigations currently available.

In spinal canal stenosis, MRI clearly demonstrates narrowing of the dural sac and compression of the neural elements by the osteoligamentous structures of the posterior vertebral arch (Fig. 8.49). Sagittal images of the spine provide similar diagnostic information to that obtained from the lateral myelogram (Figs. 8.50 and 8.51). Compared to the latter, with MRI it is possible to determine, with greater precision, the role of the intervertebral disc in the aetiology of compression of the nervous structures and to more accurately define whether compression is due to a herniated disc, stenosis, or bulging annulus fibrosus in a stenotic vertebral canal. When compression of the nervous structures is caused by constriction of the lateral portions of the spinal canal, midsagittal sections may show narrowing of the dural sac of varying entity, whereas lateral sagittal sections display a more severe compression of the neural structures (Figs. 8.51, 8.52 and 8.53).

Isolated nerve root canal stenosis may be revealed in transaxial sections, showing compression of the spinal nerve root in a narrowed radicular canal. With the scanners presently available, however, it may sometimes be difficult to obtain excellent axial images of the vertebral canal and the neural elements. In these forms of stenosis, therefore, the diagnostic capacity of MRI may not be as good as that of myelography, computerized tomography or myelo-CT.

MRI is able to demonstrate, better than any other diagnostic investigation, stenosis of the intervertebral foramen, since it allows visualization both of the walls of the neuroforamen and the nerve root within it (Fig. 8.54).

REFERENCES

ASCANI E., URSO S., MONTANARO A., PACCIANI E.: *Stenosi laterale del canale spinale: diagnosi neuroradiologica e terapia chirurgica.* Communication at the 71st SIOT (GIS) Congress, Venice, 1986.

ASZTELY M., KADZIOLKA R., NACHEMSON A.: A comparison of sonography and myelography in clinical suspected spinal stenosis. *Spine* **8**: 885, 1983.

BELL G.R., ROTHMAN R.H., BOOTH R.E., CUCKLER J.M. GARFIN S., HERKOWITZ H., SIMEONE F.A., DOLINSKAS C., HAN S.S.: A study of computer assisted tomography. Comparison of metrizamide myelography and computed tomography in the diagnosis of herniated lumbar disc and spinal stenosis. *Spine* **9:** 552, 1984.

BOLENDER N.F., SCHONSTROM N.S.R., SPENGLER D.N.: Role of myelography and computerized tomography in the diagnosis of central spinal stenosis. *J. Bone and Joint Surg.* **67-A:** 240, 1985.

CROCK H.V.: Isolated lumbar disc resorption as a cause of nerve root canal stenosis. *Clin. Orthop.* **115:** 109, 1976.

DE BERAIL A.: *Exploration radiologique du rachis lombaire normal et son application au syndrome du canal lombaire.* Thésis de Medecine, Toulose N. 176, 1976.

DVONCH V., SCARF T., BUNCH W.H., SMITH D., BOSCARDIN J., LEBARGE H., IBRAHIM K.: ‹Dermatomal somatosensory evoked potentials: their use in lumbar radiculopathy. *Spine* **9:** 291, 1984.

EISENSTEIN S.: Measurements of the lumbar spinal canal in 2 racial groups. *Clin. Orthop.* **115:** 42, 1976.

EISENSTEIN S.: The morphometry and pathological anatomy of the lumbar spine in South African Negroes and Caucasoids with specific reference to spinal stenosis. *J. Bone and Joint Surg.* **59-B:** 173, 1977.

ENGEL J.M., ENGEL G.M., GUNN D.R.: Ultrasound of the spine in focal stenosis and disc disease. *Spine* **10:** 928, 1985.

GETTY C.J.M., DIXON A.K., YOUNG A., LETTIN A.W.F. The role of computerized tomography in degenerative lumbar spine disease: a prospective trial. *J. Bone and Joint Surg.* **63-B:** 632, 1981.

JONES R.A.G., THOMSON J.L.G.: The narrow lumbar canal, a clinical and radiological review. *J. Bone and Joint Surg.* **50-B:** 595, 1968.

KADZIOLKA R., ASZTELY M., HANAI K., HANSSON T., NACHEMSON A.: Ultrasonic measurement of the lumbar spinal canal. The origin and precision of the recorded echos. *J. Bone and Joint Surg.* **63-B:** 504, 1981.

KEIM H.A., HAJDU M., GONZALES E.G., BRAND L., BALASUBRAMANIAN E.: Somatosensory evoked potentials as an aid in the diagnosis and intraoperative management of spinal stenosis. *Spine* **10:** 338, 1985.

KIRKALDY-WILLIS W.H., YONG-HING K., DE KOROMPAY V., SHANNON R.: Lumbar spinal nerve lateral entrapment: an underrated entity. *J. Bone and Joint Surg.* **63-B:** 286, 1981.

LEGG S.J., GIBBS V.: Measurement of the lumbar spinal canal by echo ultrasound. *Spine* **9:** 79, 1984.

MCCULLOCH J.A., WADDELL G.: Lateral lumbar discography. *Br. J. Radiol.* **51:** 498, 1978.

MEIRE H.B.: Diagnose des Diskusprolaps durch Ultraschallmethode entwickelt. *Med. Tribune*, 1975, 3 October: 5.

PAINE K., HUANG P.: Lumbar disc syndrome. *J. Neurosurg.* **37:** 75, 1973.

PORTER R.W., HIBBERT C.S., WICKS M.: The spinal canal in symptomatic lumbar disc lesions. *J. Bone and Joint Surg.* **60-B:** 485, 1978.

PORTER R.W., WICKS M., OTTEWELL D.: Measurement of the spinal canal by diagnostic ultrasound. *J. Bone and Joint Surg.* **60-B:** 481, 1978.

POSTACCHINI F., PEZZERI G.: CT scanning versus myelography in the diagnosis of lumbar stenosis. A preliminary report. *Intern. Orthop.* (SICOT) **5:** 209, 1981.

POSTACCHINI F.: PEZZERI G., MONTANARO A., NATALI G.: Computerized tomography in lumbar stenosis. A preliminary report. *J. Bone and Joint Surg.,* **62-B:** 78, 1980.

POSTACCHINI F., MASSOBRIO M.: *Diagnostic accuracy of computerized tomography in lumbar stenosis.* Communication at the XII ISSLS Congress, Sidney, Australia, 1985.

SCHONSTROM N.S.R., BOLENDER N.F., SPENGLER D.M.: The pathomorphology of spinal stenosis as seen on CT scans of the lumbar spine. *Spine* **10:** 806, 1985.

TSUJI H., TAMAKI T., ITOH T., YAMADA H., MOTOE T., TATEZAKI S., NOGUCHI T., TAKANO H.: Redundant nerve roots in patients with degenerative lumbar spinal stenosis. *Spine* **10:** 72, 1985.

URSO S.: Personal communication, 1986.

VERBIEST H.: *Stenosis of the bony lumbar vertebral canal.* In «*The narrow lumbar canal. Radiologic signs and surgery*». Ed. Wackenheim A. and Babin E., Springer-Verlag, Berlin-Heidelberg, New York, 1980.

VOGUE M.: *Interapophysolaminar spaces (IALS) of the lumbar spine and their utility in the diagnosis of narrow lumbar canal.* In «*The narrow lumbar canal. Radiologic signs and surgery*». Ed. Wachenheim A. and Babin E., Springer-Verlag, Berlin-Heidelberg, New York, 1980.

Chapter IX
Treatment

INTRODUCTION

Lumbar stenosis is a pathological condition with a slowly progressive course, in which two successive stages may be identified: an asymptomatic stage, in which narrowing of the spinal canal causes only a mild constriction of the dural sac; and a symptomatic stage, characterized by marked compression of the dural sac and/or the spinal nerve roots in the radicular canal. The latter stage, in turn, includes an initial phase in which symptoms and signs are relatively mild and a more advanced phase characterized by severe clinical symptomatology. Transition from one stage to the other, which is essentially determined by a progressive increase in severity of the degenerative changes in the discs and vertebrae, is strictly related to the ageing process.

In the asymptomatic stage, treatment is usually conservative. In the initial phase of the symptomatic stage, treatment may be either conservative or surgical, depending on the severity of clinical symptoms and signs and age of the patient. In the advanced symptomatic stage, management is generally surgical, except in patients who are very old and/or in poor general conditions.

CONSERVATIVE TREATMENT

In lumbar spinal stenosis conservative treatment has a less important role than in patients with disc herniation. In the latter condition, clinical symptoms and signs show a tendency to improve with time, and even disappear, probably due to the tendency of the herniated nucleus pulposus to show a progressive decrease in volume as a result of tissue dehydration. In stenosis, on the other hand, radicular symptomatology tends to show a progressive worsening with time, on account of the increase in severity of the degenerative changes related to the ageing process. In lumbar stenosis syndromes, therefore, conservative treatment is usually considered second choice or «wait and see», to be employed when surgical treatment is contraindicated due to poor general conditions of the patient or not justified on account of mildness of radicular symptoms and signs.

Conservative treatment consists in drug therapy, physiotherapy and bracing.

DRUG THERAPY

Low-back pain may be improved by anti-inflammatory non-corticosteroid drugs. For radicular symptoms, in contrast, the use of corticosteroids at low or medium dosage is more indicated, if the general conditions of the patient allow, for a maximum of two weeks. Neurotropic vitamins and gangliosides may be associated with anti-inflammatory drugs for periods of three to five weeks.

During the last twenty years, calcitonin and/or mitramicin have been employed in patients with vertebral Paget's disease presenting clinical and radiographic evidence of compression of the caudal nerve roots, and, in many cases, mild to complete improvement of the radicular symptoms have been reported (Hadijpavlov *et al.*, 1977; Herzberg and Bayliss, 1980; Douglas *et al.*, 1981). A possible explanation for the clinical effects of calcitonin, in these cases, may be that the highly vascularized pagetic bone exerts a sort of vascular theft, reducing blood flow to the vertebral nervous structures. Since calcitonin reduces the blood flow in the pagetic bone, vascularization of the nervous structures would be improved.

On the grounds of these observations, Porter and Hibbert (1983) administered salmon calcitonin (100 units, four times a week) to patients with lumbo-radicular intermittent claudication showing no evidence of Paget's disease, and found, in about one fourth of them, a significant improvement in the walking capacity after only four weeks of treatment. These therapeutic effects of calcitonin, which, however, need to be confirmed, are probably related to a reduction in the skeletal arterial blood flow induced by the hormone (Wootton, 1978) and a subsequent increase in the arterial flow in the cauda equina. Alternatively, the hormone might improve the venous blood flow, thus producing a decrease in volume of the venous epidural plexus, with subsequent increase in the oxygen supply to the cauda equina.

PHYSIOTHERAPY

It is mainly employed to relieve pain in the low back.

Physiotherapy has little or no effect upon radicular symptoms but may be effective, in the form of stimulant electrotherapy and active kinesitherapy, in the treatment of motor deficits in the lower limbs.

BRACING

The use of a corset may improve low-back pain and sometimes also radicular symptoms. Improvement of the radiated symptoms, which is, however, usually mild, is likely due to the fact that bracing reduces the dynamic stretching and compression of the caudal nerve roots, which may be produced by the articular processes and intervertebral discs during spinal movements. This interpretation is consistent with the observation that bracing leads to the greatest improvement of low-back and radicular symptoms in patients showing evidence of vertebral instability, particularly in those with degenerative spondylolisthesis.

SURGICAL TREATMENT

INDICATIONS AND CONTRAINDICATIONS

Indications for surgical treatment are based on the results of diagnostic investigations, demonstrating compression of the conus medullaris and/or cauda equina, and the presence of cord or nerve root symptoms and signs corresponding, as far as concerns level and side, to the site of compression of the spinal nervous structures.

In particular, surgical treatment is indicated:

1. In the presence of sphincteric disturbances due to compression of the conus medullaris, regardless of the severity of radicular symptoms and signs.
2. In patients with severe radicular symptoms (pain, paresthesiae, asthenia) and monoradicular or pluriradicular motor deficits.
3. In the presence of severe motor deficits and mild or discontinuous radicular symptoms, if stenosis is marked and the patient is not very elderly. In these cases, the indication for surgical treatment is based on the consideration that, with time, symptoms usually show a progressive increase in severity, not unlike the motor deficits, which the longer the duration and the greater the entity, the more likelihood they will be irreversible;
4. In patients with radicular symptoms and no neurological signs, if the symptoms have been present for more than six months and show no response to an adequate trial of conservative management. In these cases, investigations should demonstrate marked compression of the nervous structures or, in the presence of compression of mild entity, symptoms should have a precise radicular distribution with involvement of one metamer (or more metamers) in all its extent.
5. In patients with severe low-back pain and mild radicular symptoms, in whom investigations show evidence of marked compression of the nervous structures.

Conversely, surgery is not generally indicated:

1. In patients complaining of vague and imprecise radicular symptoms, when inves-

tigations demonstrate only posterior compression of the dural sac.

2. If the clinical picture is characterized only by nerve root motor deficits which, being long-standing, are likely to be irreversible. This is specifically true for subjects of advanced senile age.

3. In patients complaining of low back pain of varying severity as the main disorder, and of mild or discontinuous radicular symptoms, in the presence of investigations showing mild compression of the nervous structures. The only exception are the patients with degenerative spondylolisthesis in whom the aim of treatment may be vertebral stabilization, as well as decompression of the nerve roots of the cauda equina.

Surgical treatment is contraindicated:

1. In subjects with a narrow, but not stenotic, spinal canal.

2. In patients in whom investigations carried out for an extralumbar condition show a clinically asymptomatic stenosis.

PLANNING OF SURGERY

Surgical treatment consists in decompression of the spinal nervous structures by means of bilateral laminectomy, or monolateral or bilateral laminotomy, performed at one or more vertebral levels.

It is crucial to accurately plan the extent of decompression before surgery as it may be difficult during the operation to determine with certainty whether at a given level the spinal canal or nerve root canal are stenotic, particularly when stenosis is not severe. Lack of sufficient care in the planning of the operation may give rise to two risks, namely inadequate decompression, which would leave areas of stenosis, or too wide a decompression, which, directly or indirectly, could determine iatrogenic pathologic conditions.

Spinal canal stenosis

Surgical treatment is aimed at decompressing the nervous structures in those areas in which they are compressed. In those areas in which the spinal canal is narrow, but not stenotic, opening of the canal is not generally necessary or useful (Perugia and Postacchini, 1981).

In planning the operative treatment it is necessary to determine: the levels which need to be decompressed; the type — monolateral or bilateral — of procedure; and the usefulness of performing a vertebral fusion.

Number of levels to decompress

The stenotic levels may be distinguished, as far as concerns operative treatment, into:

a) Levels at which the need for decompression is absolute. At these levels compression of the conus medullaris or cauda equina is marked or, regardless of the severity, is responsible for clinical symptoms and signs. One to three levels may be involved.

b) Levels at which the need for decompression is relative. At these levels, compression of the spinal nervous structures is mild and asymptomatic. In most instances one level or two levels, contiguous to the area of «absolute» stenosis, are concerned (Fig. 9.1). At these levels, myelography usually reveals: a posterior indentation on the dural sac, which may be visible only on functional myelograms; lateral indentation or a mild hour-glass deformation of the dural sac on the frontal view; or medial deviation and/or partial filling of the nerve root emerging from the dural sac.

The usefulness of carrying out prophylactic decompression at the levels of «relative» stenosis stems from the evaluation of several factors, such as:

— Patient's age. In patients of advanced age, i.e. over 70 years, the need for a prophylactic decompression is less than in middle aged or early old age patients, since in the latter the chances that stenosis becomes symptomatic, due to degenerative changes related to the ageing process, are higher.

— Site of stenosis. Posterior compression of the dural sac is less likely to become symptomatic than compression of the nerve roots in the radicular canal.

— Presence of disc abnormalities. Marked bulging of the annulus fibrosus, with which time may become symptomatic, represents an indication for prophylactic

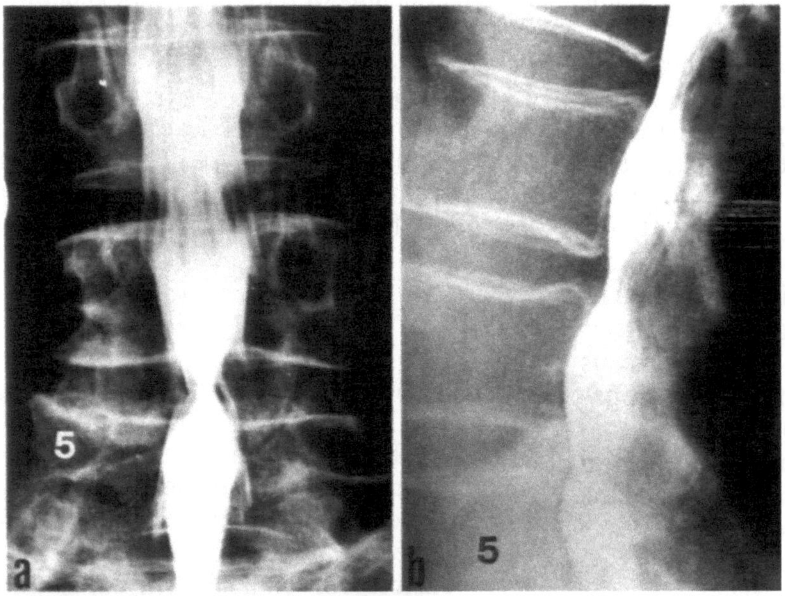

Fig. 9.1 - A 64-year-old woman with lateral and posterior radicular pain in both lower limbs. **a.** and **b.** Myelograms show lumbar stenosis at L_4-L_5 and partial filling of S_1 nerve roots at L_5-S_1: at these levels decompression is mandatory. At L_3-L_4 level, stenosis — which was asymptomatic — is also present, as indicated by the mild filling defect of the L_4 roots (**a**) and the marked posterior indentation on the dural sac (**b**): at this level, the need for decompression is relative. At L_2-L_3 a mild posterior compression of the dural sac (**b**), which was also asymptomatic, is visible; at this level, there is little need for decompression. **c.** Bilateral laminectomy from L_3-L_4 to L_5-S_1 was performed.

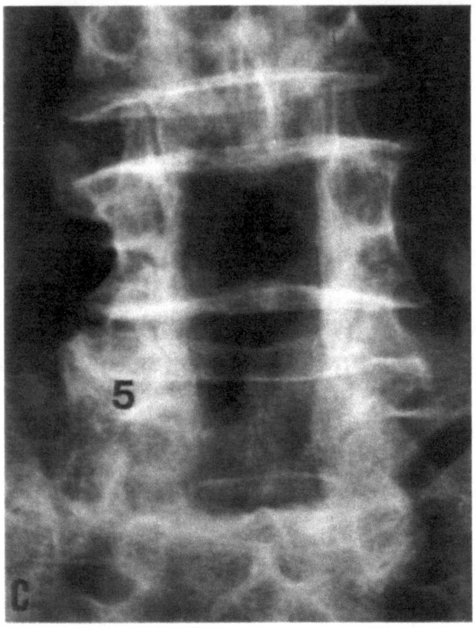

decompression. The same is true for posterior osteophytes of the vertebral body, when they are responsible for compression of the dural sac (Fig. 9.2).

— Electrodiagnostic findings. Evidence of a clinically asymptomatic compression of a nerve root tends to suggest that, with time, compression may become symptomatic.

— Vertebral stability. In the presence of instability or potential instability of the stenotic motion segment it is usually advisable as far as possible to limit the decompression. Conversely, the presence of anterior or lateral intersomatic osteophytes producing spontaneous vertebral arthrodesis, represents a guarantee against post-surgical instability. Similar observations may be made for marked narrowing of the disc space in the absence of other pathological conditions; loss of disc height, in fact, implies reduced intervertebral motion, and thus vertebral instability is highly unlikely.

In conclusion, it is not generally necessary, in very old patients, to extend laminectomy to areas of mild compression of the nervous structures in the absence of clinical disturbances and electromyographic abnormalities. On the other hand, in middle or early old age patients, decompression should be extended also to include areas of «relative» stenosis, particularly if there is no specific risk (scoliosis, spondylolisthesis, late sequelae of vertebral fractures) of postoperative instability, more particularly if vertebral stability is increased due to osteophytes connecting adjacent vertebral bodies or marked resorption of the intervertebral disc.

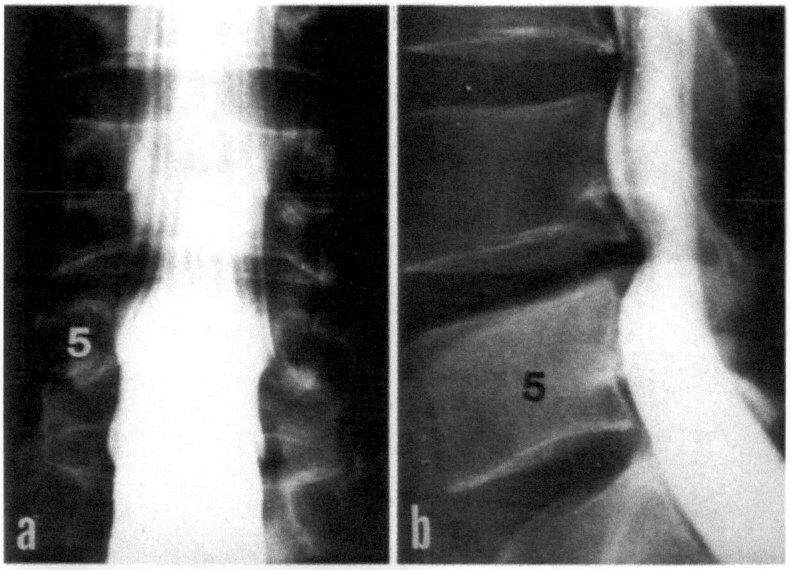

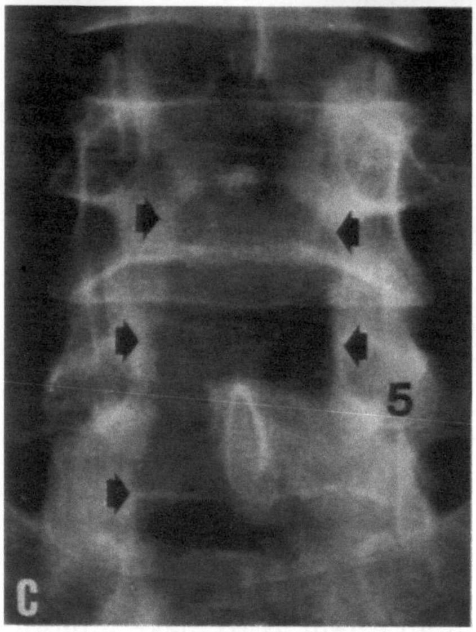

Fig. 9.2 - A-46 year-old man with right sciatic pain due to compression of the S_1 nerve root. Myelograms (**a** and **b**) showed, in addition to a slight L_5-S_1 disc herniation on the right, L_4-L_5 stenosis (which was asymptomatic) due to a marked posterior prominence of the lower bony end-plate of L_4. At surgery (**c**), L_5-S_1 disc herniation was excised and bilateral laminectomy at L_4-L_5 level (arrows) was performed.

Mono- or bilateral decompression

At those levels at which the need for decompression is absolute and stenosis is bilateral, decompression should be performed bilaterally. This is true both for patients with bilateral symptoms and/or signs, and those with unilateral symptomatology. When, at a given level, stenosis is severe and symptomatic on one side and mild and asymptomatic on the other, unilateral decomression may be considered, if discectomy is to be performed for an associated disc disease playing a significant role in the aetiology of nerve root compression. In fact, disc excision performed on one side may be sufficient to decompress the nervous structures on the opposite side. However, even in these cases, bilateral decompression is generally recommended.

At those levels at which the need for decompression is relative, the choice between unilateral and bilateral decompression should be made taking into consideration the severity of stenosis on the two sides, as well as those factors — patient's age, electrodiagnostic findings, vertebral stability — previously taken into account in determining the number of levels to decompress. As a general rule, if bilateral laminectomy is planned at the level of «absolute» stenosis, it is advisable to extend it also to the level of «relative» stenosis. On the other hand, when laminotomy is planned for the area of «absolute» stenosis, it is often sufficient to limit the decompression, for the area of «relative» stenosis, to the side of the more marked compression of the nervous structures (Fig. 9.3).

Type of decompression

The choice of the type of decompression has to be made when the spinal canal is to

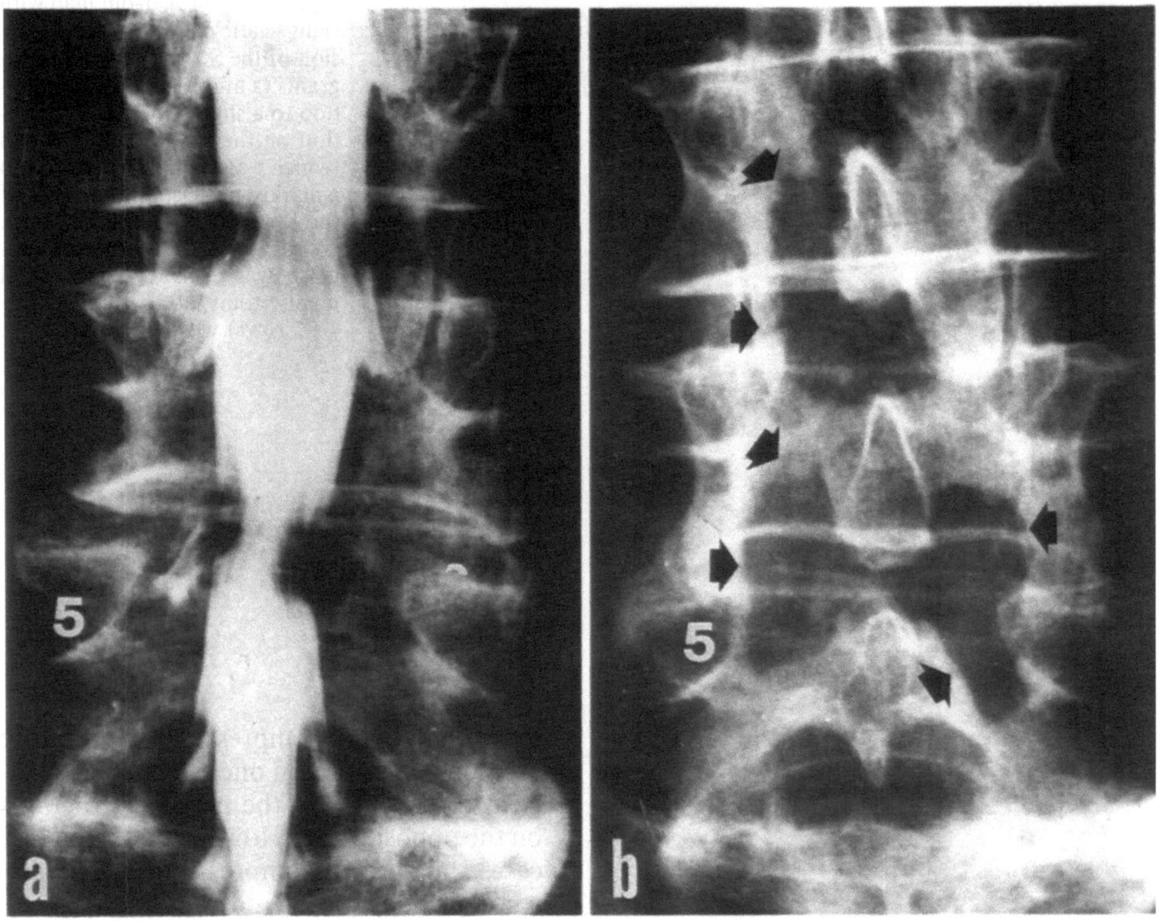

Fig. 9.3 - **a.** Symptomatic stenosis at L_4-L_5, more marked on the left, and asymptomatic stenosis at L_3-L_4. **b.** Bilateral laminotomy at L_4-L_5 and right laminotomy at L_3-L_4 (arrows) were performed.

be opened bilaterally. In these cases bilateral laminectomy or laminotomy may be carried out. Laminotomy, despite the advantage of almost completely preserving vertebral stability, may be difficult to perform when the interlaminar space is narrow or almost absent due to ossification of the ligamentum flavum. Furthermore, when laminotomy is carried out, on the same side, at two adjacent levels, also the narrow portion of lamina which should separate the two laminotomies is often removed, thus performing in effect unilateral laminectomy.

Excision of spinous processes and interspinous ligaments, that bilateral laminectomy entails, undoubtly reduces vertebral stability; not, however, to a significant degree and not to such an extent as to make a motion segment unstable, which is in itself stable.

Laminectomy, moreover, has the advantage of requiring a shorter operative time than laminotomy. In my opinion, bilateral laminectomy is preferable when bilateral decompression at more than two vertebral levels is to be performed, particularly if discectomy is not foreseen. Conversely, laminotomy is to be preferred in those patients presenting stenosis at one level or two levels, particularly when discectomy for a co-existing disc disease will probably be necessary, or when the vertebral level to be submitted to decompression is already unstable and in which spinal fusion is not planned.

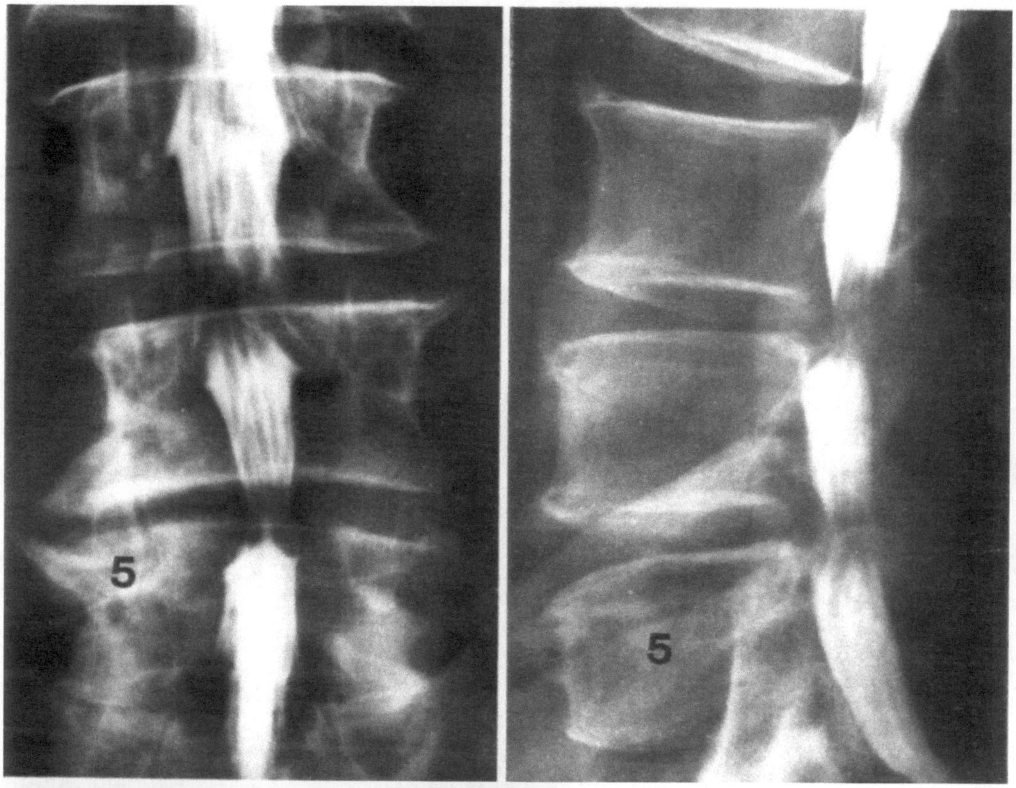

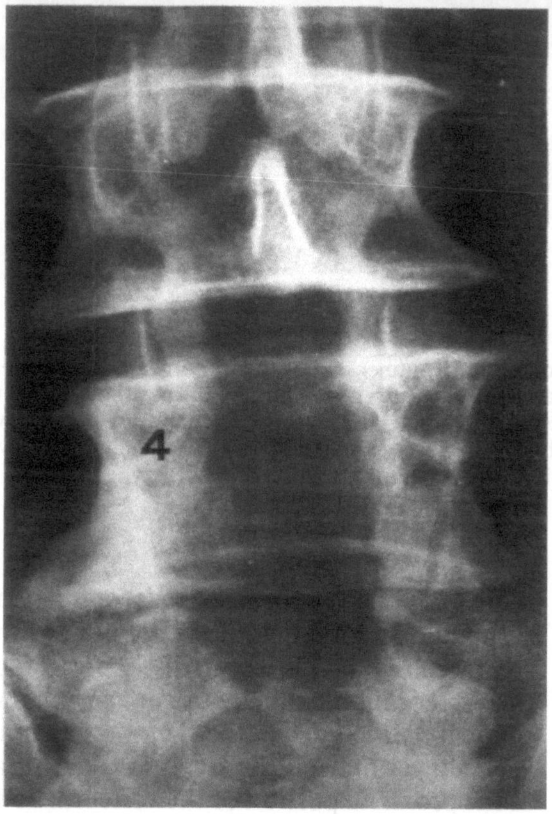

Fig. 9.4 - Myelograms show spinal canal stenosis at L_3-L_4 and L_4-L_5 levels. Laminectomy was extended proximally, as far as the middle portion of the L_3 laminae and, distally, to the caudal portion of the laminae of L_5. The neural structures were, therefore, adequately decompressed in the whole area opposite the intervertebral discs.

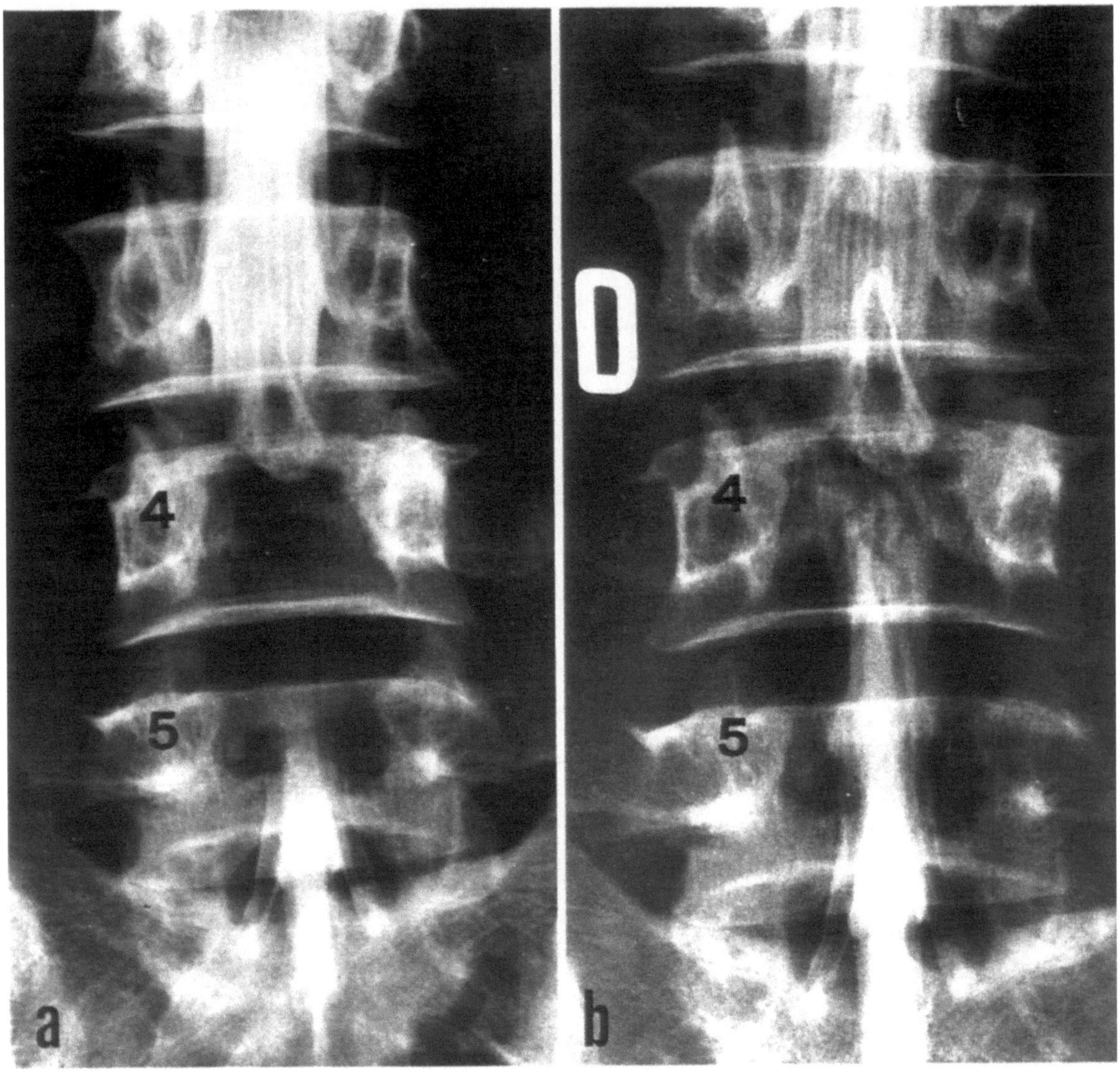

Fig. 9.5 - Inadequate decompression of the neural structures at the upper end of the stenotic area in a patient operated for L_3-L_5 spinal canal stenosis. **a.** Postoperative myelogram in semihorizontal position (10° anti-Trendelenburg) shows a persistent block of the contrast medium at L_3-L_4 level. **b.** The contrast agent flows distally in a semivertical position (50° anti-Trendelenburg); however, a partial block persists at L_3-L_4 level owing to non-removal of the distal portion of the neural arch of L_3 at surgery.

Longitudinal and transverse extent of decompression

Compression of the dural sac and spinal nerve roots usually occurs at intervertebral levels. To be adequate, therefore, decompression of the nervous structures should involve the whole area facing the intervertebral disc. That is, when performing laminectomy at more than one vertebral level, decompression should be extended, at the upper limit of the stenotic area, as far as the distal portion of the vertebral body above the most cephalad of the discs included in the stenotic area and, at the lower limit of the stenotic area, as far as the proximal portion of the vertebral body below the most caudal of the discs comprised in the area of stenosis (Fig. 9.4).

A frequent mistake, in fact, is to take decompression to the interlaminar space and not to proceed, at the level of the proximal disc, with removal of the distal portion of the inferior articular processes of the vertebra above and, at the level of the distal disc, with removal of the ligamenta flava and the basal portion of the superior articular processes of the vertebra below. As a result, areas of narrowing of the spinal canal may persist, which may be responsible for only partial relief or recurrence of radicular symptoms (Fig. 9.5).

In a transverse direction, laminectomy or laminotomy should be extensive enough to adequately decompress the dural sac and the spinal nerve roots in the radicular canal (Fig. 9.6). The optimal facetectomy is that in which the medial half, or preferably two thirds, of the superior and inferior articular processes are removed. In fact, with time, the borders of the residual portion of the articular processes tend to undergo remodeling, leading to partial reforming of the facet joint (Fig. 9.7). When facetectomy is too limited, remodeling of the borders of the articular processes may lead to recurrence of stenosis in the nerve root canal or spinal canal (Fig. 9.8). Total facetectomy, however, must be avoided not only because the far lateral portion of the articular processes is not usually responsible for compression of the nervous structures, but more particularly because total arthrectomy may lead to the risk of postoperative vertebral instability.

Vertebral fusion

Effects of laminectomy on vertebral stability

When performing bilateral laminectomy

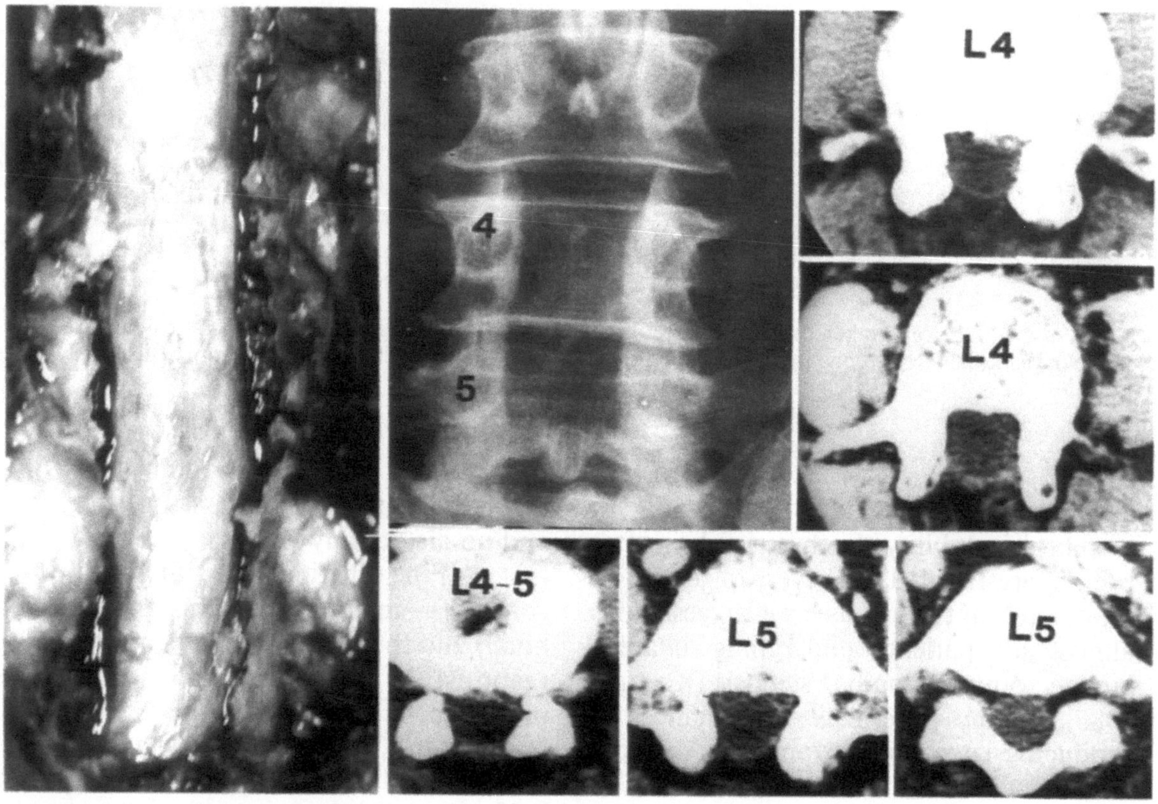

Fig. 9.6 - Left, intraoperative photograph taken at the end of bilateral laminectomy; the spinal canal should be open in the transverse direction far enough to completely expose the thecal sac and visualize the spinal nerve roots. Right, postoperative radiograph and CT scans of the same patient. CT scans confirm the adequacy of decompression of the neural structures in the transverse direction.

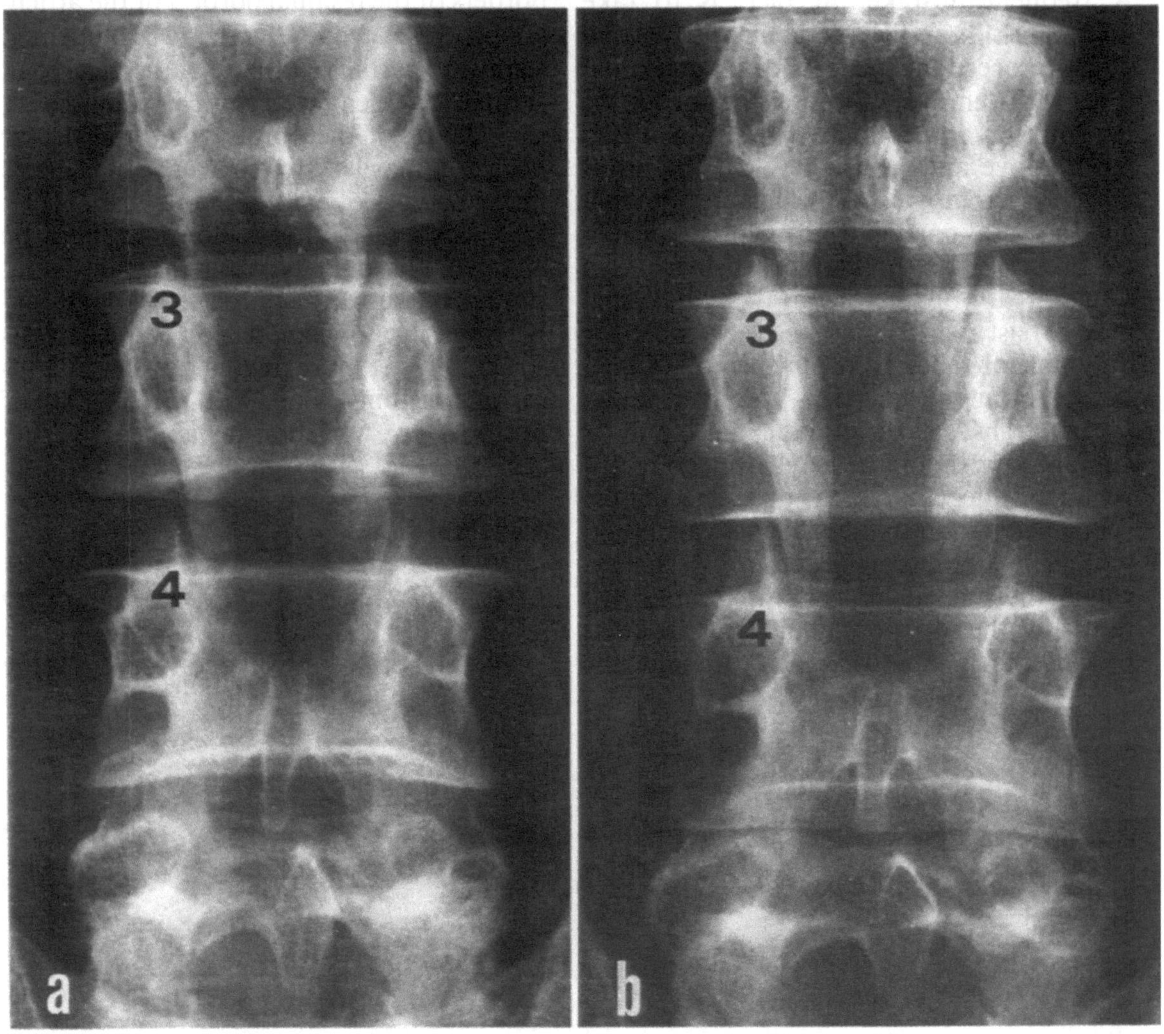

Fig. 9.7 - a. Radiograph taken one month after bilateral laminectomy performed for L_2-L_4 spinal canal stenosis. Note subtotal facetectomy, particularly on the right side. **b.** Eight months later the inferior articular processes have partly reformed.

at several levels, there is a risk of producing vertebral instability. Such a risk has often been overestimated, however, to the extent that vertebral fusion has been suggested for almost all patients undergoing bilateral laminectomy for lumbar stenosis (Kostuik, 1986). In my experience, the chances of producing iatrogenic instability are strictly related to the degree of vertebral stability prior to surgery.

When a motion segment is preoperatively stable, bilateral laminectomy does not lead to instability if the lateral one half or one third of the articular processes are preserved and no discectomy is carried out (Fig. 9.9); that is, if the functional integrity of the three columns — intervertebral disc (and vertebral body) and the two facet joints — which are responsible for vertebral stability is preserved.

Similarly, no instability usually occurs when, at an individual level, the lateral one half or one third of the articular processes on one side is preserved and no discectomy is carried out (Fig. 9.10). Functional integrity of two out of the three vertebral columns,

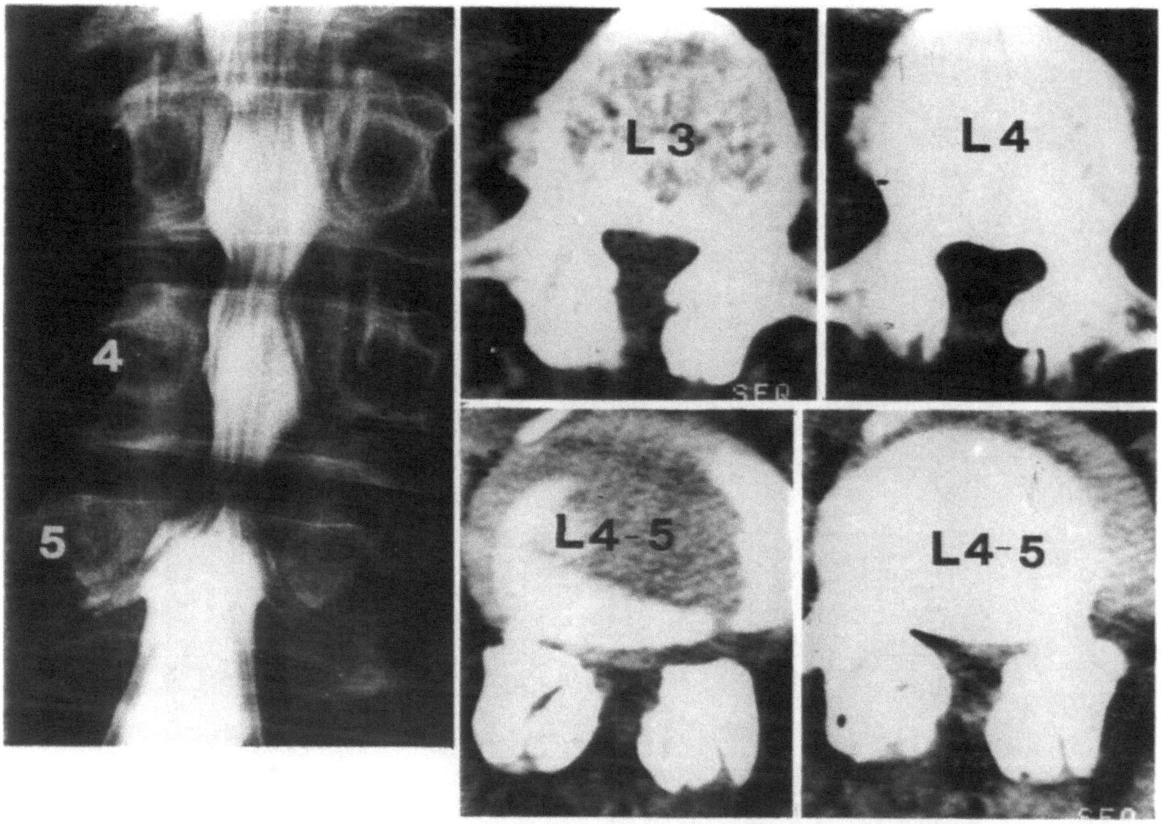

Fig. 9.8 - Myelography and CT scan performed 4 years after bilateral laminectomy from L_3 to L_5. Myelogram shows persistent compression of the neural structures at L_3-L_4 and, particularly, L_4-L_5 levels. CT scans reveal insufficient opening of the vertebral canal due to limited facetectomy at L_4-L_5 level.

is, in fact, generally sufficient to guarantee vertebral stability. Furthermore, it should be pointed out that when facetectomy is subtotal, remodeling of the residual portion of the articular process may restore a sort of joint, which contributes, even if to a lesser extent than a normal joint, to maintain vertebral stability.

Lastly, when a motion segment is stable prior to surgery, instability rarely occurs, even when, at an individual intervertebral level, bilateral total facetectomy and monolateral discectomy are carried out (Fig. 9.11). In these cases, vertebral stability is maintained by the anterolateral and residual posterior portions of the annulus fibrosus, if the latter is structurally and functionally intact. On the other hand, the chance of causing instability of a motion segment is high when bilateral facetectomy and discectomy are performed, particularly if the continuity of the posterior longitudinal ligament is interrupted along the midsagittal plane.

When a motion segment is unstable preoperatively, bilateral laminectomy extended too far laterally, or even bilateral laminotomy, may increase the instability. This is particularly true when discectomy, especially if bilateral, is performed (Fig. 9.12).

Indications to fusion

Regardless of degenerative spondylolisthesis, vertebral fusion should be planned, in addition to decompression, when the area to decompress is unstable or when bilateral laminectomy and discectomy are to be performed. In particular, the indications for spinal fusion are generally as follows: 1)

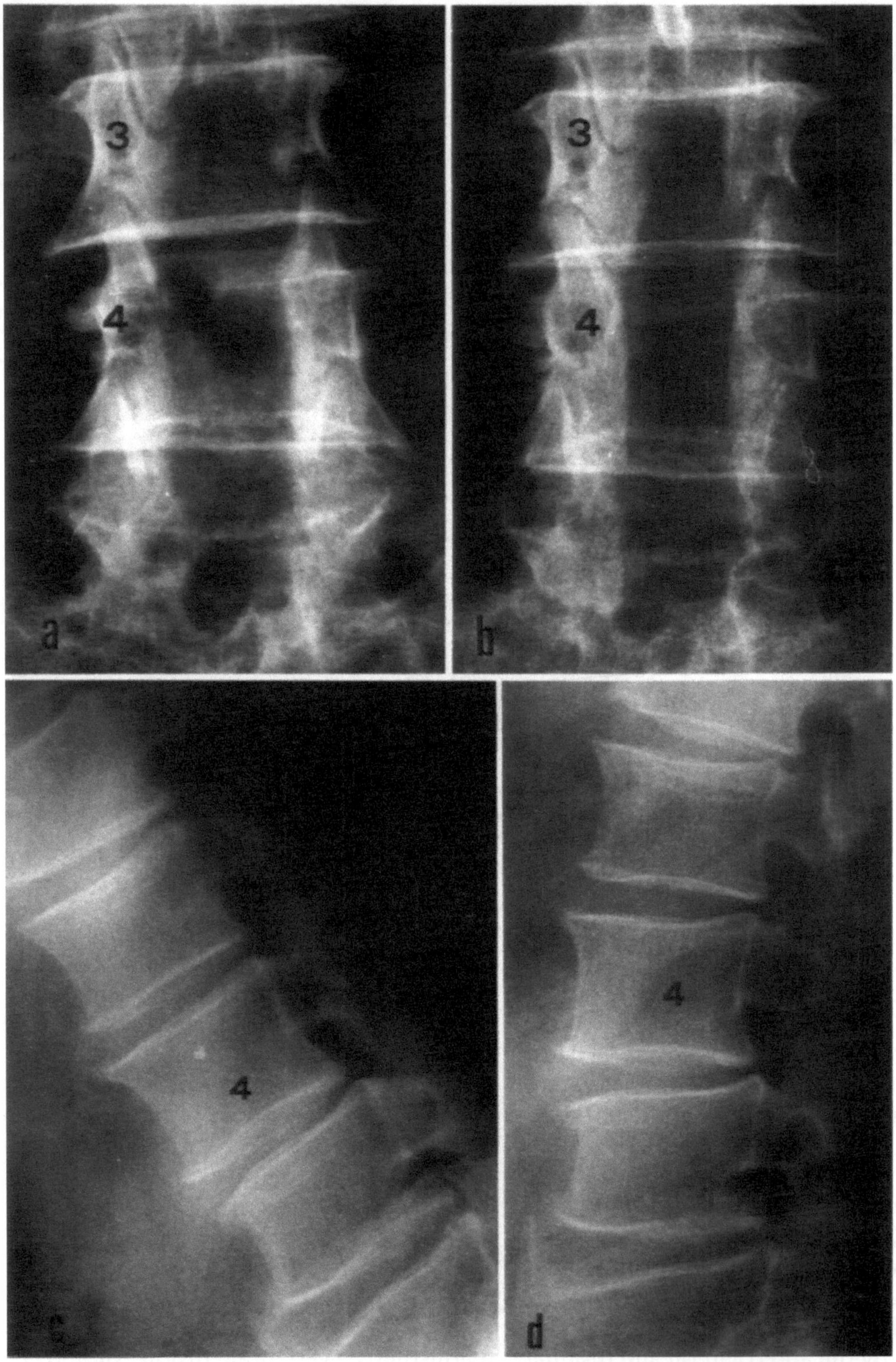

Fig. 9.9 - a. and **b.** Radiographs taken 1 month (**a**) and 3 years (**b**) after L_2-S_1 bilateral laminectomy with no discectomy; note remodelling and partial reconstitution of the articular processes. **c.** and **d.** Three years after surgery, flexion and extension radiographs of the lumbar spine reveal no evidence of vertebral instability. The mild degenerative spondylolisthesis present preoperatively in L_4, does not appear to be increased in the functional radiographs.

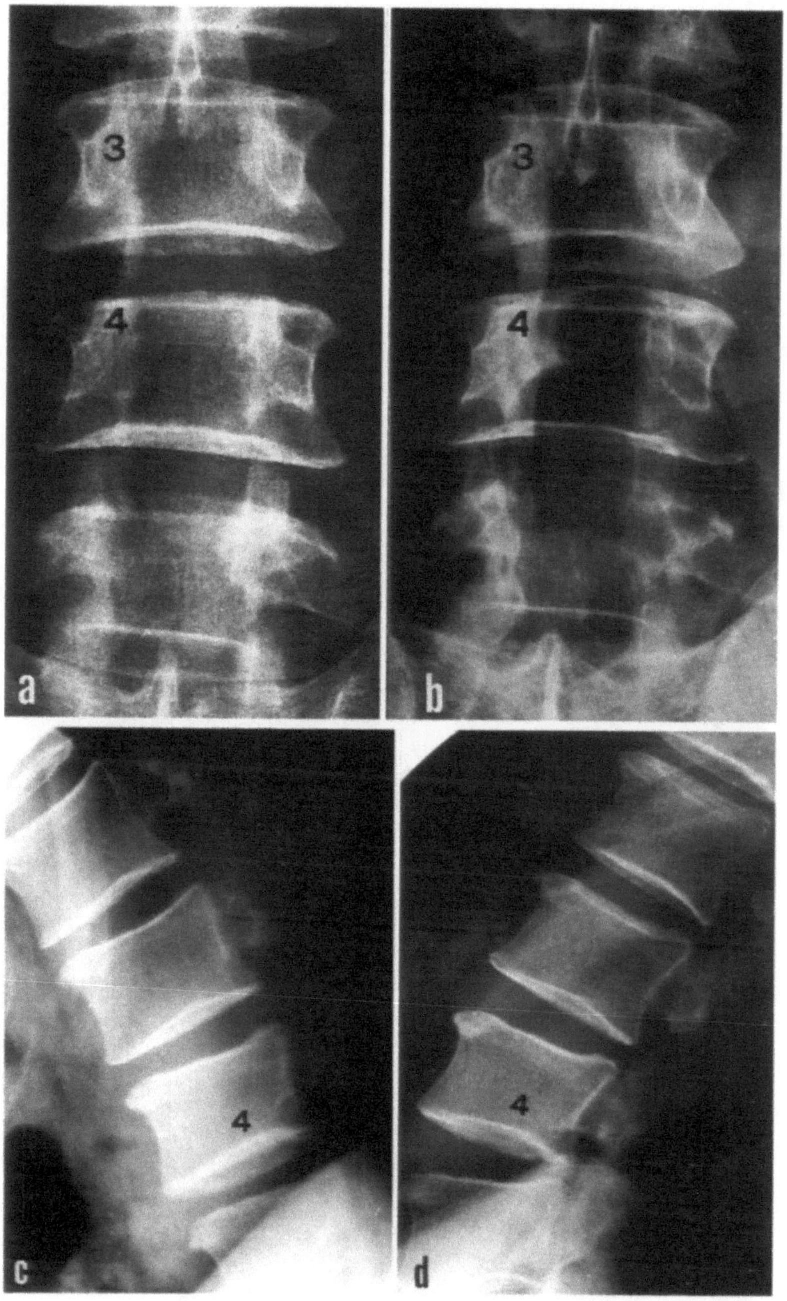

Fig. 9.10 - a. Radiograph of the lumbar spine 2 months after a wide L_2-S_1 bilateral laminectomy, associated with complete facetectomy at L_3-L_4 and L_4-L_5 levels, on the left. **b.** Six years later, remodelling and reformation of the articular processes was observed, except at L_3-L_4 level on the left. **c.** and **d.** Flexion and extension radiographs show a stable lumbar spine, even at L_3-L_4 level. The patient reported no back pain.

in patients under 70 years of age with stenosis at an unstable level, in whom bilateral laminectomy is to be carried out; 2) in young or middle aged patients with stenosis at only one level for which bilateral laminectomy has been planned and in whom discectomy will probably be necessary and it may be impossible to adequately preserve the articular processes. This may occur, in particular, for the upper lumbar levels, in which the intrinsic shortness of the laminae (which is even more marked in subjects with a narrow spinal canal) may make it difficult to decompress the nervous structures without sacrificing the facet joints.

In both cases the higher, i.e. structurally

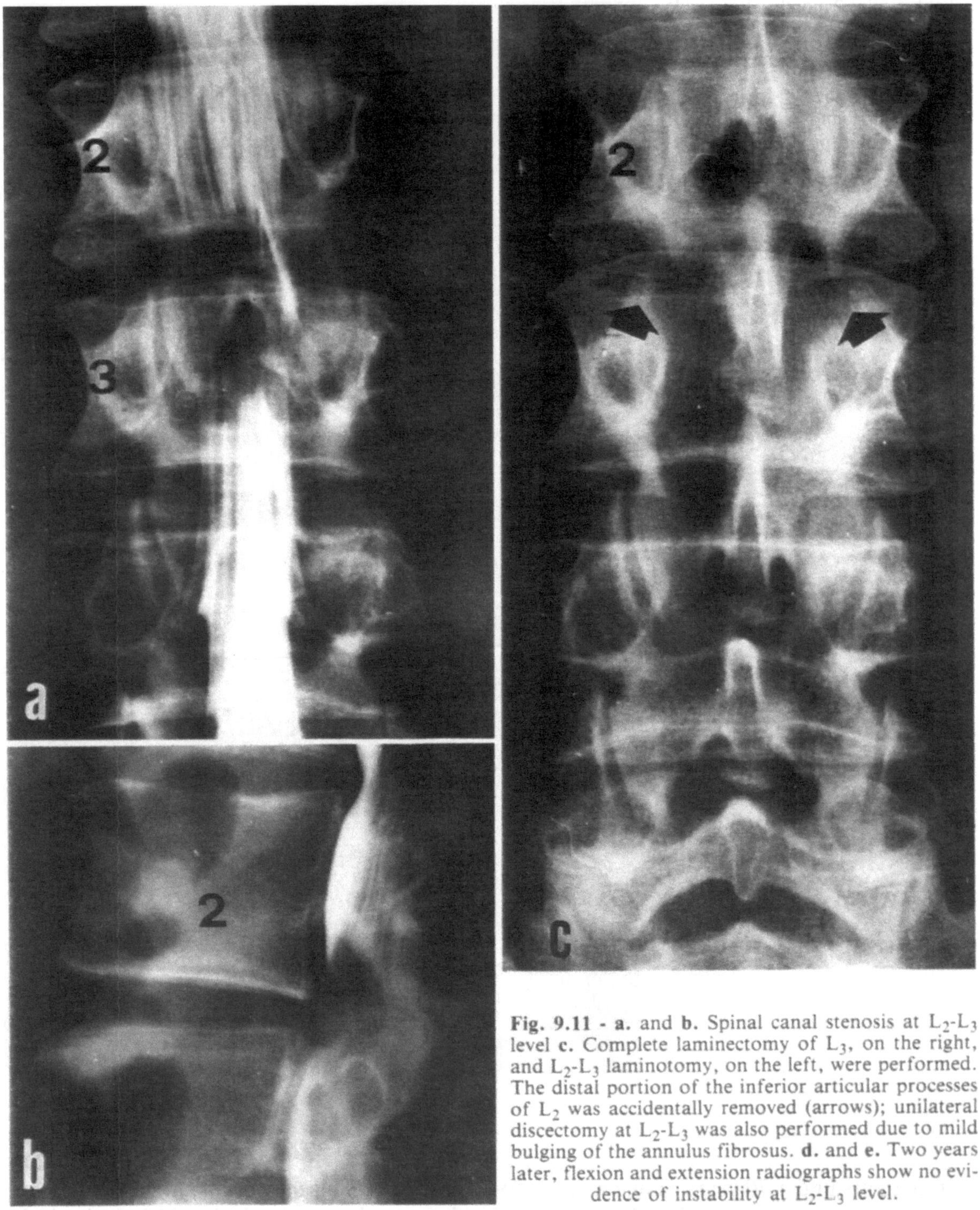

Fig. 9.11 - **a.** and **b.** Spinal canal stenosis at L_2-L_3 level **c.** Complete laminectomy of L_3, on the right, and L_2-L_3 laminotomy, on the left, were performed. The distal portion of the inferior articular processes of L_2 was accidentally removed (arrows); unilateral discectomy at L_2-L_3 was also performed due to mild bulging of the annulus fibrosus. **d.** and **e.** Two years later, flexion and extension radiographs show no evidence of instability at L_2-L_3 level.

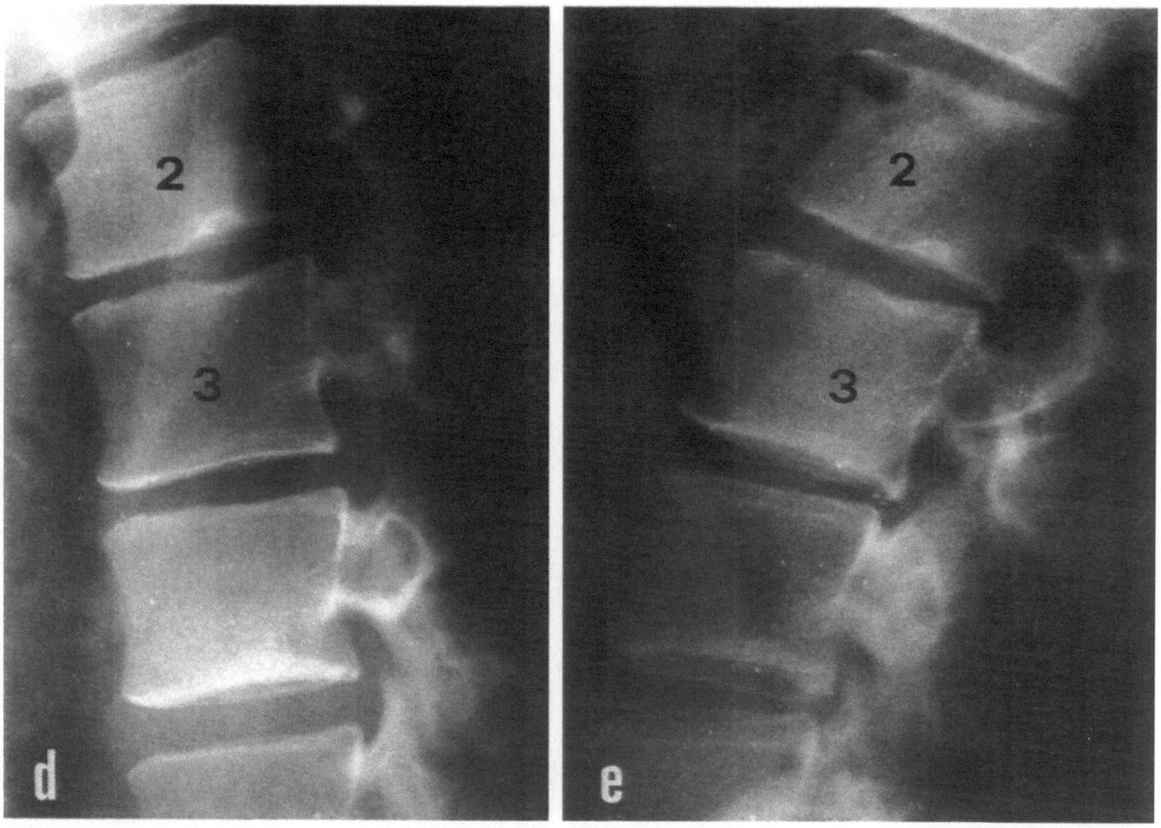

Fig. 9.11 - (continued)

intact, the intervertebral disc, the greater the need for fusion.

Planning of surgery in degenerative spondylolisthesis

Degenerative spondylolisthesis may be considered a condition of relative vertebral instability. In fact, olisthesis, which is a sign of instability, may, or may not, be associated with abnormal mobility of the slipped vertebra in flexion-extension movements of the lumbar spine. In the first instance, the olisthetic vertebra is definitly unstable, whereas in the second the instability may be considered only potential.

Planning of surgery in degenerative spondylolisthesis depends, firstly, on the presence, or not, of hypermobility of the slipped vertebra on functional radiographs and, secondly, on the degree of slipping and patient's age.

When the olisthetic vertebra is only potentially unstable, planning of the operation depends on the severity of vertebral slipping and patient age. If slipping is mild, surgery should be planned regardless of the presence of olisthesis, whatever the patient's age. In these cases, in fact, bilateral laminectomy adequately preserving the articular processes does not lead to postoperative instability (Fig. 9.13). In those patients with spondylolisthesis of moderate degree the treatment of choice is laminotomy, particularly in the absence of complete myelographic block, or bilateral laminectomy preserving the lateral one half of the articular processes (Figs. 9.14 and 9.15). In both instances, if the patient is under 60 years of age, spinal fusion should be carried out, especially when the normal, or almost normal, height of the disc below the olisthetic vertebra increases

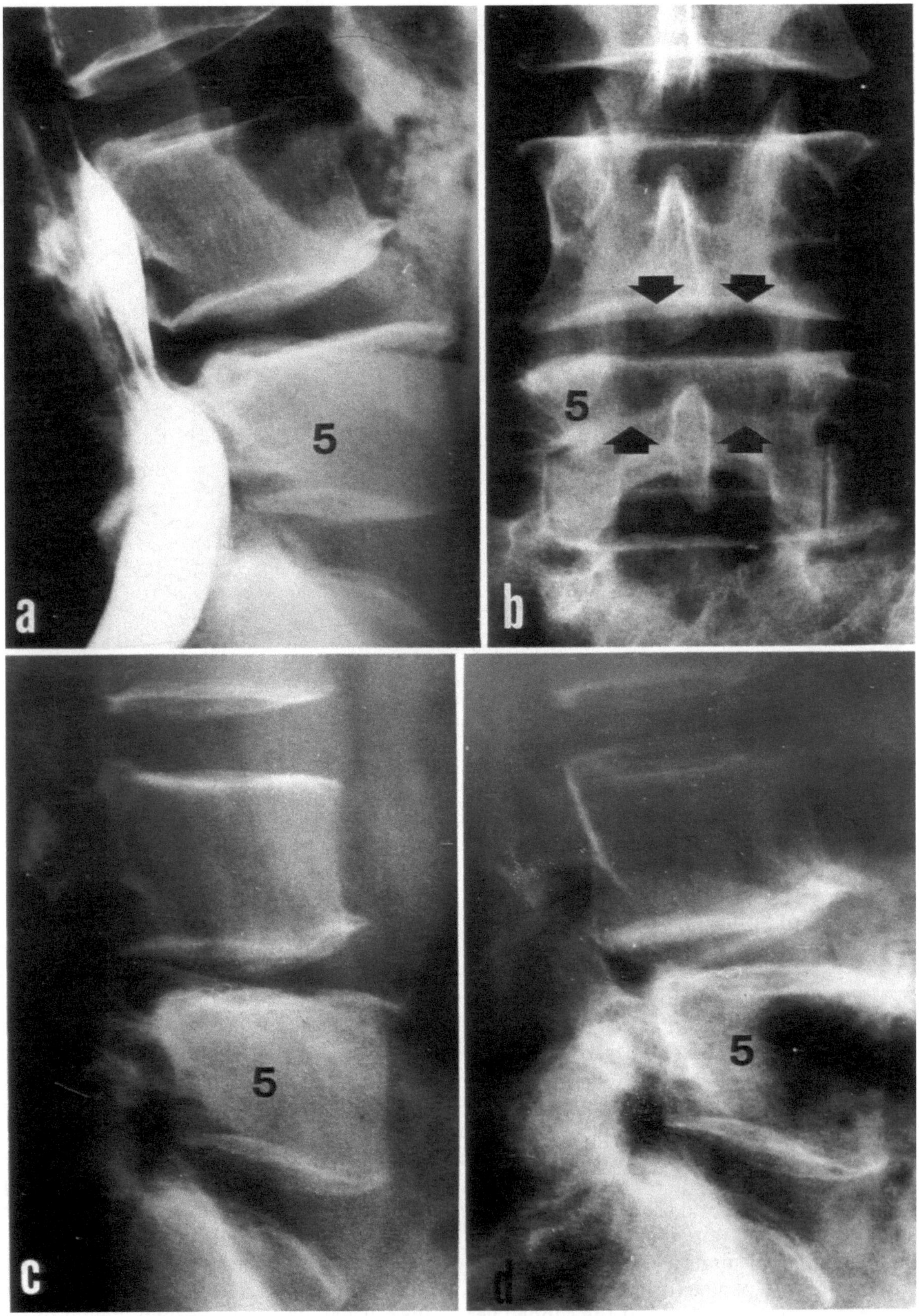
a
5
b
5
c
5
d
5

the chances of a subsequent vertebral slipping (Figs. 9.16 and 9.17). When spondylolisthesis is severe, vertebral fusion should be performed in addition to decompression, at least in patients under 70 years of age.

If the olisthetic vertebra is unstable, arthrodesis should always be carried out in addition to decompression (Fig. 9.18), the only exception being very elderly patients or patients in poor general conditions.

Isolated stenosis of the nerve root canal

Generally, in isolated stenosis of the nerve root canal, in which only one vertebral level is usually involved, lminotomy, extended distally to a varying extent depending on the site of nerve root compression, should be performed (Figs. 9.19 and 9.20).

In the presence, at any one level, of a symptomatic nerve root compression on both sides, bilateral decompression should be carried out, even if on one of the two sides radicular symptoms are mild and no neurological abnormality is present. When myelography and/or CT scan show, at any one level, bilateral nerve root compression in the presence of radicular symptoms and signs on one side only, bilateral decompression should generally be planned, especially if electrodiagnostic investigations show evidence of compression of the clinically asymptomatic nerve root, and the absence of a significant discogenic component in the nerve root compression tends to suggest that disc excision on one side may not result in adequate decompression of the nerve root on the opposite side (Fig. 9.20). Similar observations apply to patients with unilateral stenosis at two contiguous intervertebral levels. In these cases monolateral laminectomy or, preferably, two contiguous laminotomies may be performed. Bilateral laminectomy is indicated only in the presence of bilateral stenosis at two (or more) contiguous levels, when decompression of all the involved nerve roots has to be performed, but it is necessary to reduce to a minimum the operative time, which is generally shorter for a bilateral laminectomy than for multiple laminotomies.

Discectomy should generally be planned in patients in whom preoperative investigations show evidence of a bulging intervertebral disc at the stenotic level. Preoperatively, however, it is often difficult to determine the precise role played by the intervertebral disc in the aetiology of nerve root compression. In these cases, the decision of whether, or not, to carry out disc excision has to be made during surgery, on the basis of the operative findings (see page 205).

Spinal fusion is rarely needed in patients with stenosis of the nerve root canal. Arthrodesis is indicated when bilateral decompression is carried out at a preoperatively unstable level, particularly if a mono-or bilateral disc excision is performed. Fusion may also be indicated in patients complaining of longstanding low-back pain caused by disc degeneration (Crock, 1983) at the stenotic level or levels.

ANAESTHESIA

Spinal or general anaesthesia may be employed. Spinal anaesthesia, which is often preferable to general anaesthesia in patients with pulmonary disorders, may be indicated in patients with nerve root canal stenosis or single level stenosis of the spinal canal. In cases of multilevel spinal canal stenosis, in which a long surgical procedure may be poorly tolerated by the non-sleeping patient, general anaesthesia is recommended.

◄

Fig. 9.12 - Postoperative increase of a preoperative vertebral instability. **a.** Preoperative instability at L_4-L_5 level is indicated by retrolisthesis of L_4. **b.** Bilateral laminotomy, with preservation of the lateral portion of the articular processes (arrows), and bilateral discectomy were performed. **c.** Retrolisthesis showed no evidence of increase one month after surgery. **d.** At six months, retrolisthesis had considerably increased and the patient complained again of bilateral low-back and radicular pain.

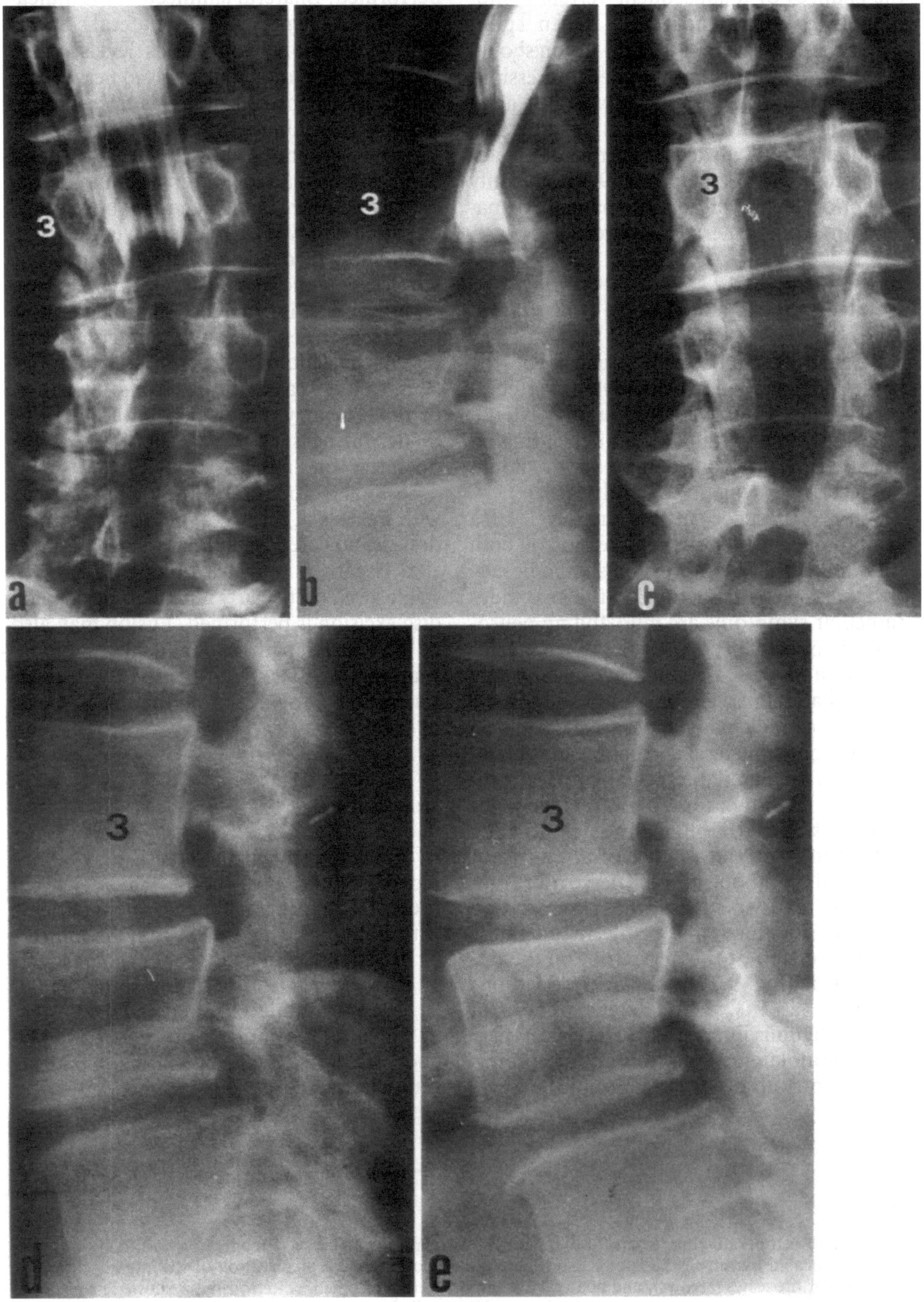
3
a
3
b
3
c
3
d
3
e

Hypotensive anaesthesia

The difficulties encountered in surgical procedures involving opening of the spinal canal are related, to a large extent, to bleeding from the bony walls of the canal and, in particular, the epidural vessels. Heavy bleeding, which hinders visualization of the nervous structures, makes the operation more difficult, prolongs the operative time and increases the risk of iatrogenic lesions to the dural sac and caudal nerve roots. Furthermore, abundant bleeding may lead to excessive blood loss and the need, or greater need, for blood replacement with all the risks that transfusional therapy involves. Operative blood loss may be reduced with controlled general anaesthesia maintaining arterial blood pressure below normal values. The advantages of hypotensive anaesthesia are observed when systolic blood pressure is decreased by at least 50 mmHg below the patient's basal values, i.e. when blood pressure is lowered, in an adult with normal arterial pressure, between 70 to 90 mmHg. With these values, Lawhon *et al.* (1984) obtained a decrease of 33% of blood loss in adult scoliotic patients undergoing spinal fusion, compared to patients submitted to normotensive anaesthesia. In my experience, a similar decrease in operative blood loss is obtained in surgical procedures involving opening of the spinal canal, particularly in long operations such as multilevel bilateral laminectomy.

Hypotensive anaesthesia, in contrast with obvious advantages, presents a 0.85% morbidity rate (Larson, 1964) due to complications of varying nature such as reactive haemorrhage, persistent hypotension, oliguria or anuria, thromboembolism, neurological and cardiovascular disturbances. Deliberate hypotension, therefore, should be avoided in patients with acute hepatic disease, renal conditions, cerebrovascular disease, arteriosclerotic heart disease or any other condition causing a significant reduction in pulmonary ventilation, cardiac output, haemoglobin concentration or oxygen saturation of arterial blood.

In patients with lumbar spinal stenosis, the anaestesiologist should be prepared to induce controlled hypotension and should warn the surgery team ahead of time when the patient's general conditions are not suitable for hypotensive anaesthesia. The surgeon should request hypotension when, upon opening of the spinal canal or during subsequent operative stages, he has to face copious bleeding from the epidural or bony vessels. The anaestesiologist should be warned in time that the operation is almost finished in order that he might slowly bring the arterial blood pressure back to normal values. Only when this has been obtained should the final haemostasis of the epidural and osseous vessels be started.

PATIENT POSITIONING

The prone position is to be preferred to the lateral posture—particularly for bilateral laminectomy — because it allows better lighting of the operative field and more adequate visualization of the nervous structures on both sides.

For operation in the prone position, a well-padded rigid frame supporting the anterior iliac crests is recommended; the frame, which allows the abdomen to be free, avoids excessive bleeding from the epidural and osseous vessels. Alternatively, the genupectoral position may be used, placing a pillow under the chest with the knees flexed at 110°-130° and the buttocks supported by a frame. In both instances, the head of the operating table should be raised

◀

Fig. 9.13 - Complete myelographic block in a woman with mild degenerative spondylolisthesis of L_3 and L_4 (**a** and **b**). Preoperative functional radiographs reveal no hypermobility of the olisthetic vertebrae. A L_3-L_5 bilateral laminectomy was performed (**c**) preserving the lateral half of the articular processes. Two years after surgery, flexion (**d**) and extension (**e**) radiographs demonstrate complete stability of the lumbar spine and no increase of olisthesis.

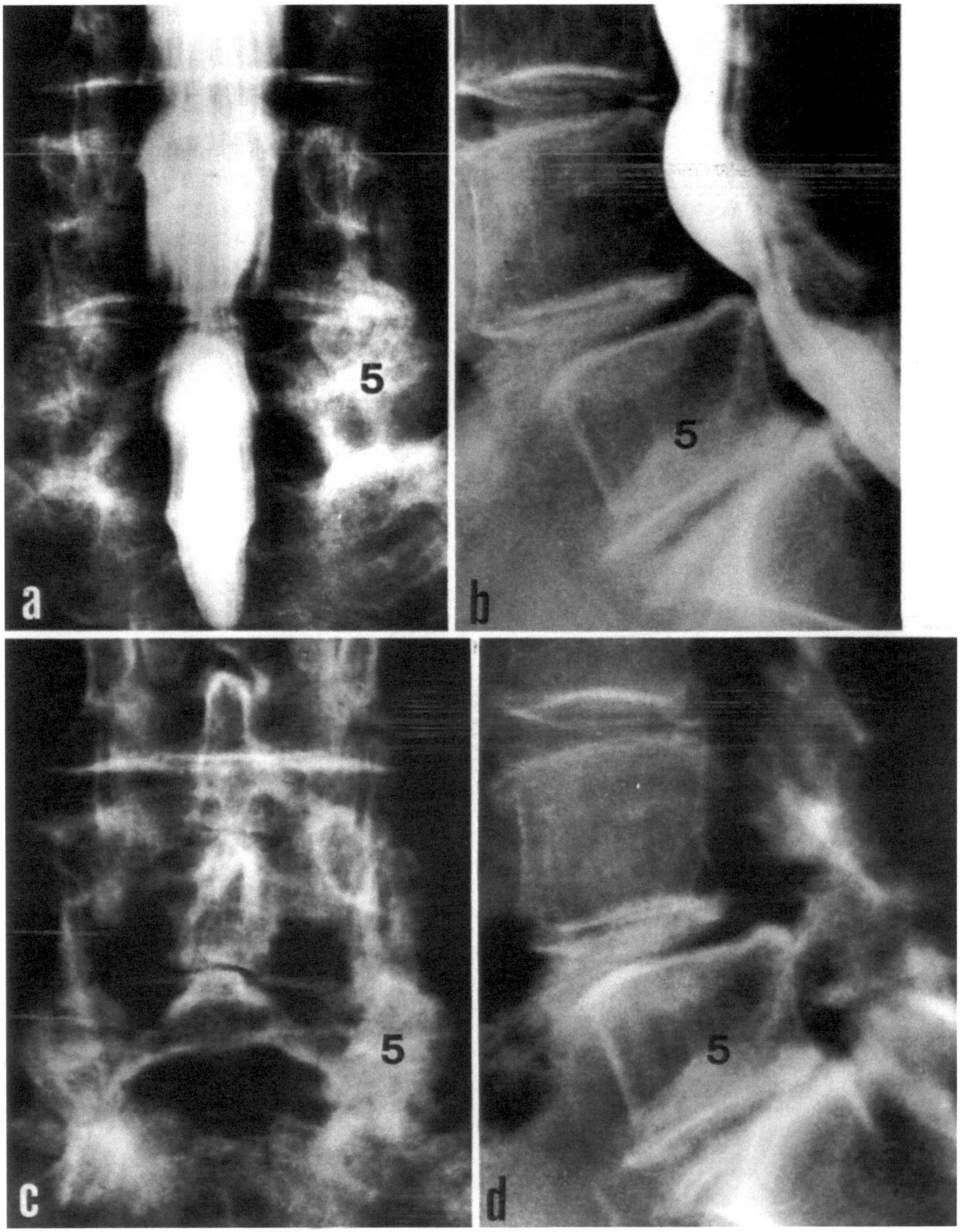

Fig. 9.14 - Degenerative lumbar stenosis at L_4-L_5 with spondylolisthesis of L_4 (**a** and **b**). Bilateral laminotomy was performed (**c**) preserving the lateral one third of the articular processes. One year after surgery (**d**) no increase was observed in slipping of L_4.

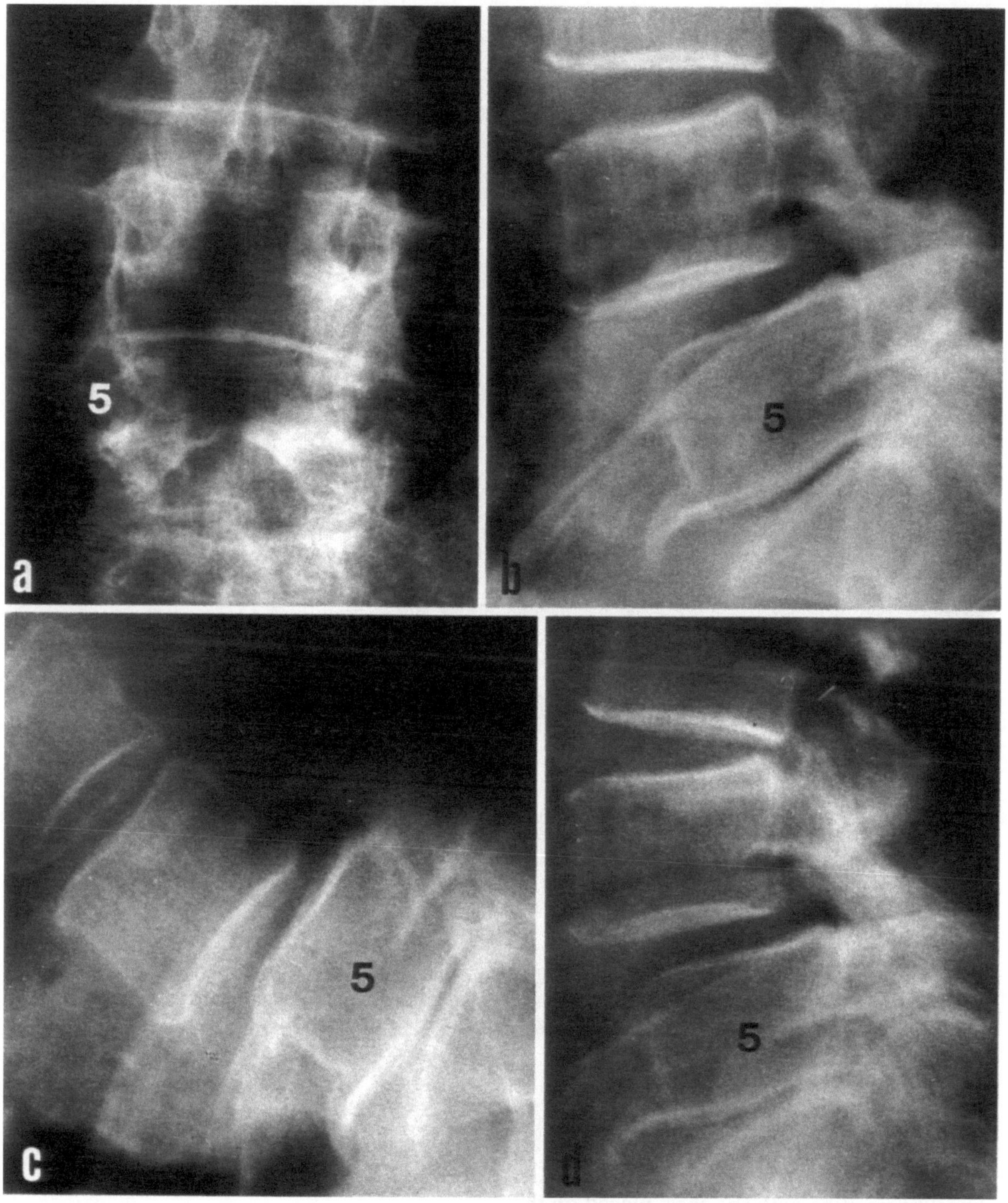

Fig. 9.15 - **a.** and **b.** Plain radiographs of a 69-year-old woman with degenerative spondylolisthesis of L_4, who had been submitted, one month previously, to bilateral laminectomy at L_4-L_5 level. **c.** and **d.** Functional radiographs, two years after surgery, show no increase in slipping of L_4 and no change in spinal flexion and extension.

(anti-Trendelenburg position) in order that the lumbar spine will be horizontal. This makes surgical manoeuvres easier and avoids stasis of brain circulation and subsequent edema, which may be responsible, in older patients submitted to general anaesthesia, for

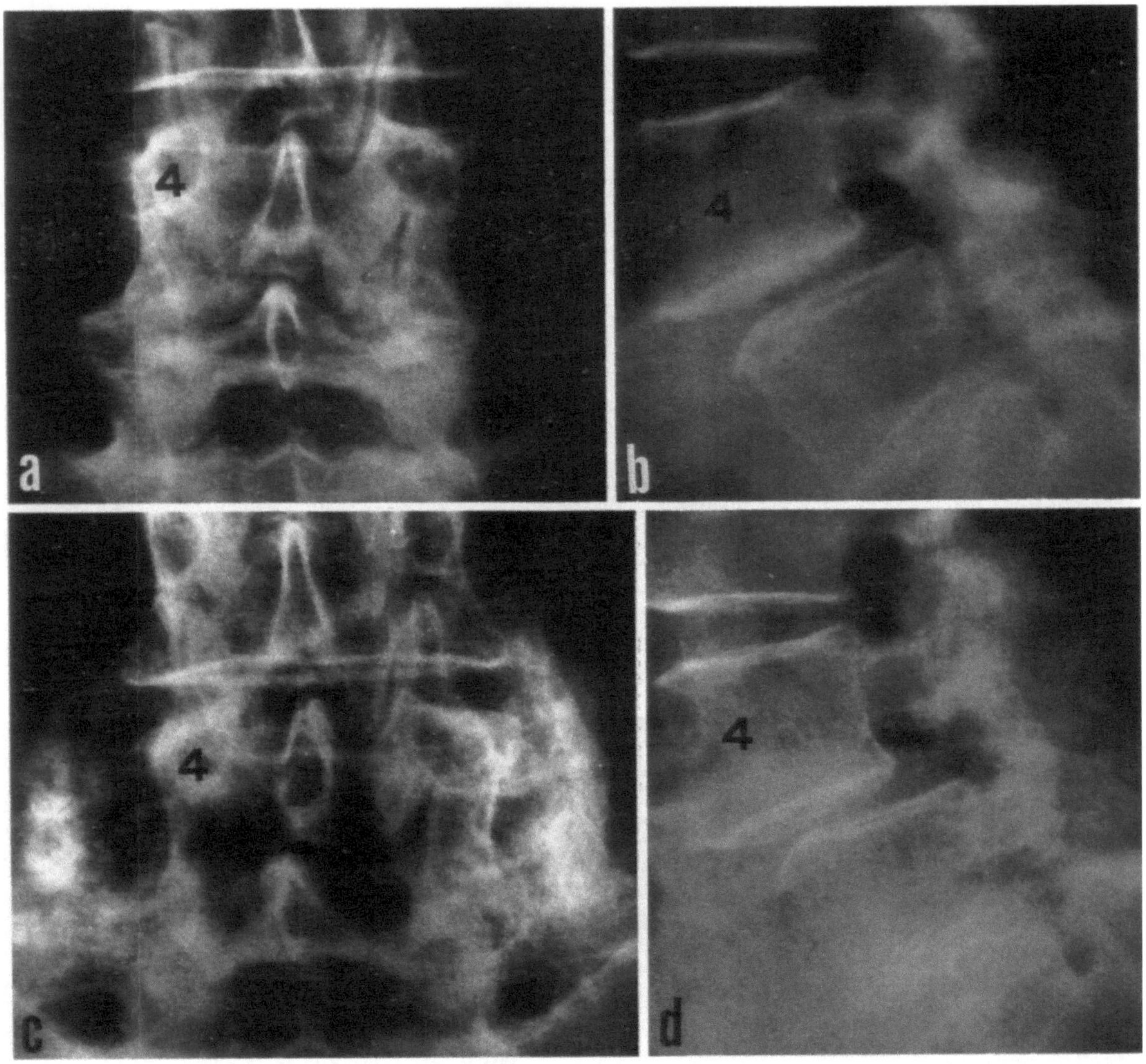

Fig. 9.16 - a. and **b.** A 54-year-old woman with degenerative spondylolisthesis of L_4 and L_4-L_5 spinal canal stenosis. **c** and **d.** Radiographs obtained 8 months after bilateral laminotomy and intertransverse fusion (**c**). A slight increase in slipping of L_4 occurred postoperatively (**d**).

postoperative confusional disturbances. Another variant to the prone posture is the kneeling position with the chest placed on the operating table angled at 90°, the knees flexed and the buttocks supported by a posterior frame. The kneeling position has the disadvantage of not reducing lumbar lordosis and, thus, not widening the interlaminar spaces. It has the advantage, however, of allowing the abdomen to be completely free and, unlike the genu-pectoral position, is well tolerated by the patient operated under spinal anaesthesia.

PREOPERATIVE IDENTIFICATION OF SPINAL LEVELS

After positioning of the patient, the interspinous spaces are palpated starting from the lumbosacral interspace in order to identify, before draping, the level or levels at which the spine is to be exposed. When identi-

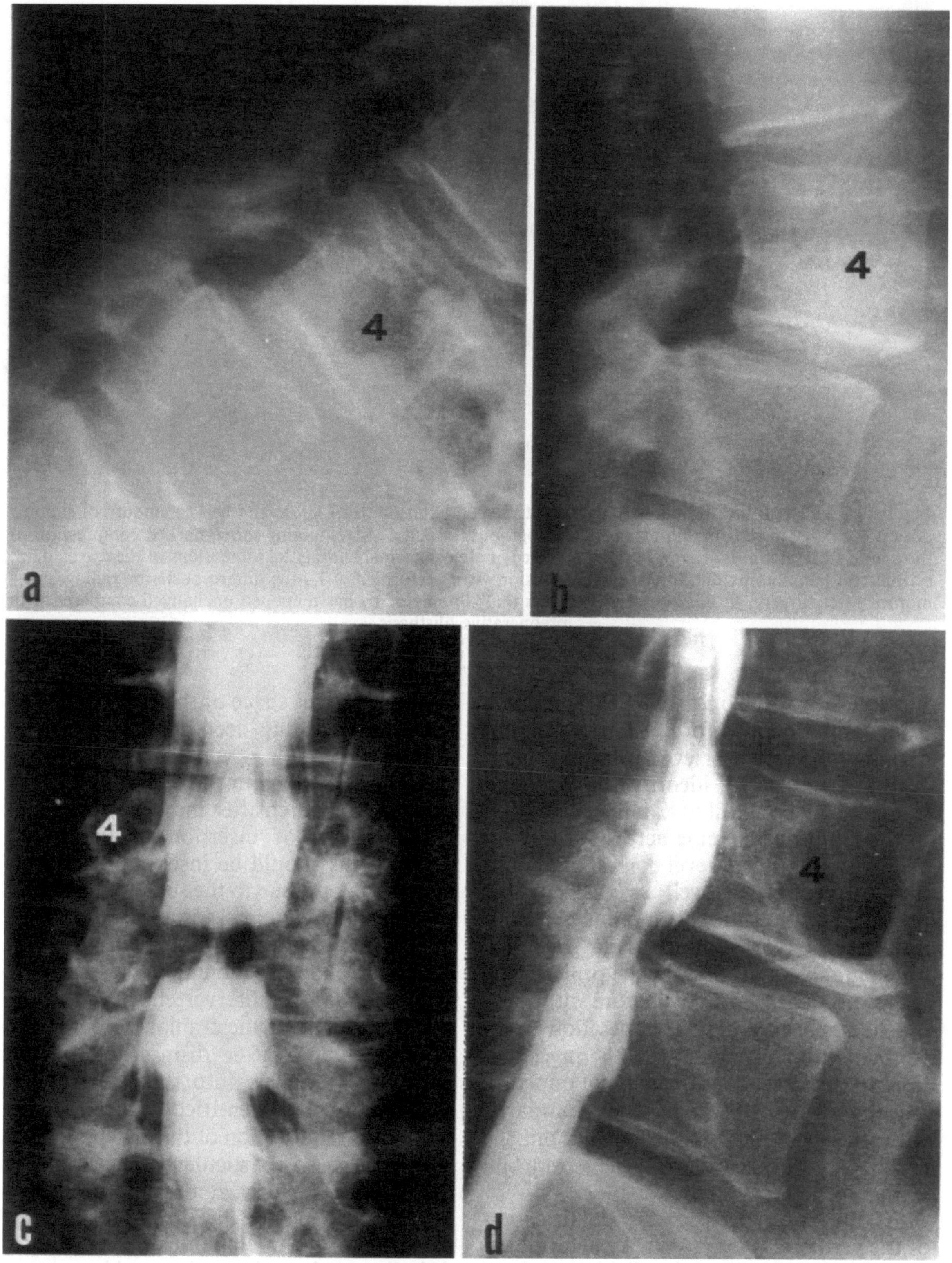

Fig. 9.17 - (legend on the following page).

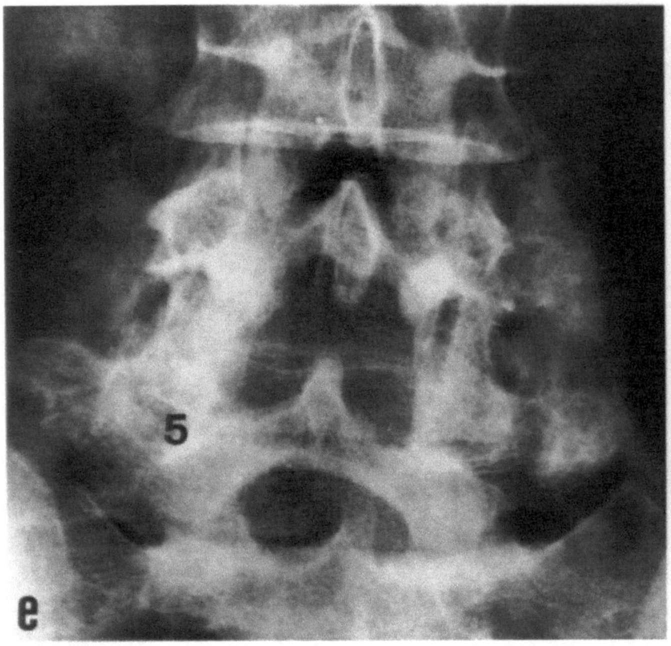

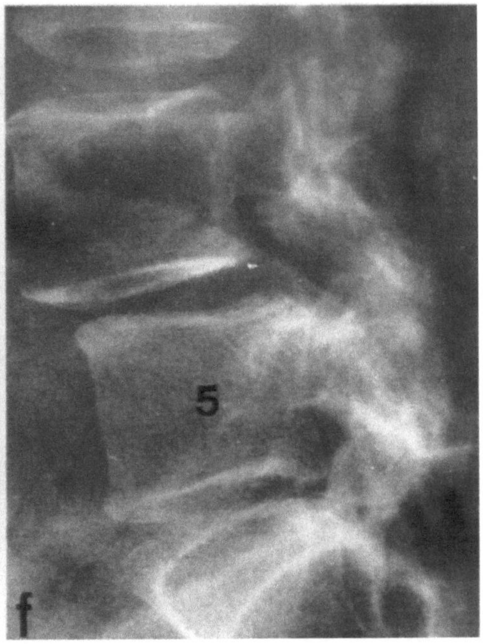

Fig. 9.17 - A 51-year-old woman with degenerative spondylolisthesis of L_4. **a.** and **b.** The amount of slipping does not change in flexion and extension radiographs. **c.** and **d.** Myelograms show marked compression of the neural structures at L_4-L_5 level, in the presence of almost normal midsagittal dimensions of the dye column. **e.** Bilateral laminotomy and intertransverse fusion were performed at L_4-L_5; antero-posterior radiograph 4 months after surgery. **f.** The lateral view shows that slipping of L_4 has remained unchanged compared with preoperative olisthesis.

fication is easy, the operative field is draped, using palpation also for definitive determination of the vertebral levels prior to skin incision. To correctly identify the vertebral levels, it may be useful to examine plain films of the lumbosacral spine before surgery, to determine the spinal level corresponding to the iliac crests, as well as the possible presence of transitional anomalies, spondylolisthesis or spina bifida occulta. Myelography may also be helpful, if the lateral myelogram is taken before withdrawing the spinal needle and the operation is performed within a few days of the investigation; in this case, the site of spinal puncture may be identified, which, when compared with the position of the needle on the myelogram, will allow one of the intervertebral spaces to be recognized.

If doubts still persist in the identification of the vertebral levels, it may be helpful, before draping the operative field, to take a lateral x-ray of the lumbosacral spine, after introducing a 19 or 20 G spinal needle into the interspinous space of the level, or one of the levels, needing decompression. Rather than a radiograph — which may be of poor quality when taken in the operating theatre — the image intensifier may be used to detect the level of insertion of the spinal needle. This should be inserted, at a given interspace, opposite to the superior end-plate of the caudal vertebra. In fact, since the laminae are orientated obliquely in a craniocaudal direction, positioning of the landmark at the level of the intervertebral disc or the lower end-plate of the cranial vertebra may lead to sliding, after disinsertion of the paraspinal muscles, into the interlaminar space above that identified by needle.

X-ray identification of the vertebral levels before surgery is particularly helpful in the presence of stenosis at the upper lumbar levels, which may be difficult to identify by palpation of the interspinous spaces, due to their distance from the lumbosacral interspace. The alternative, in these cases, is to make a long skin incision reaching the lumbosacral

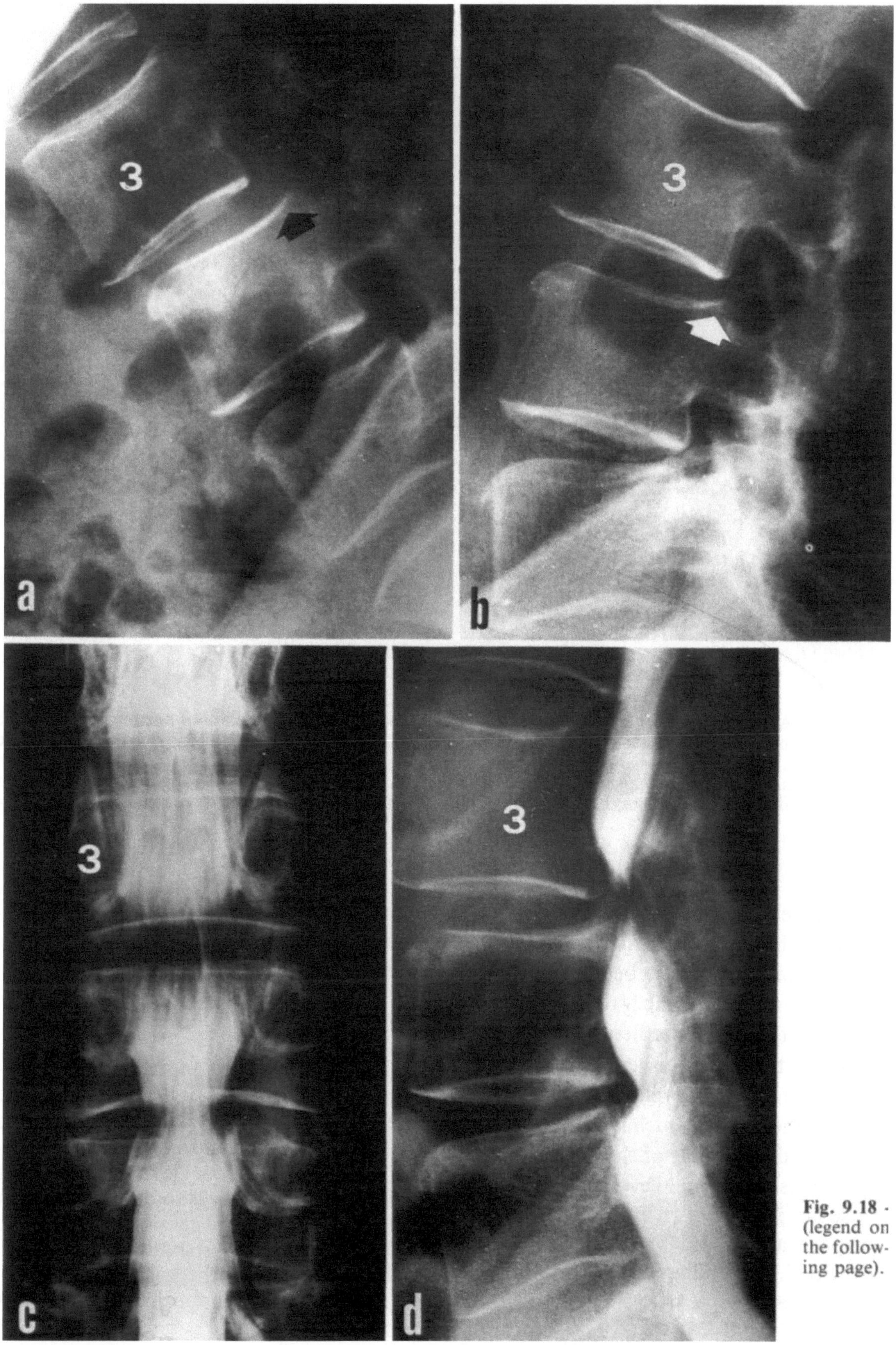

Fig. 9.18 · (legend on the following page).

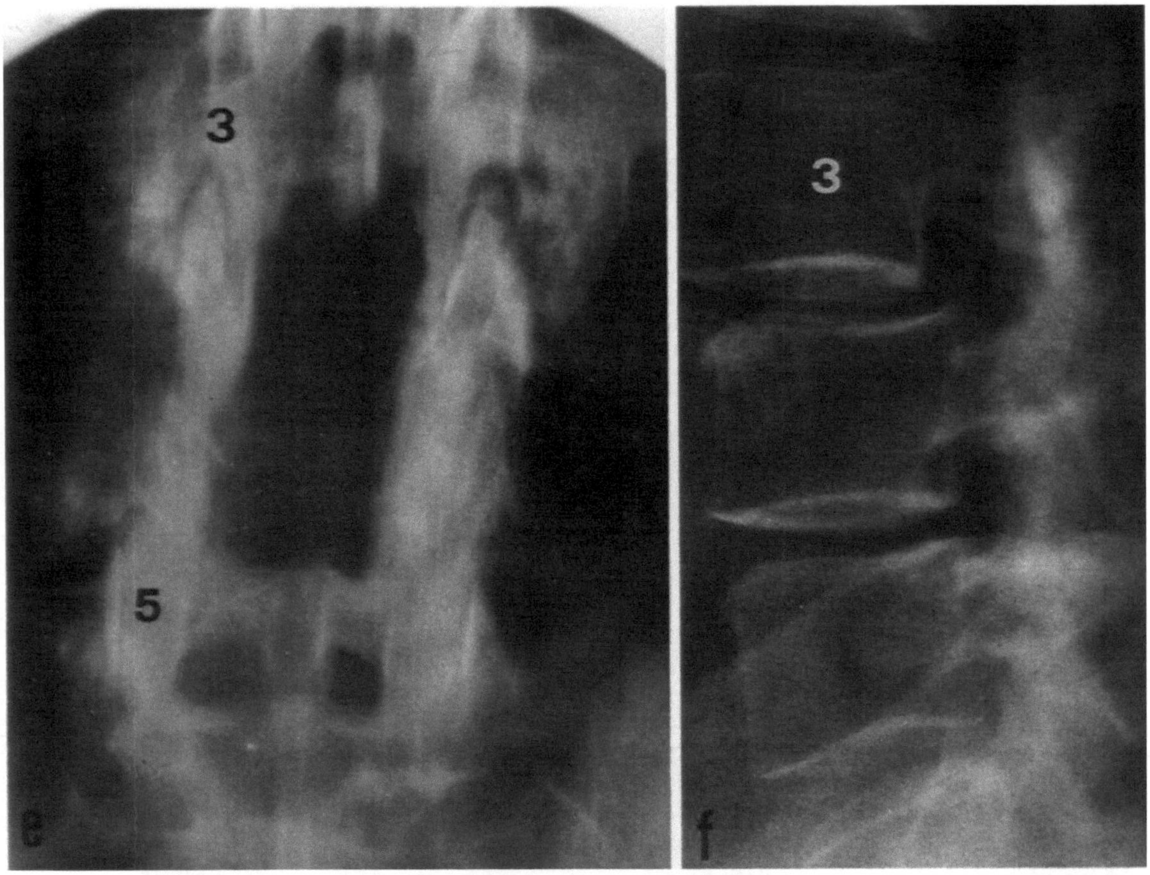

Fig. 9.18 - A 56-year-old woman with degenerative spondylolisthesis of L_3. **a.** and **b.** Functional radiographs show hypermobility of the slipped vertebra (arrows). **c.** and **d.** Myelograms show a complete block of the dye column at L_3-L_4 level and posterior protrusion of the annulus fibrosus at L_4-L_5 with partial filling of L_5 nerve root sheaths. e. Radiographic picture 6 months after L_3-L_5 laminectomy with bilateral intertransverse fusion at L_3-L_4 and unilateral fusion at L_4-L_5. **f.** Slipping has remained almost unchanged compared with preoperative condition.

interspace and to expose — damaging the paravertebral muscle to some extent — all the interlaminar spaces below the stenotic level or levels. Once the intervertebral level at which the spinal needle was inserted has been identified, a transverse line is marked on the skin with a dermographic pen at the level of the needle, which is then withdrawn to proceed to draping of the operative field. In the presence of multilevel stenosis, a transverse line is also drawn at the level of the interspace above and/or below that earlier identified, depending on the number of stenotic levels.

SURGICAL TECHNIQUE

Bilateral laminectomy

Skin incision and superficial haemostasis

The skin is incised on the midline. If decompression has to be performed at a single intervertebral level, skin incision runs from the interspinous space above to that below the intervertebral level involved. If bilateral laminectomy is to be carried out at one or more levels, the incision extends from the cranial edge of the spinous process above, to the caudal edge of the spinous process below that of the vertebra, or the group of ver-

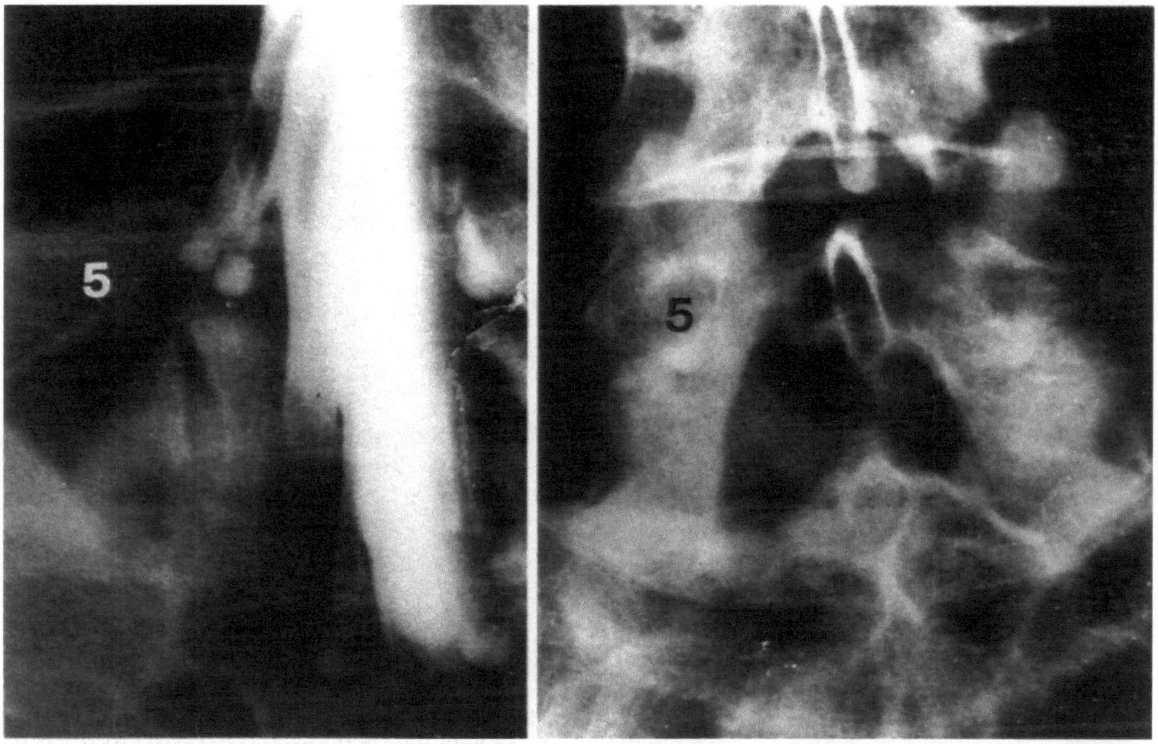

Fig. 9.19 - Isolated stenosis of the right S_1 nerve root canal. Laminotomy, extending one centimetre beyond the L_5-S_1 disc, was performed. The disc, which appeared to be degenerated but not herniated, was excised.

tebrae, needing decompression. The superficial layer of subcutaneous tissue is cut with the original skin incision. Dermal and subdermal vessels may be cauterized or preferably clamped together with a small portion of surrounding tissue; clamps (usually placed at a distance of approximately one centimetre from each other) are then turned outwards of the surgical wound and held together with an elastic band anchored to the surgical drape. This step makes haemostasis of the superficial vessels very rapid and avoids cauterization, which, when excessive, may damage the derma and superficial subcutaneous tissue with the subsequent possibility of delayed healing of the skin. The remaining portion of subcutaneous tissue is then incised. If the latter is very thick, the deep portion may be detached from the supraspinous ligament and adjacent portions of the thoracolumbar fascia with a dry sponge. One or two Adson retractors may be applied, if necessary, to widen the exposure of the fascial plane. Subcutaneous vessels are coagulated until the operative field is free from blood. Cauterization may be carried out rapidly and precisely using a sucker in the bleeding areas. In this and the subsequent operative stages a sucker of medium calibre should be used, whereas a thin aspiration cannula must be employed for epidural vessels to avoid damage to the nervous structures.

Disinsertion of paraspinal muscles

The thoracolumbar fascia is incised starting on the side of operator immediately adjacent and parallel to the tip of the spinous processes and interspinous ligaments, using a plain knife or, preferably, an electric cautery knife (Fig. 9.21). Frequently, the tip of the spinous processes may be palpated, but is not visible, particularly in subjects with well developed paraspinal muscles. In these

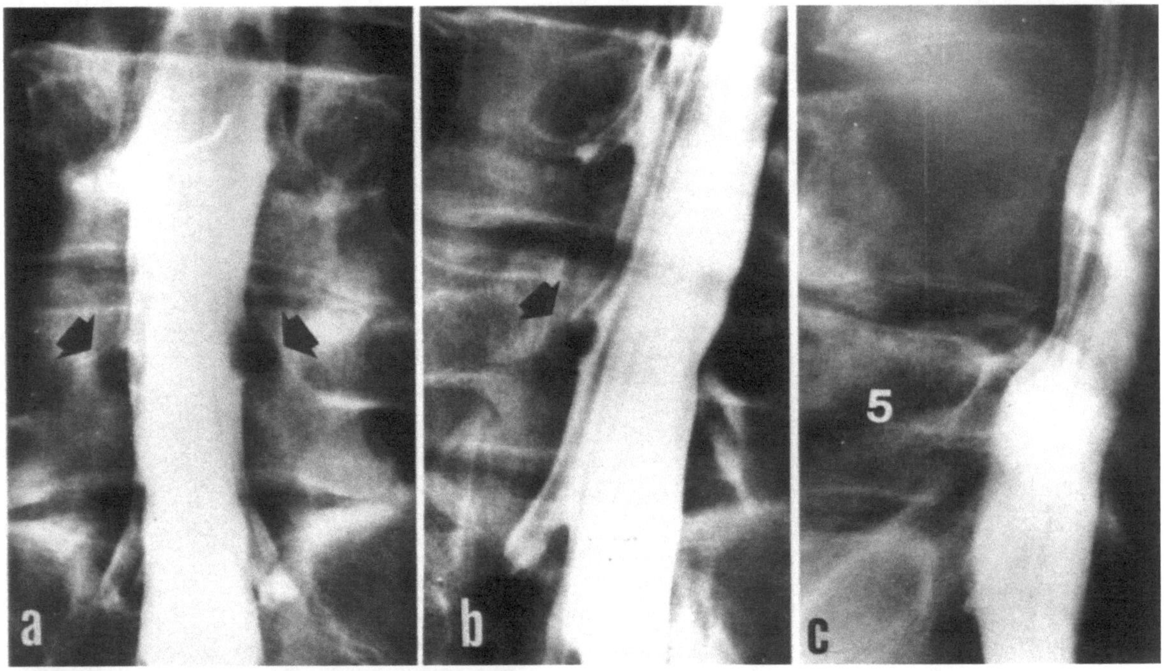

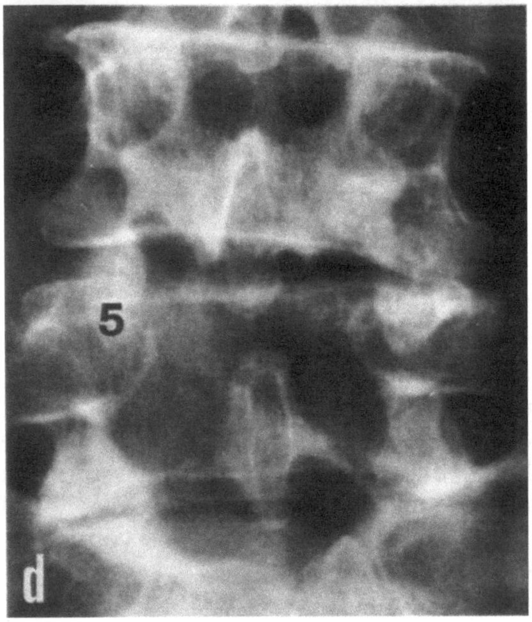

Fig. 9.20 - Isolated stenosis of the nerve root canal of L_5 on both sides in the presence of retrolisthesis of the L_4 vertebra (**a, b** and **c**). The patient complained of L_5 radicular syndrome only on the right. A wide bilateral laminotomy was performed (**d**), with decompression of the L_5 nerve roots as far as the entrance of the intervertebral foramen. The L_4-L_5 disc was not excised.

instances, the fascia may be erroneously incised along the median line or one may inadvertently pass over the opposite side. To avoid this, the assistant operator should press down the paraspinal muscles on his side using a periosteal elevator applied against the outer surface of the spinous processes in order that these are clearly visible to the operator (Fig. 9.21). The latter may carry out this same manouvre on his side, while incising the fascial layer.

Disinsertion of the paraspinal muscles starts from the most cranial of the exposed vertebrae. A broad periosteal elevator is introduced deep to muscle mass and allowed to slip along the outer surface of the spinous process and lamina to strip the spinal muscles from the spine to the lateral margin of the apophyseal joints (Fig. 9.22). Dry sponges are then packed, using the periosteal elevator, beneath the muscle mass (Fig. 9.23). This manoeuvre is aimed both at disinserting the paraspinal muscles from the lateral portion of the laminae and the facet joints, and arresting bleeding from the posterior branches of the lumbar arteries and veins. When spinal muscles are correctly separated, without stripping the periosteum and penetrating the muscle mass, very little bleed-

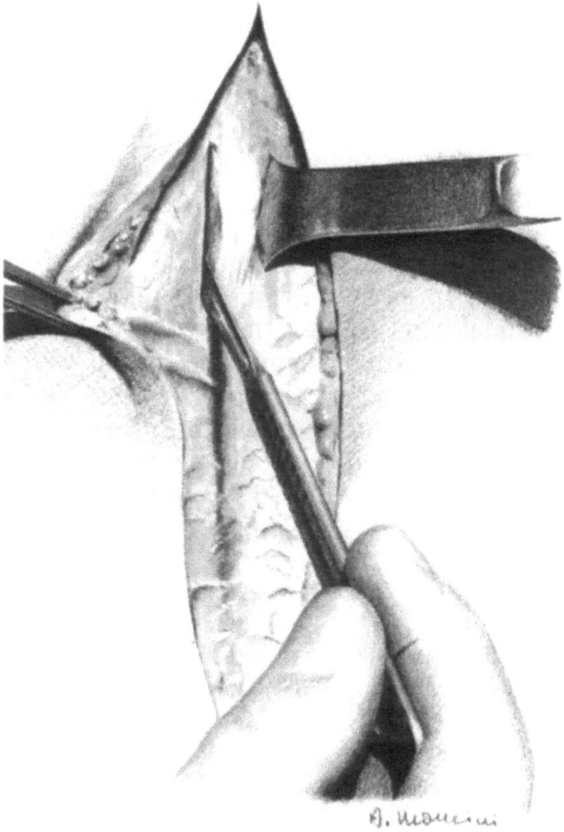

Fig. 9.21 - Incision of the thoracolumbar fascia with a plain or electric cautery knife. The latter may be used for sectioning the insertions of the paraspinal muscles to the laminae and the spinous processes. During incision of the fascia, it may be helpful if the assistant presses down the paraspinal muscle mass on the opposite side with a periosteal elevator to better expose the tip of the spinous processes, in order to section the fascia in close proximity to the latter.

ing occurs and is, usually, very well controlled following insertion of dry sponges, which are temporarily left in place. The same manoeuvres are then performed on both sides at all the vertebral levels to be exposed (Fig. 9.23). Sponges packed at the level of two contiguous vertebrae are subsequently removed and, while retracting the muscle mass, the residual musculo-tendinous attachments to the base of the spinous processes and interspinous ligaments are sectioned using a diathermy knife or scissors. Disinsertion of muscles from the two contiguous vertebrae and intervertebral space is completed with periosteal elevator. At this stage, care should be taken not to penetrate with the elevator into the interspinous ligament, because it is possible to enter the spinal canal and damage the dural sac. Care should also be taken not to slip with the periosteal elevator on the outer surface of the apophyseal joints and pars interarticularis in order to avoid injury to the stems of the posterior branches of the lumbar arteries resulting in copious bleeding, which may be difficult to control due to the lateral position of the vessels. After separation of the spinal muscles at two contiguous vertebral levels, dry sponges are again packed into the depth of the wound and the vertebrae and intervertebral spaces below are then exposed. Subsequently, while remaining on the same side of the patient, the paraspinal muscles on the opposite side are dissected, with the help of the assistant retracting the muscle mass.

At this stage, one or two self-retaining retractors, depending upon the length of the wound and the number of exposed vertebrae,

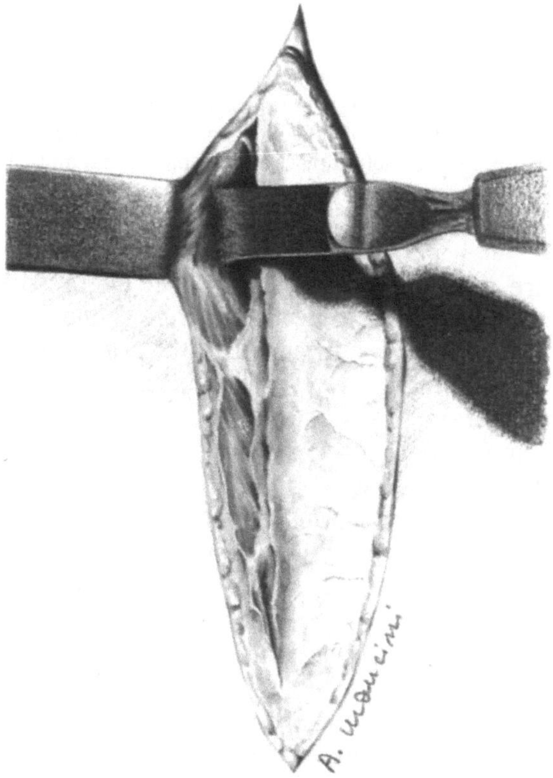

Fig. 9.22 - Disinsertion of the paraspinal muscles with a periosteal elevator, starting from the most cranial of the vertebrae exposed.

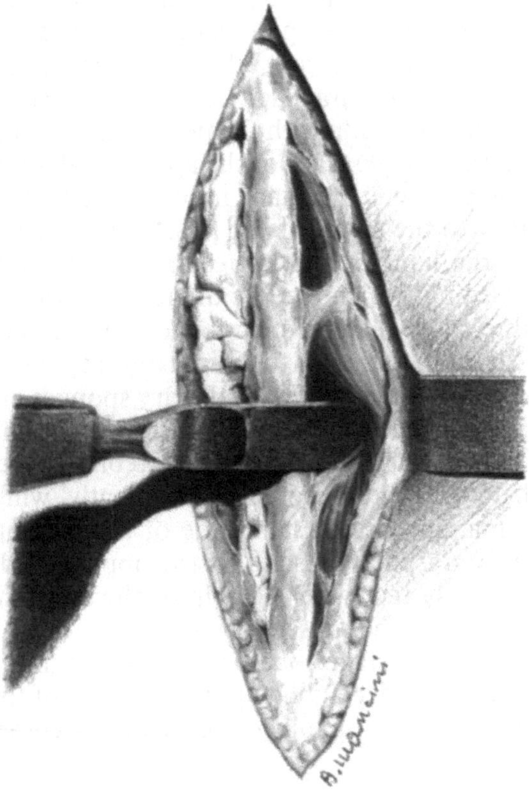

Fig. 9.23 - Gradually as the paraspinal muscles are detached, dry sponges are packed deep to the muscle mass. At the end of muscle disinsertion on one side, the sponges are left in place and the paraspinal muscles on the opposite side are detached.

are applied and fixed in place. Retractors should be inserted deep enough to remain adherent to the skin surface and not impede surgical manoeuvres. After insertion of the retractors, haemostasis is completed, and remnants of muscle and fat tissue still adherent to the laminae, posterior joints and yellow and interspinous ligaments are removed with gouge forceps or a large curette.

Opening of spinal canal

After the yellow and interspinous ligaments have been exposed, the vertebrae included in the operative field are identified by locating the lumbosacral interspace, if this has been exposed, counting the spinous processes starting from the fifth lumbar, or referring to a landmark applied preoperatively. Identification, at this stage, of the individual vertebrae is extremely important, because, once the spinous processes have been removed and laminectomy started, it becomes exceedingly difficult to identify the vertebral levels.

When a single intervertebral level has to be decompressed, the cranial half of the spinous process of the distal vertebra and the caudal half or two thirds of the spinous process of the proximal vertebra as well as the interspinous ligament are resected. Resection of the spinous processes, using a sharp angled bone biter, should be carried out as far as their base (Fig. 9.24). Removal of the spinous processes is then completed with a

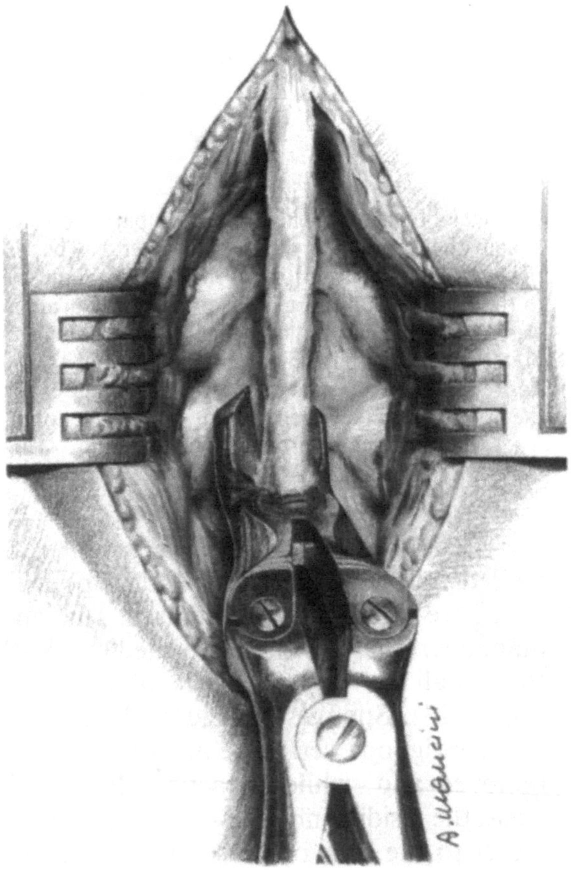

Fig. 9.24 - After installing the self-retaining retractor the spinous processes are cut at their base with an angled bone biter and removed. Removal of the residual portion of the base of the spinous processes is then completed with a gouge forceps.

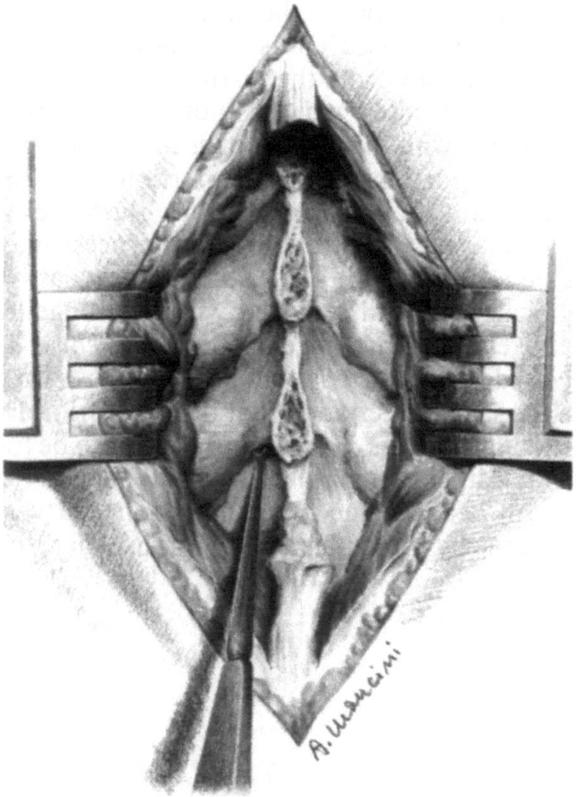

Fig. 9.25 - Disinsertion of the ligamentum flavum from the anterior surface of the distal portion of the lamina. This manoeuvre starts from the medial end of the lamina and then proceeds laterally. A small curette should be used to penetrate between the lamina and the ligamentum flavum. Detachment of the ligamentum is carried out for as far as possible beneath the lamina. The portion of the lamina from which the ligamentum has been detatched can progressively be excised as the manoeuvre proceeds.

large gouge forceps. Bleeding from the cut surface of the cancellous bone, when copious, may be controlled using bone wax applied with the tip of a dissector and then compressed against the bone surface with the finger or a small clamp-held compress. A small curette is used to detach the ligamentum flavum from the deep surface of the proximal laminae, starting medially near the base of the spinous process, and proceeding laterally as far as the articular processes (Fig. 9.25). The curette should be introduced between the ligament and bone and maintained constantly in contact with the latter to avoid damage, either by compression or tearing, to the underlying nervous structures. Laminectomy is initiated in the medial portion of the laminar arch, that is, at the level of the posterior angle of the spinal canal, which is not occupied by the dural sac (Fig. 9.26). The lamina can be removed with a small gouge forceps, or a punch rongeur when the spinal canal is markedly stenotic. Laminectomy is then continued, alternately on one side and the other, after the ligamenta flava have been further stripped with a curette from the residual portion of the laminae. The ligamenta flava are subsequently detatched from the proximal border of the laminae of the distal vertebra starting from the most medial portion. The cut edge of the ligament is picked up with a forceps or a fine-toothed Kocher, sectioned vertically with

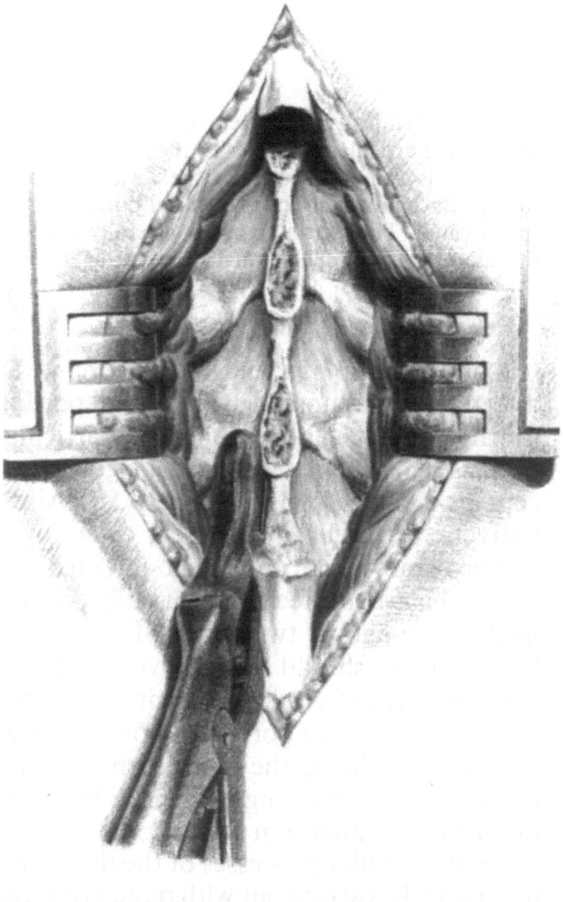

Fig. 9.26 - Laminectomy performed by gouge forceps. Excision of the lamina is started in close proximity to the interlaminar angle, where the width of the spinal canal is greater, and is then continued laterally.

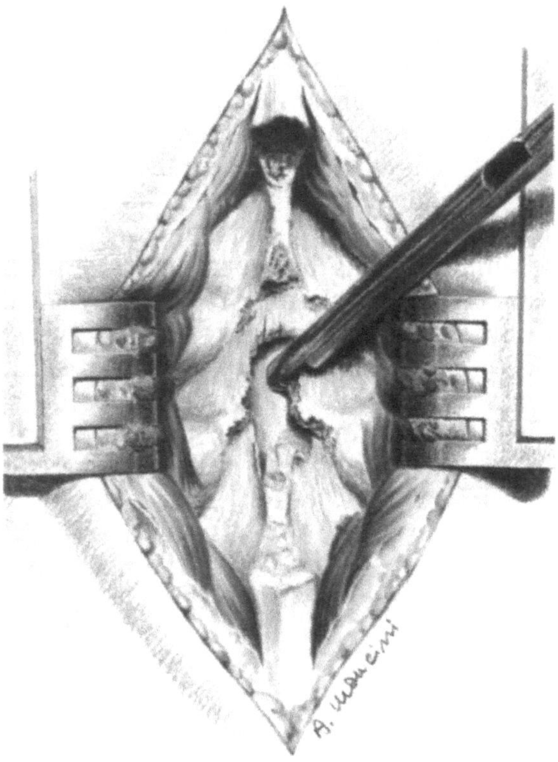

Fig. 9.27 - Removal of the lateral portion of the laminae and the articular processes by the punch rongeur. The latter is generally used alternately with the gouge forceps during opening of the central portion of the spinal canal. The rongeur only is generally used for the lateral portions of the canal, which are narrower.

scissors or the tip of a fine knife and removed as extensively as possible. The lateral portion of the laminae and the inferior articular processes may be removed using a gouge forceps or a punch rongeur (Fig. 9.27) Alternatively, a chisel may be used, orienting it in a proximo-caudal and medio-lateral direction. Whatever the technique, usually only the medial one-half or two thirds of the articular processes should be removed. When a chisel is used, after osteotomizing the articular process, the cut portion of bone is elevated with the tip of the instrument and removed, after sectioning of the residual portion of the ligamentum flavum. Removal of superior articular processes of the distal vertebra may be carried out with punch rongeur or chisel. Use of the latter, however, exposes to greater risks than with the inferior articular processes, on account of the proximity of the nerve root to the superior facet. If the rongeur is used, it is advisable to begin facetectomy from the tip of the superior articular process, which is not in such direct contact with the nerve root as the middle and distal portions. Residual portions of ligamentum flavum attached to the anteromedial border of the articular process may be stripped with a curette or, more easily, picked up and removed with the rongeur, together with adjacent bone. If a chisel is used, osteotomy should be carried out with the same direction as that of the inferior articular process. Facetectomy may also be total, rather than partial, if a posterolateral fusion between the two laminectomized vertebrae has been planned. In this instance, the

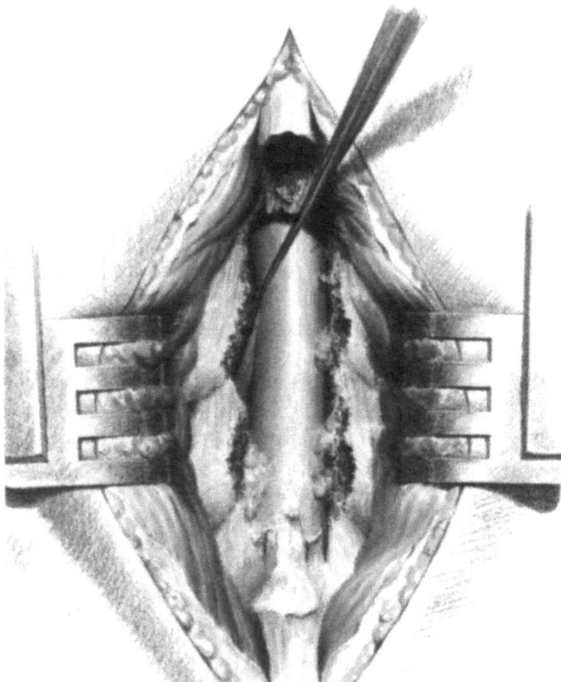

Fig. 9.28 - Exploration of the intervertebral discs and spinal nerve roots in the radicular canal. After removal of the laminae and the medial half of the articular processes, the intervertebral discs are identified and palpated with a blunt probe to determine their consistency and degree of posterior prominence. The mobility of the spinal nerve roots is then evaluated, and a right angled blunt probe is used to determine whether the roots are compressed in the radicular canal or the neuroforamen.

pars interarticularis of the proximal vertebra is exposed and osteotomized transversely. The articular capsule of the apophyseal joint is then sectioned and the inferior articular process is removed, levering with a curved chisel introduced into the joint space. The superior articular process of the distal vertebra may be removed with the rongeur or osteotomized transversely immediately above the pedicle.

When complete bilateral laminectomy of a vertebra (or two or more vertebrae) and partial laminectomy of the vertebrae above and below are to be performed, the interspinous ligament located distally to the vertebra submitted to complete laminectomy is sectioned with a knife and the spinous process of this vertebra is removed with a sharp angled bone cutter together with the distal half of the spinous process of the vertebra above. The spinous process of the vertebra below may not be included in spinectomy, because, since it is located caudally to the intervertebral space, it does not usually hinder partial laminectomy of the vertebra to which it belongs. If this does not occur, however, the spinous process may subsequently be removed with gouge forceps to the extent required.

Decompression is performed with the technique described, taking certain precautions. Laminectomy should be initiated at the level of the intervertebral space in which compression of the nervous structures is less marked. Lesser narrowing of the spinal canal, in fact, makes it easier to expose the dural sac, which serves as a guide for continuation of decompression in the narrower area. After the laminae of the vertebra requiring complete laminectomy have been entirely resected, the ligamenta flava above this vertebra are removed with gouge forceps or punch rongeur, without previously stripping them from the laminae. Decompression of the nerve root in the radicular canal may easily and rapidly be performed with the surgeon staying on the same side, particularly when stenosis is severe. Therefore, if nerve root decompression has to be carried out at several levels, after removal of the laminae, decompression of the nerve roots on one side and excision of the medial portion of the articular processes on the opposite side, it may be helpful for the surgeon to change side with respect to the patient to complete opening of the nerve root canal on the opposite site. Laminectomy, at the level of the intervertebral spaces located at the extremities of the stenotic area, should be continued until it is certain that the nervous structures are no longer compressed. However, it is better to abound in extending laminectomy proximally and distally than to leave stenosis in areas for which decompression had been planned preoperatively.

Exploration of intervertebral discs and spinal nerve roots

The spinal canal is opened laterally until the nerve roots emerging from the dural sac are visualized. The nerve root and dural sac are then retracted medially and the disc is exposed at each of the intervertebral levels included in the area of laminectomy. To identify the intervertebral discs it should be borne in mind that the lowest two lumbar discs are usually located at the level of, or distally to, the emergence of the spinal nerve root from the theca, whereas the second and third discs are usually located cranially to the emerging root. The disc can generally be recognized by its whitish colour and, more particularly, by its fibrous consistency, contrasting with the bony hardness of the vertebral body. Consistency of the annulus fibrosus is tested with a blunt probe (Fig. 9.28). If the annulus is hard in consistency, the disc should not be entered, even when it protrudes posteriorly. Discectomy is carried out only when the intervertebral disc is herniated or, in the absence of a true herniation, it is soft in consistency and easily depressed by the probe.

A right-angled blunt probe is then used to evaluate the width of the nerve root canal. If the instrument passes freely along the nerve root and this is easily movable, it is not necessary to open the nerve root canal beyond the emergence of the root from the dural sac. On the other hand, if difficulty is encountered in introducing the probe into the nerve root canal, this should be opened with the punch rongeur until complete decompression of the root is obtained. It is important to adequately free the spinal nerve root even if this implies complete excision of the articular processes, because persistent compression of the nerve root may lead to unsatisfactory results. Bilateral complete foraminectomy at a single intervertebral level is rarely necessary. However, one should not hesitate to carry it out if this is required for adequate decompression of the nerve root, since vertebral instability which might result can be eliminated by a spinal fusion performed in a subsequent operation, which is technically simpler than repeat exploration of the spinal and nerve root canal, when a bilateral laminectomy has already been performed.

According to McNab (1977), it may, at times, be necessary to remove the pedicle when, on account of resorption of the underlying disc, this causes compression of the spinal nerve root in the intervertebral foramen (kinking of the pedicle). In my experience, this is only very occasionally necessary since the spinal nerve root is not usually compressed by the pedicle, even if the underlying disc shows evidence of marked resorption.

Some authors, in order to decompress the nerve root in the intervertebral foramen without sacrificing the outer half of the articular processes, suggest removing the posterolateral portion of the vertebral body, delimiting ventrally the neuroforamen, with a chisel (Wiltse *et al.*, 1976). This, however, is a technically difficult surgical manoeuvre, which exposes the nerve root to the risk of injury. This should be employed only in particular circumstances and, specifically, in the presence of marked osteophytosis of the vertebral body, responsible for compression of the nerve root within the intervertebral foramen.

Excision of posterior osteophytes of the vertebral body

Posterior osteophytes of the vertebral endplates do not usually need to be excised when bilateral laminectomy is performed, as in most cases opening of the spinal canal is sufficient to adequately decompress the nervous structures. However, when the osteophyte invades one half, or more, of the spinal canal in the sagittal direction, it may be useful to excise it, if the outgrowth impinges on the nerve root emerging from the dural sac, producing a kind of kinking. Before excising the osteophyte, or the osteophytes of two adjacent vertebral bodies, discectomy should be carried out, removing the posterior annulus fibrosus as far as possible. Osteophytectomy is perfomed with a curved chisel, starting laterally to the nerve root and proceeding towards the midline, first on one side and then on the other. Definitive regularization of the vertebral border may then be accomplished with a long, small-sized gouge forceps.

During surgical manoeuvre, the dural sac and emerging nerve root must be adequately protected with a supple retractor. At the end of the procedure, bone wax is applied over the cut bony surface to arrest bleeding.

Control of deep haemorrhage

During lamino-arthrectomy and exploration of the spinal nerve roots and intervertebral discs, the operative field should be maintained bloodless by sucking with an aspiration cannula in the sites where the surgeon is working. Bleeding from cut bone surfaces is generally mild and does not usually require haemostasis with bone wax. Similarly, haemorrhage from the epidural venous plexus, mostly coming from small vessels, rarely requires coagulation. Bleeding from large epidural vessels may be controlled in two ways: by applying. in the bleeding areas, small pieces of haemostatic material gently compressed with a moistened patty; or by identifying the bleeding vessels and coagulating them with low-voltage current or, preferably, with a bipolar coagulator, which avoids the risk of damage to the nervous structures.

As laminectomy proceeds, in the areas in which the spinal canal has already been opened, the dural sac and the lateral walls and floor of the spinal canal are covered with moistened patties to control bleeding from small epidural vessels. When an intervertebral disc has to be explored and disc tissue excised, it may be useful, if bleeding hinders surgical manoeuvres, to pack small patties cranially and caudally to the disc space to reduce the accumulation of blood on it.

At the end of the operation — after arterial blood pressure has been brought back to normal values — there must be no significant bleeding from deep vessels in the operative field. Should this not be the case, all bleeding vessels must be meticulously identified and cauterized. Formation of a submuscular haematoma compressing the nervous structures may, in fact, lead to the risk of serious postoperative neurological complications. To avoid this, suction drainage should consistently be applied, unless a deliberate opening of the dural tube has been made or a tear has occurred, from which cerebrospinal fluid may leak as a result of aspiration.

Opening of dural sac

Myelographic evidence of redundancy of caudal nerve roots represents, according to some authors (Tsuji *et al.*, 1985), an indication for opening of the thecal sac. The aim would be to eliminate the compression exerted by a dural tube which has become relatively tight for hypertrophied spinal nerve roots. Two methods may be used for opening of the thecal envelope. One implies sectioning of only the dural layer with preservation of the arachnoid membrane, the integrity of which does not allow cerebrospinal fluid to leak out. Subsequently, the dural sheet may be fixed, or not, to the deep portion of the paravertebral muscles with silk sutures and the arachnoid membrane covered with a thin layer of fat tissue. Alternatively, both the dura and arachnoid may be incised, after accurate haemostasis of epidural, bony and muscular vessels and application of moistened sponges along the internal surface of the paraspinal muscles, to avoid penetration of blood within the thecal sac. A dural plasty using fascia (thoracolumbar fascia or fascia lata) or liophilized dura is then performed with continuous silk sutures.

In my experience, there is no need to open the dural sac in patients with redundant caudal nerve roots. Redundancy of spinal nerve roots is, in fact, a relatively frequent finding at autopsy in subjects who during their lifetime had been asymptomatic. Furthermore, the presence or not of redundant nerve roots does not seem to influence the results of decompression, nor has opening of the thecal sac been shown to give significantly better results than bone decompression alone. With incision of only the dura mater, however, there is a risk of complications, such as fistula or spinal extradural cyst.

Two other conditions may require opening of the dural sac: a myelographic block of uncertain interpretation as concerns aetiology, and chronic inflammatory changes of the arachnoid membrane. Opening of the thecal sac, aimed at excluding intradural pathological conditions, should always be performed when there is no evidence of extradural conditions (bony or discal in nature) of such entity to justify a myelographic block. Arachnoiditis of the cauda equina is extremely rare in patients with lumbar spinal stenosis, particularly in those not previously submitted to surgical treatment. The condition may be suspected when the dura is opaque and fibrous in consistency and does not pulsate. In these cases, one may open only the dural sheet leaving the arachnoid membrane intact (Crock, 1983) or also open the latter releasing the individual nerve roots, preferably using the operative microscope, from adhesions with the arachnoid and other intrathecal nerve roots (Johnston and Nathney, 1978). It should be pointed out, however, that the clinical results of radicular neurolysis are very often unsatisfactory, particularly when arachnoiditis represents the main pathological condition responsible for neurological symptoms and signs.

Prevention of epidural scar formation

To avoid the fibrous membrane, which forms in the area of laminectomy between the dural sac and muscle layer following organization of deep haematoma, from causing compression of the nervous structures, it is advisable to cover the dural tube and exposed nerve roots with a layer of fat tissue. A fat tissue graft will, in fact, maintain its vitality and isolate the nervous structures, from submuscular fibrous tissue (Langenskiold and Kiviluoto, 1976; Jacobs *et al.*, 1980). This procedure also has the advantage of making any further surgery in the area of laminectomy much easier.

The graft of fat tissue, which should be at least 0.5 mm in thickness, may be taken from subcutaneous tissue at the surgical wound or, in thin subjects, from the iliac region through a second skin incision. The only drawback, in both cases, is the possible formation of postoperative subcutaneous haematoma in the site of removal. This may be avoided by filling, at least partially, the dead space left by the excised fat tissue with haemostatic sponge and carefully suturing the dermis to the underlying fascia.

Wound closure

In those areas in which the spinous processes have been removed, the paraspinal muscles of the two sides are approximated in the midline by interrupted sutures of slow-resorbing material (Fig. 9.29). Stitches should not be excessively tight in order to avoid muscle ischemia. In these areas, the thoracolumbar fascia is closed with interrupted, plain or mattress, sutures using large-calibre non-resorbing material. Alternatively, a continuous suture may be performed, which has the advantage of being more rapid and better closing the fascial layer (Fig. 9.29). In the sites where the spinous processes have been preserved, the thoracolumbar fascia is anchored to the supraspinous ligament with interrupted sutures, first on one side and then on the other, or with mattress sutures passing through the fascia on both sides and the interspinous ligament.

The formation of a haematoma between the subcutaneous tissue and thoracolumbar fascia may be avoided by passing a few sutures both in the deep and middle subcutaneous layers and the fascia. Four to eight of these sutures are generally sufficient, depending on the length of the surgical wound. Subcutaneous closure is completed with interrupted sutures passing through the deep part of the dermis in order to ensure good closure of the skin borders.

The skin is closed by simple interrupted or mattress sutures, or a continuous intradermic suture with fine slow-resorbing or non resorbing material. Intradermic suture has the advantage of producing a more esthetic skin scar but also involves, when not correctly performed, greater risk of delayed wound healing on account of the formation of cutaneous fistulae due to giving way of stitches in the presence of subcutaneous serous accumulation.

Spinal fusion

When posterolateral vertebral fusion is to be performed in association with opening of the spinal canal, a longer skin incision is needed than that for decompression alone. For an anthrodesis L_4-L_5 or L_4-S_1, incision should extend at least from L_3 to S_1.

Paraspinal muscles, after disinsertion from posterior elements of the spine, are stripped from the outer surface of articular processes and the transverse processes. When this is completed, dry sponges are tightly packed in the latero-vertebral gutters to control bleeding. Laminectomy is then carried out, after which the transverse processes and ala of the sacrum, and the external surface of the articular processes, pedicles and partes interarticulares are meticulously decorticated, using gouge forceps, Cobb periosteal elevator and curved curettes of varying size. Bone graft is obtained from the iliac crest through the midline skin incision or a second incision. In the former instance, the postero-superior iliac spine and the adjacent portion of the iliac crest are exposed after dissection of subcutaneous tissue from the fascial plane. With this type of access, a suprafascial haematoma easily develops, which may delay wound healing. For this reason, it is preferable to obtain the bone graft through an additional skin incision at the level of the posterior third of the iliac crest, in an oblique direction from above to below and from inside to outside. This direction, since

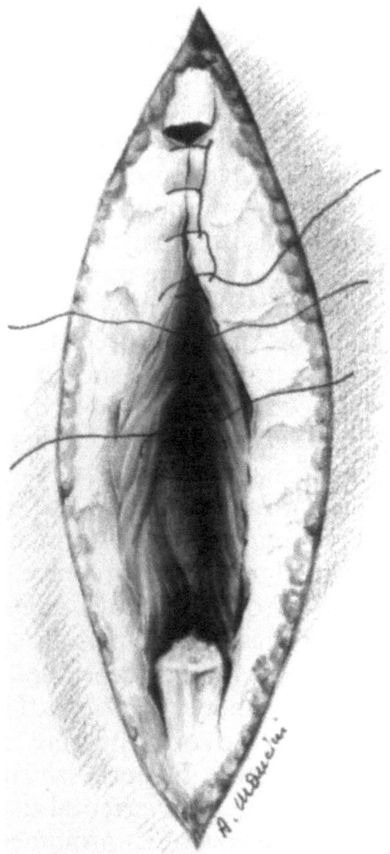

Fig. 9.29 - Muscular and fascial suture. The paraspinal muscles are brought together with interrupted stitches anchoring at least the dorsal two thirds of the muscle layer. A continuous suture is used to close the thoracolumbar fascia.

it is parallel to the course of the cutaneous nerves, involves less risk of formation of neuromas from sectioned nerve branches.

Bone graft material, obtained by the usual technique, is packed in the latero-vertebral gutters, the fragments of cancellous bone being placed more deeply with respect to those of cortical bone. Prior to suturing paraspinal muscles, a thin layer of fat tissue or haemostatic material should be placed over the dural tube and spinal nerve roots to avoid the possibility that bone fragments, passing from the lateral gutters to the site of laminectomy, may compress the nervous structures.

Laminotomy

Laminotomy — a term equivalent to that of hemilaminectomy — consists in the removal of the caudal portion of the lamina of one vertebra and the cranial portion of the lamina of the vertebra below, associated with excision of the medial portion of the articular processes, respectively inferior and superior, of the two vertebrae.

Skin incision, for unilateral laminotomy at a single level, extends from the cranial border of the spinous process of the proximal vertebra to the caudal border of the spinous process of the distal vertebra. The incision should not exceed 5 to 7 cm in length. As for bilateral laminectomy, dermal-subcutaneous vessels, rather than coagulated, may be grasped with clamps, which are then turned outwards the surgical wound. The thoracolumbar fascia is incised with the electric cautery knife parallel, and in immediate proximity, to the spinous processes, which may be more easily identified if the

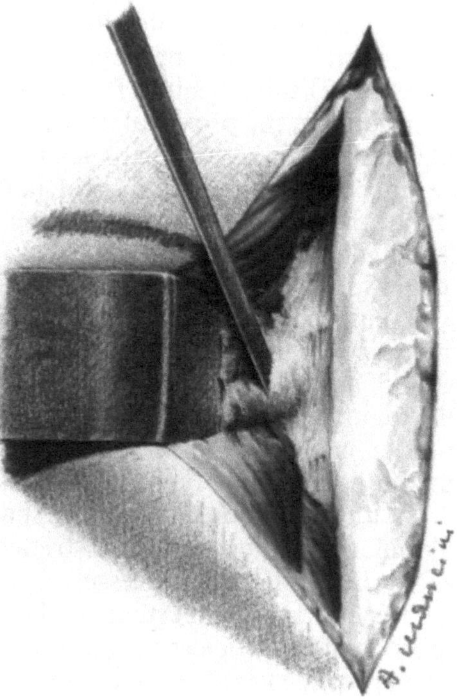

Fig. 9.30 - Resection of the medial half of the inferior articular process of the proximal vertebra using a chisel. Osteotomy should reach the articular surface. The base of the articular process is then sectioned transversely and the medial half removed, levering with the chisel.

assistant operator depresses the paraspinal muscles of the opposite side with a periosteal elevator (see page 200).

Gradually as the paravertebral muscles are disinserted from the bone surface, dry sponges are packed into the osteo-muscular space, in order to control bleeding from deep vessels and to better strip the muscle mass as far as the lateral portion of the articular processes. A Taylor retractor is installed with the tip placed against the external surface of the articular processes. The retractor may be held by an assistant or by a metal weight of some two kilos left hanging at the side of the patient and anchored to the surgical drape.

The ligamentum flavum is detached with a small curette from the deep surface of the proximal lamina, the distal third of which is progressively excised with a thin gouge forceps gradually as the ligamentum is disinserted. When the inferior articular process is markedly hypertrophic, its medial half may be resected with a chisel (Fig. 9.30). This manoeuvre, if correctly done, does not expose the nervous structures to the risk of injury on account of the protection provided by the superior articular process of the vertebra below. The ligamentum flavum is then disinserted from the proximal border of the distal lamina. This allows the punch rongeur to be introduced under the distal lamina, about one third of which is initially removed.

The ligamentum flavum, detached from the distal lamina and retracted proximally, may be removed in different ways: gripping it with a Kocher and cutting it with scissors, sectioning it with a fine knife, excising it in small fragments with a rongeur (Fig. 9.31). The latter manoeuvre is the most suitable when the ligamentum flavum is markedly thick and the interapophysolaminar space is developmentally narrow or constricted by hypertrophied articular processes, as often occurs in nerve root canal stenosis. The medial portion of the articular processes and the lateral part of the ligamentum flavum inserted on it is subsequently removed (Fig. 9.32). In the presence of marked narrowing of the nerve root canal, it is advisable to begin facetectomy from the inferior articular process and then proceed distally, using small 45° angled punch rongeurs, which, compared with the 90° angled rongeurs, penetrate more easily beneath the articular process and are less traumatic for the spinal nerve root. When marked hypertrophy of the articular processes makes it difficult to carry out facetectomy, the posteromedial portion of the inferior articular process may be removed with a gouge forceps, chisel or high speed drill, thereafter using the punch rongeur to complete the arthrectomy.

In both this and the successive surgical stages, the operative field should be maintained as bloodless as possible by using a small-calibre sucker and, if necessary, patties or pieces of haemostatic material gently packed beneath the proximal and distal lamina. This makes surgical manoeuvres easier, particularly in the presence of copious bleeding from epidural vessels which have become ectasic due to chronic compression in a stenotic nerve root canal.

Facetectomy should be extended laterally to expose the nerve root emerging from the dural sac. Retracting the dural sac and nerve root medially, the intervertebral disc is exposed and the degree of its prominence and consistency is evaluated. Excision of disc tissue is not usually necessary when the disc, though showing a slight posterior prominence, is hard-fibrous in consistency and does not appear to compress the spinal nerve root. If any uncertainty exists, however, it is better to proceed with discectomy rather than risk leaving a disc protrusion responsible for even mild compression of the nerve root. In isolated stenosis of the nerve root canal, there is generally no risk, in fact, of causing iatrogenic vertebral instability, particularly when stenosis, and therefore laminotomy, is unilateral.

Once the intervertebral disc has been explored, laminotomy of the distal vertebra is enlarged and the medial portion of the base of the superior articular process is removed with a punch rongeur or fine chisel to expose the spinal nerve root as far as the medial surface of the pedicle. A blunt probe is then used to evaluate the width of the distal portion of the lateral recess and the neuroforamen, proceeding, if the latter appear to be stenotic, with the lamino-facetectomy until complete decompression is achieved of the

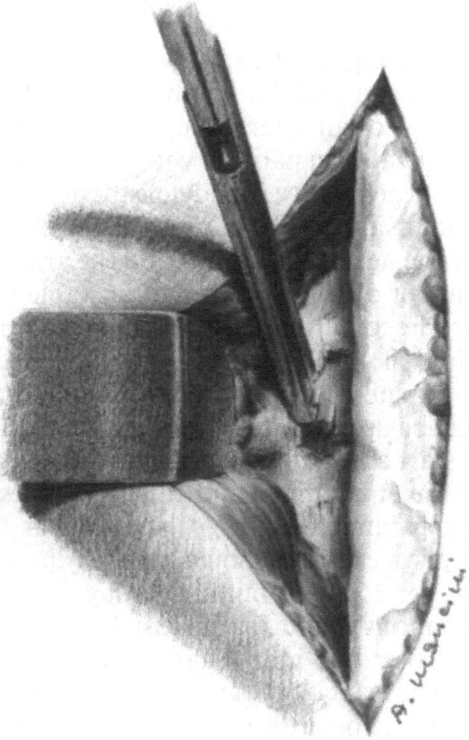

Fig. 9.31 - Excision of the ligamentum flavum, previously detatched from the distal lamina, by a punch rongeur.

nerve root, which should be entirely mobile at the end of the operation.

After thorough irrigation of the surgical field with saline, the thoracolumbar fascia is closed with interrupted or continuous sutures using slow-resorbing material. To avoid superficial haematomas, the deeper layer of subcutaneous tissue may be anchored to the fascial plane with two or three sutures before closing the superficial layer.

Microsurgery

Most of the difficulties encountered in laminotomy are related to poor lighting of the operative field, particularly when a short skin incision is made. These difficulties may be overcome with the use of a cold frontal light or an operative microscope.

The microscope provides not only excellent lighting of the deep surgical field, but allows a better and more detailed visualization of the anatomical structures and, thus, surgical manoeuvres are more precise and less traumatic to the nervous structures. Furthermore, by providing vertical lighting, a very short skin incision, not exceeding 3-4 cm, can be made for a single level laminotomy, and thus paraspinal muscle disinsertion can be limited to the area comprised between the distal half of the cranial vertebra and the proximal half of the caudal vertebra. This reduces muscle fibrosis in the operative area to a minimum and the functional damage which may result.

The microsurgical and macrosurgical techniques for laminotomy are very similar in as much as the same instruments are needed, with the exception of the paraspinal muscle retractor, which should be as narrow as possible, on account of the short skin incision. Particularly suitable for this purpose is a Taylor retractor about half or one third

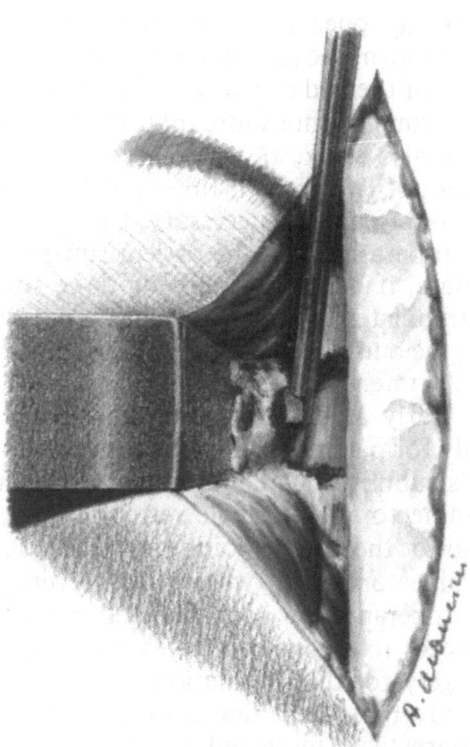

Fig. 9.32 - Removal of the medial half of the articular processes and the distal lamina with rongeur. Laminofacetectomy should expose the nerve root along the entire length of the radicular canal.

in width of the standard instrument. The main technical differences concern removal of the proximal lamina, which is performed with a punch rongeur rather than a gouge forceps, and the excision of ligamentum flavum, which is preferably sectioned in an L-shaped fashion with the tip of a fine knife and then removed with the rongeur.

With the microscope placed at the level of the intervertebral disc and used at low magnification (4 or 6x), it is generally possible to expose the spinal nerve root for the entire length of the radicular canal. Even decompression in the intervertebral foramen is, however, usually easy, if the microscope is placed more distally or is inclined in a slightly caudal direction.

POSTOPERATIVE TREATMENT

The patient is left in the supine position for 4 to 6 hours after surgery to favor maintenance of hemostasis until sufficiently resistant clots are formed. On the first postoperative day, once the suction drainage has been withdrawn, the patient is invited to sit on the edge of the bed as many as five times a day, each time for not more than 10 minutes; he may also walk, if he wishes, for 5 to 10 minutes, two to four times a day, with the aid of a frame, if necessary. On the second postoperative day, the patient starts to ambulate, if he has not already done so, and is stimulated to walk 4 to 8 times a day, limiting the out-of-bed period to 10 to 15 minutes each time.

Early ambulation is recommended not only for patients with nerve root canal stenosis submitted to laminotomy or unilateral laminectomy at a single vertebral level, but also for those undergoing multilevel bilateral laminectomy, in whom the severity of postoperative low back pain does not usually exceed, to a considerable extent, that after surgery for disc herniation.

Over the next few days, ambulation is progressively increased, the standing period being limited to 15 to 20 minutes each time. The patient is usually discharged between the fourth and tenth postoperative day.

It is generally advisable (though not strictly necessary) to fit patients submitted to spinal arthrodesis with a rigid brace for four to eight weeks, depending on the patient's age and the number of fused levels. The use of an external support is particularly indicated in patients with moderate to severe degenerative spondylolisthesis, in whom solid fusion may be more difficult. The younger the age of the patient and the greater the number of fused levels and unstable the arthrodesed vertebrae, the longer immobilization should be.

In subjects in middle or early old age it may be useful, after removal of the stitches, to start an exercise programme aimed at activating abdominal and gluteal muscles, and at regaining mobility of the lumbar spine. Physical exercises should generally be carried out for 15 to 30 minutes a day in the first two months and for at least 15 minutes for a further two months.

The exercise programme is then stopped, except in the presence of persistent low-back pain. The use of a corset, in patients submitted only to decompressive surgery, is unnecessary, except in rare cases of considerable postoperative back pain related to segmental vertebral instability.

COMPLICATIONS

Complications may be either vertebral or extravertebral. As far as concerns the former, the most frequent are intraoperative tears of the thecal sac and nerve roots, or spinal cord injuries. Postoperative extravertebral complications include urinary retention, intestinal ileus and thromboembolic disease.

Vertebral complications

Tears in the dural sac occur most often in areas of severe stenosis, in which the epidural fat tissue is thin or absent and adhesions may be present between the thecal sac and the bony walls of the spinal canal or the ligamenta flava. Dural tears are usually produced either while gaining access to the spinal canal, that is before an extensive portion of the dural sac, which serves as a guide for the execution of laminectomy, has been exposed, or when, with clumsy manoeuvre, the ligamenta flava are torn from the bone insertions. Thecal injury may consist in a dural tear with no involvement of the arachnoid membrane, through which the spinal nerve root may be seen, or a full-thickness tear through which cerebrospinal fluid may leak. In the former instance, it is usually sufficient to cover the injured area with haemostatic sponge, whereas in the second the thecal defect must be repaired. Even a small full-thickness tear, in fact, may result in the formation of a fistula with subsequent risk of meningitis or a spinal extradural cyst, which may be responsible for compression of the dural sac or the spinal nerve roots in the extrathecal course.

Dural tears should be repaired with continuous suture employing 5-0 or 6-0 silk. However, when the thecal defect is too wide or irregular to allow approximation of the borders, the use of a fascial graft from the fascia lata or lumbosacral fascia may be necessary. Fascial graft is sutured to the dura with interrupted silk stitches, after trimming, if needed, the edges of the tear. After closure of the dural defect, the firmness of the repair is tested by performing the Valsalva manoeuvre with the patient in the anti-Trendelenburg position or by asking the anaestesiologist to increase to a maximum the respiratory excursions. After surgery, the patient is kept in a horizontal position for 3 to 7 days, depending on the size of the tear and the strength of the repair.

Nerve root or spinal cord deficits may become apparent after surgery because of operative trauma to the neural elements (excessive or too prolonged retraction with metallic instruments or compression by the punch rongeur) or inadequate haemostasis, during or at the end of the operation, resulting in compression of the nervous structures by an epidural haematoma.

Nerve root deficits tend to occur more frequently in older than in younger subjects and in patients with nerve root canal stenosis compared with those with spinal canal stenosis. This is probably due to the fact that in old patients nerve roots are less resistant to surgical trauma. This is greater when the root is exposed along its whole intraspinal course as in nerve root canal stenosis, rather than for a short course, at the level of the exit from the dural sac, as is generally sufficient in stenosis of the spinal canal. In old patients, moreover, intraoperative bleeding is often more copious than in the younger subjects and the compressive effects of a haematoma on the nerve root are greater when these are no longer protected by the bony walls of the vertebral canal.

The nerve root which most frequently shows a postoperative deficit is L_5, followed by L_4 and S_1. The more frequent involvement of L_5 compared to the other lumbar nerve roots is due to the fact that the L_4-L_5 level is the most frequently found to present stenosis in the lumbar area and that the innervation of the muscles supplied by L_5 nerve root is less pluriradicular than that of the other muscles in the lower limb.

Postoperative nerve root deficits may be partial or complete. Usually a partial deficit occurs, which improves considerably or disappears with adequate physical therapy within two to four months after surgery. Prior to surgery, the involved nerve root may be functionally normal, or show a deficit of varying severity; the former occurrence is rare, whereas the latter is relatively frequent, the greater the preoperative deficit the higher the chances of increase of the deficit after surgery. The evolution of a radicular palsy is unpredictable. In most cases, the involved root shows no, or only a mild, functional recovery. The cases with the most severe prognosis are those in which there is no evidence of active muscle contraction four to six weeks after surgery. Otherwise the deficit tends to regress progressively during the first postoperative months. One year after surgery there is no longer any reasonable possibility of a significant improvement in muscle deficit.

Spinal cord complications may occur when decompressive surgery is carried out at the upper two lumbar levels, containing the caudal portion of the cord. These complications consist in paralytic sphinteric disturbances, usually related only or mainly to the bladder, and impotence. Spinal cord dysfunction, similarly to nerve roots deficits, may be transient or permanent and when there is a tendency to recovery, this occurs within four to six months after surgery.

Little is known about the incidence of neurological complications in patients submitted to surgery for lumbar spinal stenosis. Only Verbiest (1977) and Reale *et al.* (1978) have reported the observation of postoperative neurological disturbances absent preoperatively or an increase in preexisting abnormalities. Reale *et al.*, however, do not indicate the percentage of patients with neurological complications, whereas Verbiest reports on 7 cases observed in a series of 147 patients with spinal canal stenosis. Of the seven patients, five showed nerve root deficits, one had an increase in severity of a preexisting micturition disorder and another presented a radicular deficit associated with impaired micturition. Most of these patients presented a severe constriction of the spinal canal and two of them showed no recovery of neurological disturbances.

The author has observed 6 postoperative complications in a series of 166 cases of lumbar spinal stenosis.

In the two patients with stenosis of the spinal canal, a preoperative severe longstanding motor deficit of L_5 nerve root became worse. The patients were 64 and 67 years old, respectively. In both cases, no particular difficulty had been encountered during surgery and bleeding had not been more copious than usually. In both patients the deficit improved during the first six postoperative months reaching the same degree as that present preoperatively.

Postoperative radicular deficit was complete in one of the four patients with nerve root canal stenosis and partial in two; in all three, the L_5 nerve root was involved, which preoperatively showed a mild or no deficit. In the fourth case, a marked increase in severity of a mild preoperative deficit of L_4 root was observed. In all patients, the operation had been difficult due to abundant bleeding from bony and epidural vessels; in three cases an L_4-L_5 discectomy had been performed in addition to decompression of L_5 root in the radicular canal. In the patient with paralysis of the L_5 nerve root, the motor deficit showed no improvement. In the others, the deficit disappeared completely, or almost completely, after three to six months.

Extravertebral complications

Urinary retention is not rare, particularly in old patients; catheterization sbould be carried out and, if still persistent one week after surgery, drugs should be given to stimulate bladder musculature. The occurrence of an intestinal ileus is less frequent and is usually overcome within two to three days with a rectal probe, possibly also associated with drugs aimed at enhancing intestinal peristalsis. Deep venous thrombosis in the lower limbs may sometimes be observed when the patient is forced to stay in bed for many days before and/or after surgery (Choudhury and Taylor, 1977).

REFERENCES

Choudhury A.R., Taylor J.C.: Occult lumbar spinal stenosis. *J. Neurol. Neurosurg. Psych.* **40:** 506, 1977.

Crock H.V.: *Practice of spinal surgery.* Springer-Verlag, Wien, New York, 1983.

Douglas D.L., Duckworth T., Kanis J.A., Jefferson A.A., Martin J.J., Russel R.G.G.: Spinal cord dysfunction in Paget's disease of bone. Has medical treatment a vascular basis? *J. Bone and Joint Surg.* **63-B:** 495, 1981.

Hadijpavlov A.B., Tsoukas G.M., Siller T.N., Danais S., Greenwood F.: Combination drug therapy in treatment of Paget's disease of bone. *J. Bone and Joint Surg.* **59-A:** 1045, 1977.

Herzberg L., Bayliss E.: Spinal-cord syndrome due to non-compressive Paget's disease of bone: a spinal artery steal phenomenon reversible with calcitonin. *Lancet*: 13, 1980.

Jacobs R.R., McClain O., Neff J.: Control of postlaminectomy scar formation. An experimental and clinical study. *Spine* **5:** 223, 1980.

Johnston J.D.H., Nathney J.B.: Microscopic lysis of lumbar adhesive arachnoiditis. *Spine* **3:** 36, 1978.

KOSTUIK J.P.: *Posterior instrumentation for multiple level instability.* Presented at the 7th AOA International Symposium, Chicago, 1986.

LANGENSKIOLD A., KIVILUOTO O.: Prevention of epidural scar formation after operation on the lumbar spine by means of free fat transplant. *Clin. Orthop.* **115:** 92, 1976.

LARSON A.G.: Deliberate hypotension. *Anesthesiology* **25:** 682, 1964.

LAWHON S.M., KAHN III A., CRAWFORD A.H., BRINKER M.S.: Controlled hypotensive anesthesia during spinal surgery. A retrospective study. *Spine* **9:** 450, 1984.

MCNAB I.: *Backache.* Williams and Wilkins. Baltimore, 1977.

PERUGIA L., POSTACCHINI F.: La patologia stenotica lombare. *Giorn. Ital. Ortop. Traumat.*, suppl. vol. 10, n. 2, 229, 1984.

PORTER R.W., HIBBERT C.: Calcitonin treatment for neurogenic claudication. *Spine* **8:** 585, 1983.

REALE F., DELFINI R., GAMBACORTA D., CANTORE G.P.: Congenital stenosis of lumbar spinal canal: comparison of results of surgical treatment for this and other causes of lumbar syndrome. *Acta Neurochir.* **42:** 199, 1978.

TSUJI H., TAMAKI I., ITOH T., YAMADA H., MOTOE T., TATEZAKI S., NOGUCHI T., TAKANO H.: Redundant nerve roots in patients with degeneration lumbar spinal stenosis. *Spine* **10:** 72, 1985.

VERBIEST H.: Results of surgical treatment of idiopathic developmental stenosis of the lumbar vertebral canal. A review of twenty-seven years' experience. *J. Bone and Joint Surg.* **59-B:** 181, 1977.

WILTSE L.L. KIRKALDY-WILLIS W.H., MCIVOR G.W.D.: The treatment of spinal stenosis. *Clin. Orthop.* **115:** 83, 1976.

WOOTTON R., REEVE J., SPELLACY E., TELLEZ-YUDILEVICH M.: Skeletal blood flow in Paget's disease of bone and its response to calcitonin therapy. *Clin. Sci. Molec. Med.* **54:** 69, 1978.

Chapter X
Results of treatment

NATURAL HISTORY

Little is known about the evolution of an untreated lumbar stenosis syndrome. The only published data are those of Porter *et al.* (1984), who reviewed 169 patients (mean follow-up 2.2 years) with a radicular canal stenosis syndrome, most of whom (81%) had not undergone treatment. At the last follow-up, 78% of the patients still complained of radicular symptoms, but in almost all cases (90%) symptoms had improved or were so mild as to require no treatment. It should be pointed out, however, that in the vast majority of the patients there was no evidence of neurological deficits (motor, sensory or reflex changes) and that in no instances was clinical diagnosis confirmed by diagnostic investigations, such as EMG, CT scan or myelography. This study although indicating that a nerve root canal stenosis syndrome not associated with neurological deficits tends to improve with time or at least not to worsen, does not help to determine the natural course of those cases showing neurological signs of nerve root compression, usually present in patients undergoing surgery.

The present author was able to follow up, for 3 to 9 years, 11 patients with lumbar stenosis who had not undergone treatment. All patients, at the time of diagnosis, had a monoradicular or pluriradicular deficit of muscle strength, sensory sensibility and/or reflex activity; in all patients myelography and/or CT scan showed evidence of lumbar stenosis and displayed (myelography), or led to suspect (CT scan), compression of at least one caudal nerve root. There was an indication, in all cases, for surgical treatment, which, however, was not carried out because of refusal, and/or the poor general conditions, of the patients. Of the eleven patients, five had spinal canal stenosis and six nerve root canal stenosis.

Of the patients with stenosis of the spinal canal (3 males and 2 females, aged 58 to 74 years), three had a combined radicular syndrome and two an intermittent radicular syndrome. The duration of symptoms, at the time of diagnosis, ranged from one to three years. Neurological deficits were monoradicular in three cases and pluriradicular in two. In three cases, only one lumbar level (L_4-L_5) was involved, whereas in two cases stenosis was present at two adjacent levels (L_2-L_4 and L_3-L_5, respectively). The mean follow-up in these patients after diagnosis was 3.4 years. Symptoms remained unchanged in two cases, improved in one and worsened slightly in two. Neurological deficits were unchanged in four patients and had partially improved in one.

Patients with nerve root canal stenosis (4 males and 2 females) were 46 to 68 years old. The radicular syndrome was continuous in two cases, combined in three and intermittent in one. Symptoms had been present, at the time of diagnosis, for 8 months to 2 years. In four cases the L_5 nerve root was involved and in two the S_1 root. At the last follow-up — after a mean period of 4.2 years from the time of diagnosis — three patients considered that radicular symptoms were almost unchanged, two reported a significant improvement and three a complete relief of radiated symptoms.

Analysis of this group, although limited, of patients with untreated lumbar stenosis responsible for neurological changes indicates that, at least at medium-term, symptoms and signs tend, in nerve root canal stenosis, to remain unchanged or improve and, in spinal canal stenosis, to remain unchanged or worsen.

The spontaneous improvement of a radicular canal stenosis syndrome may be ascribed to two different factors: the changes which the intervertebral disc may undergo with time and the reduction of the patient's physical activity resulting from the radicular symptoms. A posterior protrusion of the intervertebral disc may play a primary role in the aetiology of nerve root canal stenosis. The progressive dehydration which may occur in a degenerated nucleus pulposus may lead to a decrease in the size of a posterior disc protrusion and, thus, a progressive reduction of the nerve root compression. The decrease of physical activity, on the other hand, may lead to a reduction in the attrition between the nerve root and the walls of a stenotic radicular canal and, thus, a decrease in inflammatory changes in the nerve root and the consequent radiated symptoms.

These same factors may explain the spontaneous improvement of an untreated spinal canal stenosis syndrome. Worsening, instead, is presumably due to the progressive increase of vertebral degenerative changes and the consequent compression of the caudal nerve roots.

CONSERVATIVE TREATMENT

Like the natural history, the results of conservative treatment of lumbar spinal stenosis are not well known.

Of the two patients reported by Jones and Thomson (1968) one, complaining of radicular pain and showing multiple disc protrusions on myelography, improved, whereas the other, who had a lumbo-radicular intermittent claudication and myelographic evidence of a narrow spinal canal, showed no significant improvement.

Tile *et al.* (1976),in14 cases of stenosis of the spinal canal (4 developmental and 10 degenerative, 6 of whom associated to spondylolisthesis) treated with conventional conservative therapy, obtained unsatisfactory results (poor or fair) in 78%. Excellent results were only observed in patients with developmental stenosis, whereas poor results were obtained in almost all the patients with a degenerative spondylolisthesis. However, the clinical symptoms and signs, the severity of compression of the caudal nerve roots as detected on myelography and the length of follow-up are not described for any of these cases. Similar considerations are valid for the some 150 patients with degenerative spondylolisthesis treated with conservative measures by Rosenberg (1976); most of these patients, however, had mild clinical symptoms which, although not significantly improved by conservative therapy, were not sufficiently severe to require surgical treatment.

Of the 23 patients submitted to conservative treatment by Hasue *et al.* (1977), improvement of symptoms, particularly of the low-back and radicular pain, was observed in over half the cases, but almost none showed an improvement of neurological deficits, when present; in most of these patients, myelography revealed evidence of only posterior or posterolateral compression of the dural sac. Lee *et al.* (1978) obtained satisfactory results in only one out of the six patients with developmental stenosis of the spinal canal submitted to conservative treatment.

As far as treatment with calcitonin is concerned, of the 41 patients with intermittent claudication in the series of Porter and Hibbert (1983), 11 showed lasting improvement both of radicular symptoms at rest and walking capacity. Before treatment most of the improved patients (almost all males) had shown a walking capacity of less than one mile and complained of pain and paresthetic disturbances, which involved both the lower limbs and extended below the knee. It should be pointed out, however, that most of these patients did not show neurological deficits and that myelography (when performed) mostly showed, at least as far as the cases report appears to indicate, a relatively mild compression of the spinal nervous structures. These observations would seem to throw some doubt on the efficacy of calcitonin treatment in patients with neurological signs of compression of one or more caudal nerve roots, as is the case in most of the patients complaining of a typical intermittent claudication due to lumbar spinal stenosis.

In my experience, patients with marked stenosis of the spinal canal (complete or almost complete myelographic block) do not improve or show only temporary relief following conventional conservative treatments. In contrast, patients with a spinal canal stenosis responsible for a posterior or posterolateral compression of the dural sac, in the absence of significant nerve root compression in the radicular canal, often show a significant improvement with drug or physical therapy. This holds true also for isolated stenosis of the nerve root canal: if narrowing is marked, and as such is responsible for significant neurological changes, conservative treatment does not usually produce any appreciable improvement, particularly when stenosis is essentially or exclusively bony in nature; in contrast, when narrowing is mild and/or a disc protrusion is involved in the aetiology of nerve root compression, conservative treatment (or even the absence of any form of treatment, as noted for non-treated patients) may lead to a significant improvement of clinical symptoms and signs.

SURGICAL TREATMENT

REVIEW OF THE LITERATURE

Many authors have attempted to analyze the results of surgical treatment of lumbar stenosis. Some, however, do not provide a precise definition of the term stenosis and, thus, of the nature of the pathological conditions included in the clinical series. It is therefore difficult to compare the results in the different series, also because there are various definitions, sometimes contrasting, of the concept of stenosis. These difficulties are further increased by the lack of uniformity in the postoperative clinical evaluation of patients and the qualitative definition of the results. Lastly, it should be pointed out that, in some series, no distinction is made between patients not previously submitted to spine surgery and patients previously operated upon, in whom results may be negatively influenced by the earlier surgical treatment or treatments.

In spite of these considerations, the data emerging from the various clinical series are in agreement as far as concerns the high proportion of satisfactory results in patients treated surgically.

Spinal canal stenosis

Of the 29 patients (with degenerative or, in some instances, probably combined, stenosis) reported by Teng and Papateodorou (1963), 25 showed a significant clinical improvement, but only 18 (62%) were asymptomatic at long-term follow-up.

Of the 17 patients in the series of Scapinelli (1973), twelve (70%) obtained a complete disappearance of preoperative symptoms and three (of whom one with a paralyzing sciatica) marked improvement of symptoms but only partial recovery of motor deficits; the remaining two showed no clinical improvement. Most of these patients presented a relative stenosis in the sense of Verbiest (see page 49).

In the series of Tile *et al.* (1976), satisfactory results were observed in 83% of the 18 patients with developmental stenosis and 82% of the 29 cases of degenerative stenosis (with or without spondylolisthesis).

Paine (1976) analyzed the results of surgical treatment in 150 patients with spinal stenosis alone and in 119 in whom stenosis was associated to herniation of the nucleus pulposus. In the former group, the highest proportion of satisfactory results was found in patients with degenerative stenosis (79%) and the lowest in those with developmental stenosis (62%). Conversely, in the latter group, the highest proportion of satisfactory results was recorded in patients with developmental stenosis (89%) and the lowest in those with combined stenosis (74%). In the group of patients with degenerative stenosis, the percentage of satisfactory results was higher in the cases in which only one level or two levels were involved and decompressed, compared to those in which decompression was carried out at three or more vertebral levels; furthermore, the greater the sagittal dimensions of the spinal canal as measured on the lateral myelogram, the better the results obtained.

Of the 92 patients observed by Verbiest (1977) for periods of follow-up varying between one and twenty years, 62 (68%) were completely relieved of preoperative symptoms and neurological deficits. In the remaining 29 cases, low-back pain was the most frequent persisting symptom (18 cases); none of the 29 patients complained of radicular pain, but in 10 cases sensory and/or motor deficits persisted. The highest rate of complete recovery of preoperative symptoms and signs was obtained in cases with pure absolute stenosis; i.e. with the form showing the most marked narrowing of the bony vertebral canal, whereas the patients showing the least favourable results were those with pure relative stenosis (for definition see page 49).

In the series of Dick *et al.* (1977), more than 80% of the patients showed a clinical improvement. Of the two achondroplastic dwarfs included in the series (both previously unsuccessfully operated upon), one had no improvement of preoperative paraplegia and disturbances in micturition despite extensive decompression from T_{10} to the sacrum, whereas in the other disturbances in micturition and radicular pain were relieved after laminectomy of the last two thoracic vertebrae. Similarly, in the two cases of achondroplastic stenosis reported by Alexander (1969), which were submitted to extensive decompressive laminectomy as far as the last thoracic vertebrae, only a partial improvement of symptoms and signs was obtained.

Hasue *et al.* (1977), in a follow-up of 58 patients for at least six months, observed complete relief of the preoperative symptoms and signs of stenosis in 52% of the cases and partial improvement in 36%. Results were excellent in 55% of the 20 patients with a radicular syndrome, in 61% of the 31 with intermittent claudication and in none of the 7 with multiple radicular paralysis, 5 of whom, however, showed partial improvement.

In the series of Getty (1980), composed of 31 patients, the results were good in 55% of the cases, fair in 20% and poor in 16%. Four of the 31 patients, who had previously undergone bilateral laminectomy at multiple levels, were operated on due to a persisting stenosis of the nerve root canals; the clinical results improved in two cases, but remained unchanged in the other two.

Surin *et al.* (1982), in a review of 22 patients with degenerative lumbar spinal stenosis followed-up for an average period of 2.5 years, found the results to be satisfactory in 19 cases (86%), in only 8 of whom, however, was an excellent outcome reported. In agreement with the findings of Paine (1976), the rate of unsatisfactory results was higher when three or more vertebral levels were involved and the sagittal dimensions of the spinal canal were less than ten millimeters, than in the presence of mild stenosis involving only one or two lumbar levels.

In the series of San Martino *et al.* (1983), comprising 20 patients with spinal stenosis (in some cases, probably only of the nerve root canals) associated to lumbar scoliosis, the results were rated as excellent in 80% of the cases and good in 20%.

Boccanera *et al.* (1984) in a series of 25 patients with spinal canal stenosis, found an improvement of symptoms and signs in the lower limbs in 84% of the cases, but completely satisfactory results in only 32%. Of the 5 cases, who had previously undergone discectomy, 3 obtained poor results.

Tsuji *et al.* (1985) reported on a series of 50 surgically treated patients with degenerative lumbar stenosis, most of whom presented a redundancy of the caudal nerve roots. Surgical treatment led to a marked improvement of symptoms and signs in 36% of the cases and a moderate improvement in 57%. Although no significant relationship was found between the degree of nerve root redundancy and quality of the results, the patients with a considerable improvement had more frequently presented with a mild or no redundancy than with a marked redundancy of the nerve roots.

Degenerative spondylolisthesis

Several authors have selectively analyzed the results of surgical treatment in degenerative spondylolisthesis. Rosenberg (1976) carried out follow-up studies on 26 patients, of whom 11 had been submitted to monolateral or bilateral laminotomy and partial arthrectomy, and 15 to bilateral laminectomy. Satisfactory results were obtained in only 54% of the patients in the first treatment group, whereas considerable improvement of symptoms was obtained in all patients in the second group. Similar results are reported both by Cauchoix *et al.* (1976), who found satisfactory outcomes in 85% of 26 patients submitted to bilateral laminectomy associated or not with arthrectomy, and Epstein *et al.* (1983) who, in 60 operated patients, obtained excellent results in 41 (67%), good results in 12 (20%) and poor outcomes in 7 (13%) (the seven patients had a long history of symptoms in the lower limbs, were obese and/or diabetic and showed osteoarthritic disorders of varying entity in the hips and knees).

In spite of agreement between the various clinical series, the influence that the lateral extension of decompression and the vertebral fusion have on the results of surgery still gives rise to some controversy. Reynolds and Wiltse (1979) obtained satisfactory results in 78% of the patients who had undergone laminectomy and partial arthrectomy and in only 33% of those submitted to total arthrectomy. Dale and Rowe (1985), however, reported almost opposite results. In almost all the series, an increase in vertebral slipping ranging from 33% to 100% was observed after bilateral laminectomy, but in none of the series was a significant relationship found between the increase in olisthesis and the presence or severity of postoperative low-back pain. Feffer *et al.* (1985), however, observed a significantly higher proportion of satisfactory results in patients undergoing posterolateral fusion in addition to decompression, compared to those who were submitted to decompression alone. Hanley (1986), in a series of 20 patients treated with a combination of decompressive laminectomy and distraction arthrodesis with short Harrington rods, achieved satisfactory results in 85% of the cases. In 14 cases, the anterior slipping increased by 1 to 3 millimetres after the operation, but in none did olisthesis exceed that seen on preoperative flexion radiographs. In only one patient, with a poor result, did spondylolisthesis significantly increase after surgery.

Nerve root canal stenosis

Epstein *et al.* (1972), in an analysis of the results of surgical treatment in 15 cases of isolated nerve root canal stenosis, found excellent or good results in 73% and 20% of the patients, respectively. A similar proportion (93%) of satisfactory outcomes is reported by Choudhury and Taylor (1977), who obtained complete relief of preoperative symptoms in 86% of 28 operated patients. The 9 cases reported by Tile *et al.* (1976) all had excellent results. Venner and Crock (1981), in 45 patients with narrowing of the nerve root canal of S_1 (98%) or L_5 and S_1, obtained complete relief of preoperative symptoms in 62% of the cases and partial relief in 24%; overall, 84% of the patients considered the operation to be worthwhile and 91% showed an improvement in radicular symptoms.

AUTHOR'S SERIES

Material

During the period 1974-1986, the author has operated on, or has participated in the surgical treatment of, 109 cases of spinal canal stenosis, 54 cases of isolated nerve root canal stenosis and 3 patients with isolated stenosis of the intervertebral foramen. The results reported here concern 97 cases of spinal canal stenosis, 43 cases of nerve root canal stenosis and 2 cases of isolated stenosis of the intervertebral foramen, all observed at follow-up for at least one year after surgery.

Of the patients with spinal canal stenosis 65 were males and 32 females, ranging in age from 32 to 73 years (mean 56 years). The type of stenosis and the levels involved are reported in Tables 10.I and 10.II. The duration of radicular symptoms ranged, at the time of surgery, from 4 months to 9 years. The type of preoperative clinical pattern and the frequency of clinical symptoms and signs are reported in Tables 10.III and 10.IV. Bilateral laminectomy was performed in 85% of the cases: the remaining patients underwent monolateral laminectomy (4%), or monolateral or bilateral laminotomy (8%) at one or more vertebral levels. In 17 cases, discectomy was carried out at a single level due to the presence of a herniated disc or marked

Table 10.I

TYPE OF STENOSIS IN 97 CASES OF SPINAL CANAL STENOSIS

Primary stenosis	congenital developmental	1 14
Secondary stenosis	simple degenerative degenerative associated with spondylolisthesis post-traumatic	21 9 2
Combined stenosis	developmental and simple degenerative developmental and degenerative associated with spondylolisthesis	38 10
Mixed stenosis	developmental and combined	2

Table 10.II

STENOTIC LEVELS IN 97 CASES OF SPINAL CANAL STENOSIS

No. of levels	**Stenotic levels**	**No. of cases**
1 level	L2-L3 L3-L4 L4-L5	3 4 17
2 levels	L2-L4 L3-L5	5 24
3 levels	L1-L4 L2-L5 L3-S1	5 23 2
4 levels	L1-L5 L2-S1	10 2
5 levels	L1-S1	2

posterior bulging of the intervertebral disc.

Of the 43 patients with isolated stenosis of the nerve root canal, 27 were males and 16 females with an age range of 36 to 67 years (mean 45 years). The vertebral levels involved and the type of preoperative clinical pattern are reported in Tables 10.V to 10.VII. Diagnosis of stenosis was made preoperatively from myelography and/or CT scan in 22 cases, and intraoperatively in 21 cases. In 12 of these 21 cases, all of whom had undergone myelography but only 4 a CT scan, a preoperative diagnosis of disc herniation was made. At surgery, the intervertebral disc, at the involved level or levels, did not display

Table 10.III

TYPE OF PREOPERATIVE CLINICAL PATTERN IN 97 CASES OF SPINAL CANAL STENOSIS

Type of syndrome		**No. of cases**
Continuous radicular syndrome	acute chronic	13 18
Intermittent syndrome		21
Combined syndrome		45

Table 10.IV

FREQUENCY OF CLINICAL SYMPTOMS AND SIGNS IN 97 CASES OF SPINAL CANAL STENOSIS

Symptoms and signs	**No. of patients**	**%**
Low back pain	78	(80)
Radicular pain at rest	71	(73)
Sensory deficits at rest	44	(45)
Claudicatio intermittens	66	(68)
Motor deficits	82	(85)
Reflex changes	59	(61)

Table 10.V

STENOTIC LEVELS IN 43 PATIENTS WITH ISOLATED STENOSIS OF THE NERVE ROOT CANAL

No. of levels	**Stenotic levels**	**No. of cases**
1 level	L2-L3 L3-L4 L4-L5 L5-S1	2 (U*) 2 (U) 22 (15U, 7B*) 12 (8U, 4B)
2 levels	L3-L4 L4-L5	2 (1U, 1B)
	L4-L5 L5-S1	3 (1U, 2B)

U = unilateral; B: bilateral.

Table 10.VI

TYPE OF CLINICAL PATTERN IN 43 PATIENTS WITH ISOLATED STENOSIS OF THE NERVE ROOT CANAL

Type of syndrome		**No. of patients**
Continuous radicular syndrome	acute chronic	9 16
Intermittent syndrome		6
Combined syndrome		12

Table 10.VII
FREQUENCY OF CLINICAL SYMPTOMS AND SIGNS IN 43 PATIENTS WITH ISOLATED STENOSIS OF THE NERVE ROOT CANAL

Symptoms and signs	No. of patients	%
Low back pain	32	(74)
Radicular pain at rest	36	(84)
Sensory deficits at rest	27	(63)
Claudicatio intermittens	18	(42)
Motor deficits	29	(69)
Reflex changes	13	(30)

evidence of herniation but showed a more or less marked bulging of the annulus fibrosus; the nerve root canal showed narrowing of varying entity, which appeared to be responsible in itself, or in association with the posterior disc bulging, for the nerve root compression. In the remaining 9 cases, in which diagnosis was made at surgery, myelograms or CT scans (the latter carried out in only 3 cases) were negative or uncertain; at surgery, performed on the basis of the clinical-electromyographic findings, nerve root canal stenosis of varying entity was found, which was associated in 4 cases with bulging of the annulus fibrosus. Surgical treatment, in nerve root canal stenosis, consisted of a wide laminotomy or unilateral laminectomy, associated with partial or total facetectomy. In 14 cases, laminectomy was performed bilaterally at a single vertebral level. Disc excision was carried out at a single level in 32 cases and at two levels in one. Discectomy was not performed in the remaining 10 cases.

The L_4-L_5 neuroforamen was involved in both cases of isolated stenosis of the intervertebral foramen; stenosis was unilateral in one case and bilateral in the other. In the former case total facetectomy and discectomy were performed on the side of the stenosis. In the patient with bilateral stenosis, facetectomy was complete on one side and partial on the opposite side; the intervertebral disc was not entered.

Evaluation of the results

The last follow-up, intended as that to which the results reported are referred, was performed 1 to 10 years after surgery (mean 4.2 years) in patients with spinal canal stenosis, and 1 to 7 years after surgery (mean 3.1 years) in those with nerve root canal stenosis.

Evaluation of the results was based on the subjective score of the patient and an objective score given by the examiner.

For subjective evaluation, patients were asked to fill in a questionnaire in which they were invited to express their opinions regarding the overall result of surgery using a scale of 0 to 100, with 0 corresponding to the preoperative condition and 100 to complete relief of symptoms. In the questionnaire, patients were also asked to assign an analytical improvement score for each of the following symptoms: lumbar pain, radicular pain, paresthesiae and claudication.

In turn, the examiner, assigned a score of 0 to 100 based on three parameters: range of motion of the lumbar spine, positivity of nerve root tension tests (SLRT and femoral nerve stretching test), entity of motor deficits, when present, (evaluated on a scale of 0 to 5) compared to preoperative degree of muscle weakness. For patients with no preoperative motor deficits the highest scores for the first two parameters were 40 and 60, whereas for patients with a preoperative muscle weakness the highest scores were, respectively, 30, 40 and 30. The mean of the patient's overall subjective score and the examiner's objective score represented the final improvement score.

Result were rated as excellent when the final score fell within the range of 81 to 100 points, good when the score was between 61 and 80, fair when it was between 41 and 60, and poor when the score was 40 points or less.

Spinal canal stenosis

Overall results

In spinal canal stenosis the results of surgery were satisfactory in 81% of the cases

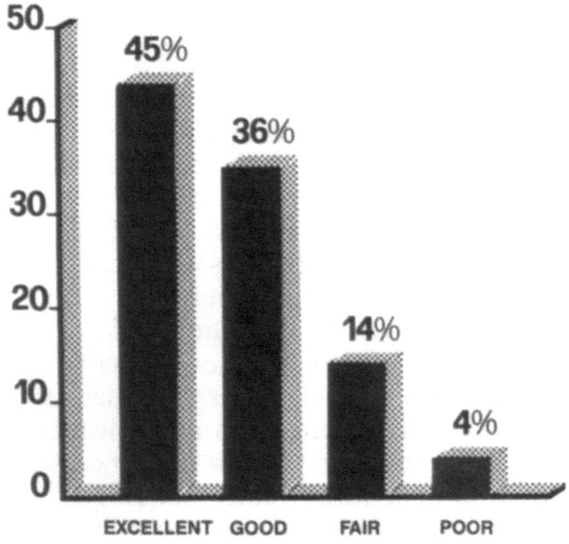

Fig. 10.1 - Overall results of operative treatment in 97 cases of spinal canal stenosis.

and unsatisfactory in 18% (Fig. 10.1).

The quality of the result did not appear to be influenced by the type of stenosis or the number of levels involved, but was found to be strictly related to the severity of compression of the nervous structures as evaluated on myelography or MRI and the degree of preoperative motor weakness.

Satisfactory results were obtained in 87% of the 60 patients with marked compression of the nervous structures (complete myelographic block or the equivalent on MRI), and in only 73% of the 37 patients with less severe compression (partial block, or posterior or lateral indentations on the dural sac, upon myelography, or the equivalent on MRI). However, in most patients with severe preoperative radicular deficits, symptoms disappeared or were considerably relieved by surgery, whereas motor deficits showed only a partial, or no, improvement.

Eight patients had previously undergone surgery for lumbar disc herniation: 5 at levels not involved in stenosis and 3 at the stenotic level or at one of the stenotic levels (Figs. 10.2 and 10.3). Results, in the first five, were satisfactory in 4 cases and unsatisfactory in one, whilst of the other 3 patients, two showed good, and one fair, results. In two patients, who had previously undergone decompressive laminectomy, repeat surgery was necessary, respectively, 1 and 4 years later, to extend laminectomy to areas of stenosis which were asymptomatic at the time of the first operation; the final results were satisfactory in both cases.

In 56 patients submitted to bilateral laminectomy, flexion-extension radiographs of the lumbar spine were obtained at least one year after surgery. In 31% of the 45 patients who did not show a degenerative spondylolisthesis preoperatively, one or more vertebrae included in the area of laminectomy showed a slight hypermobility ranging from 5% to 10%. This occurred particularly at the levels at which extensive lateral decompression or total unilateral or bilateral facetectomy had been performed. In no case, however, did the increase in mobility appear to be related to the presence, or severity, of postoperative low back pain.

In 13 patients with degenerative spondylolisthesis, flexion-extension radiographs were obtained after surgery. In 9 cases (only 4 of whom had undergone posterolateral fusion) the degree of vertebral slipping was equal to that observed preoperatively. The remaining 4 showed an increase in olisthesis ranging from 5% to 10% (Fig. 10.4). None of the four patients had undergone spinal fusion and three showed a hypermobility of the olisthetic vertebra in preoperative dynamic radiographs.

Analytical results

Low-back pain of varying severity was present preoperatively in 78 patients; in three of these, back pain represented the main symptom and was associated with sciatic scoliosis. The result of surgery, as far as concerns low-back pain, was satisfactory in 52% of the cases and unsatisfactory in 49% (Fig. 10.5).

In many of the patients with unsatisfactory results, preoperative low-back pain was of mild entity and the fair or bad outcome only indicates the poor, or lack of, improvement in back pain after surgery. In no case, however, did back pain increase in severity

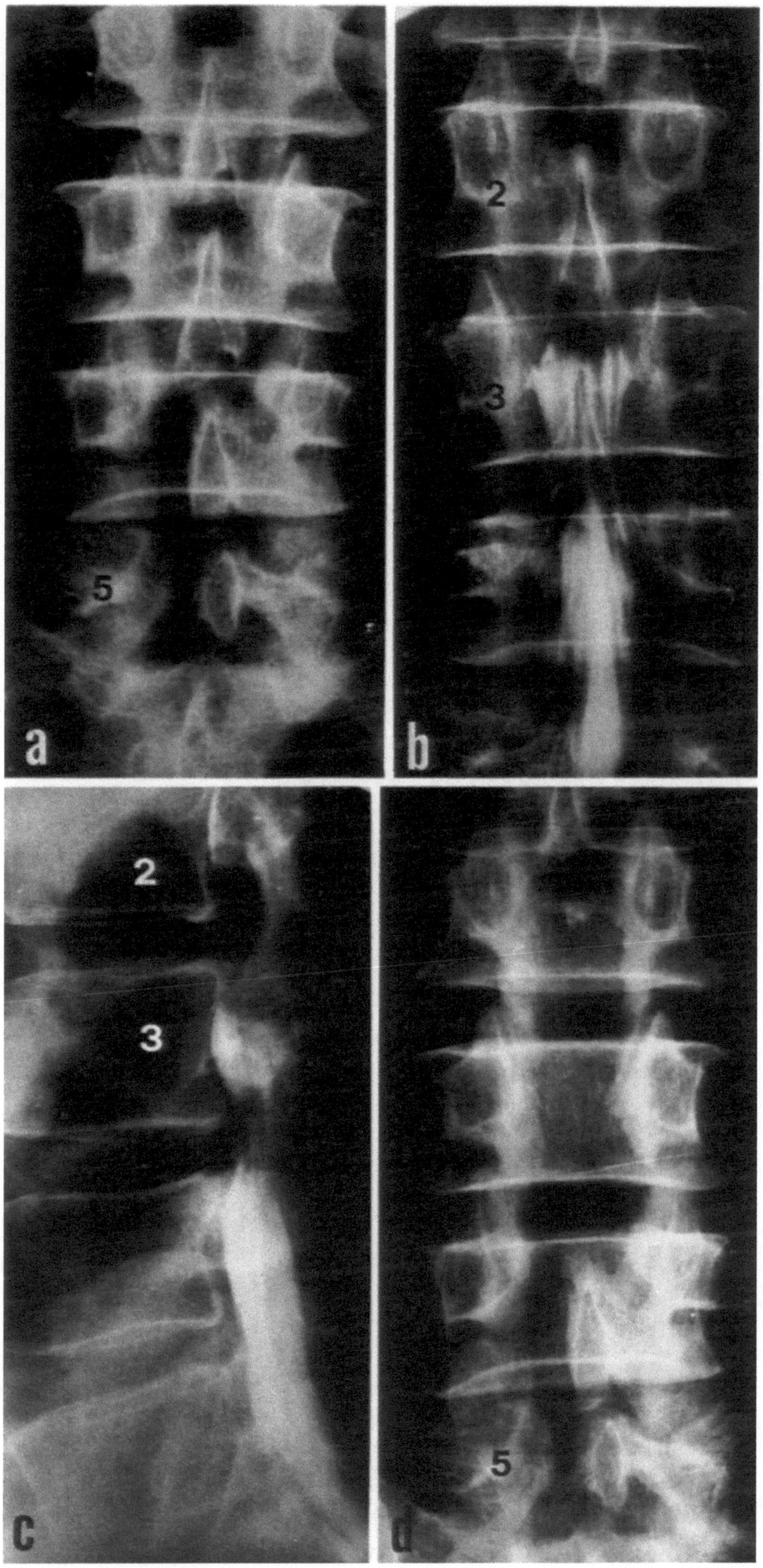

Fig. 10.2 - Spinal canal stenosis in a patient previously submitted to surgery elsewhere for suspected disc herniation, diagnosed preoperatively only on clinical grounds. **a.** Anteroposterior radiograph after the operation shows a right laminectomy of L_5. **b.** and **c.** One year after surgery, myelograms show a complete block of the dye column at L_2-L_3 level and an hour-glass deformation of the dural sac at L_3-L_4. **d.** Bilateral laminectomy of L_2 and L_3 was performed. The second and third lumbar disc showed only mild posterior bulging of the annulus fibrosus.

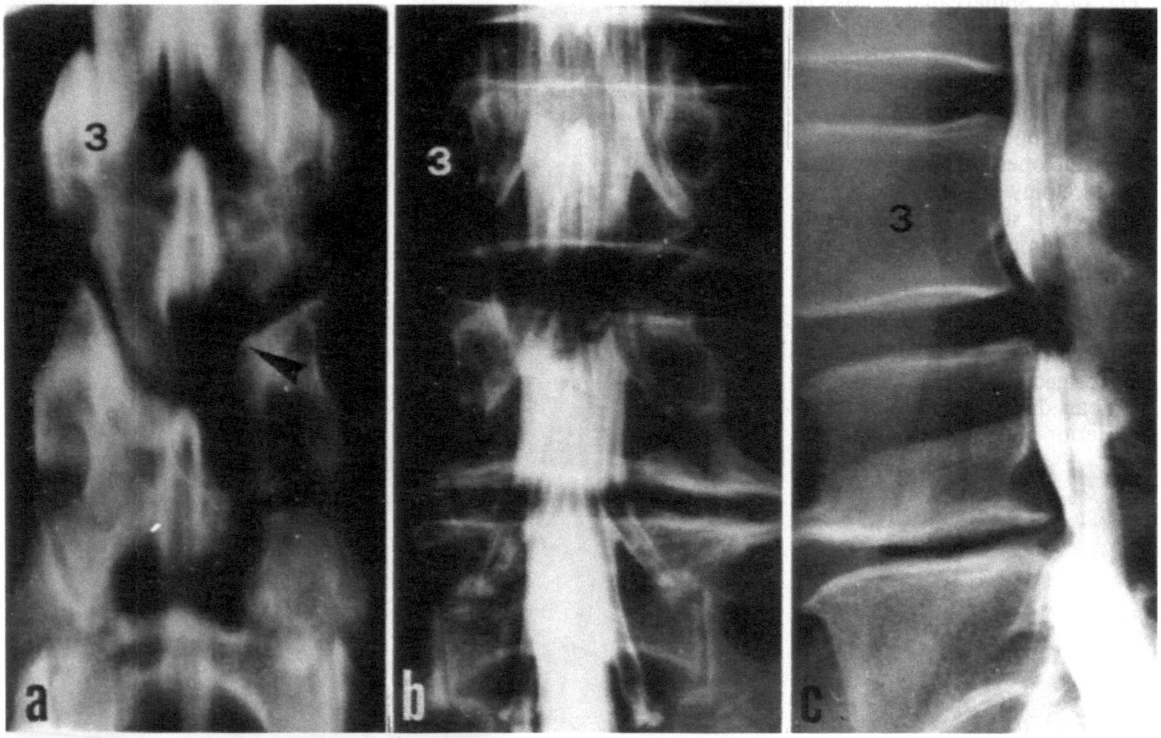

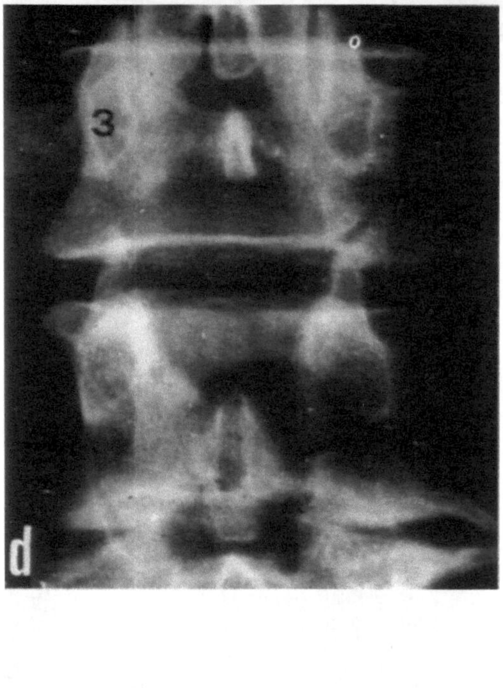

Fig. 10.3 - This patient had been submitted 8 years earlier to surgery for left L_3-L_4 disc herniation. He had no symptoms for 7 years after surgery. Since 3 months he had been complaining of low-back pain and bilateral crural pain which was more severe on the left. **a.** Antero-posterior radiograph at the time of clinical observation. **b.** and **c.** Myelograms show an almost complete block of the contrast column at L_3-L_4 level. **d.** Antero-posterior radiograph after the second operation, which confirmed the preoperative diagnosis of combined spinal canal stenosis at L_3-L_4 level.

after surgery. No significant relationship was found between the type of stenosis or the number of decompressed lumbar levels and the results of surgery. Similarly, no relationship was detected between the type of decompression (laminotomy, unilateral laminectomy, bilateral laminectomy) and the severity of postoperative low-back pain. Of the 19 patients with degenerative spondylolisthesis, only 14 presented significant preoperative low-back pain; the results of surgery were satisfactory in 9 of the 14 cases and unsatisfactory in 5. In only four of the 14 patients was posterolateral fusion associated with decompressive laminectomy; final results were satisfactory in all four.

Radicular pain at rest. The results of surgery were satisfactory in 87% of the cases (Fig. 10.6). Only one patient with poor result, after one year of well being, had a recurrence of radicular pain both at rest and during walking, in the absence of any evidence of

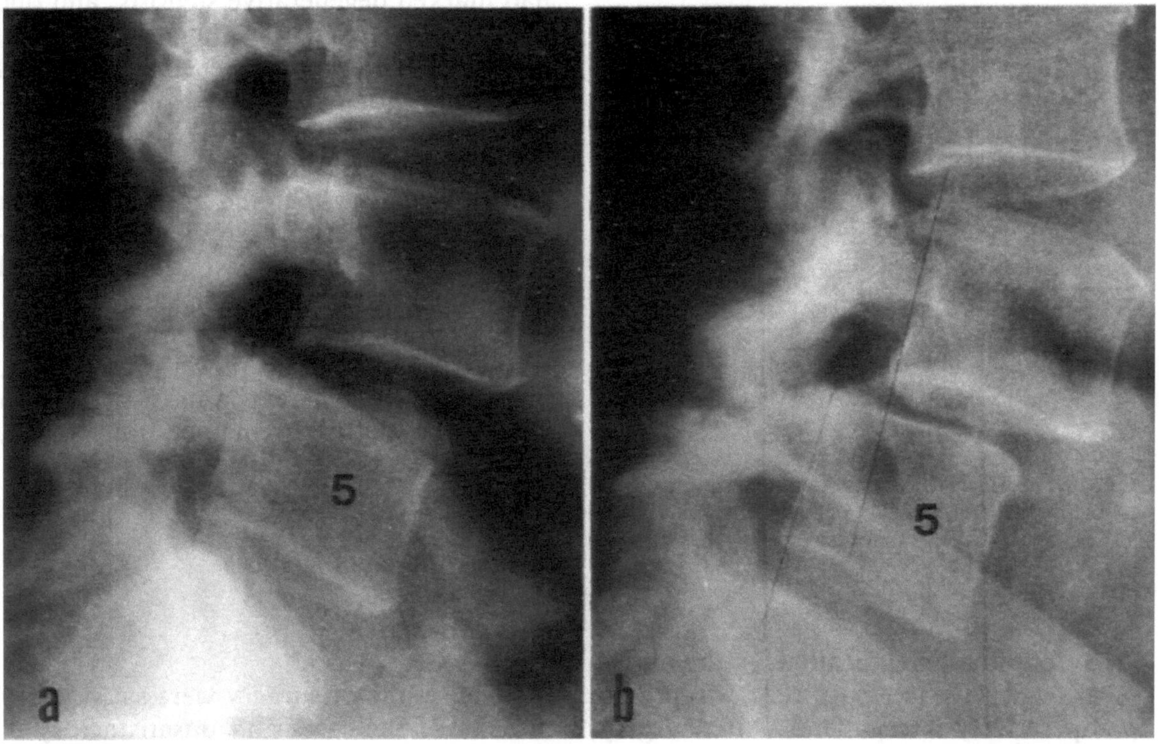

Fig. 10.4 - Increase of olisthesis after bilateral laminectomy at L_4-L_5 in a patient with degenerative spondylolisthesis of L_4. **a.** Preoperative radiograph. **b.** Eight months after surgery.

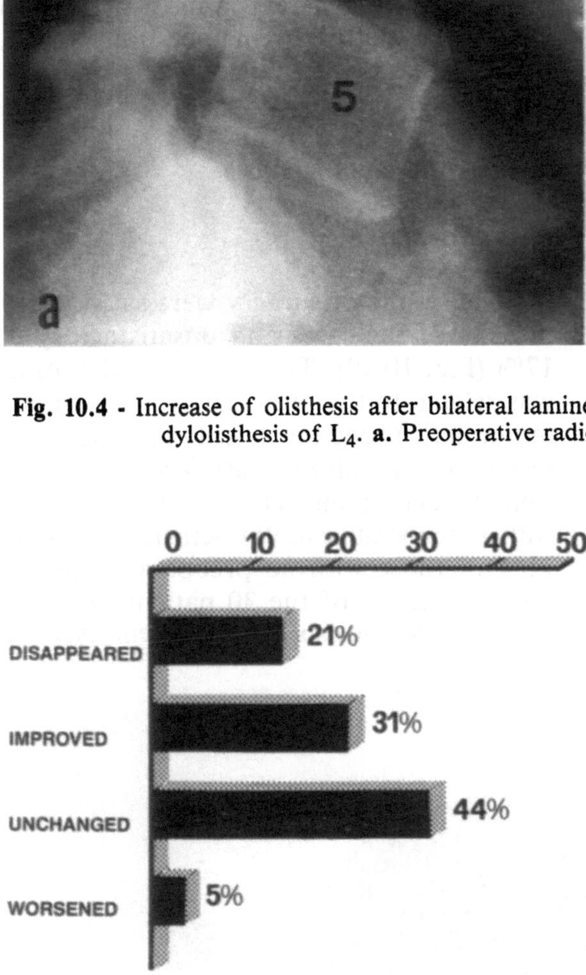

Fig. 10.5 - Effect of surgical treatment upon low-back pain in 78 patients with spinal canal stenosis, who preoperatively complained of back pain.

a herniated disc or areas of persistent stenosis on CT scans.

Subjective sensory disturbances (paraesthesia and hypoaesthesia) decreased to a satisfactory extent in 70% of the cases (Fig. 10.7). In 5 patients, with poor final results, hypoaesthesia had not improved, or was only slightly relieved after operation. In four of these cases, sensory disturbances had been present for more than two years at the time of surgery.

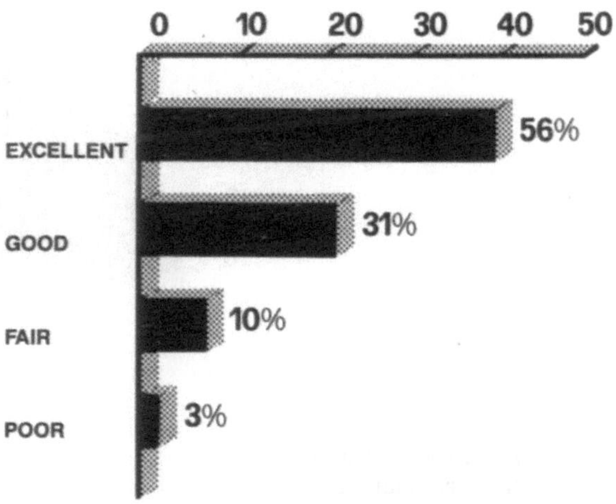

Fig. 10.6 - Effects of surgical treatment upon radicular pain at rest in spinal canal stenosis (71 cases).

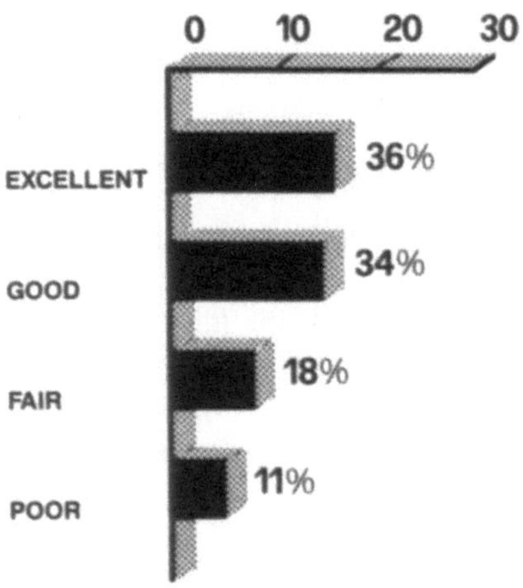

Fig. 10.7 - Effects of surgical treatment upon subjective sensory disturbances in patients with spinal canal stenosis.

Intermittent claudication, in the above-mentioned sense (see page 102), was present preoperatively in 66 patients. After surgery, claudication had disappeared in 74% of the cases and had improved in 20% (Fig. 10.8). Of the four patients in whom intermittent claudication remained almost unchanged, two complained of asthenia in the lower limbs, one of unilateral radicular pain and one of both asthenia and pain. Two of the four patients had, respectively, developmental and combined stenosis of mild entity; one had marked degenerative stenosis; and one presented severe combined lumbar stenosis, associated with cervical stenosis, which was responsible for mild clinical signs of compression of the spinal cord.

Motor deficits, monoradicular or pluriradicular, were found preoperatively in 82 patients. After surgery, deficits had disappeared in 48% of the cases, had improved in 26% and had remained unchanged in 27% (Fig. 10.9). In most patients in the first and second group, muscle power was 3 or 4, preoperatively, whereas in most patients in whom the deficits remained unchanged, preoperative muscle power was 1 or 2.

Nerve root canal stenosis

Overall results

The results of surgery were satisfactory in 83% of the cases and unsatisfactory in 17% (Fig. 10.10). The quality of the result was related to the presence of preoperative motor deficits and the severity of stenosis detected at operation. Satisfactory results, were, in fact, obtained in 90% of the patients with a preoperative motor deficit, and in only 71% of those with no preoperative motor loss. Similarly, of the 30 patients with intraoperative findings of severe stenosis, 87%

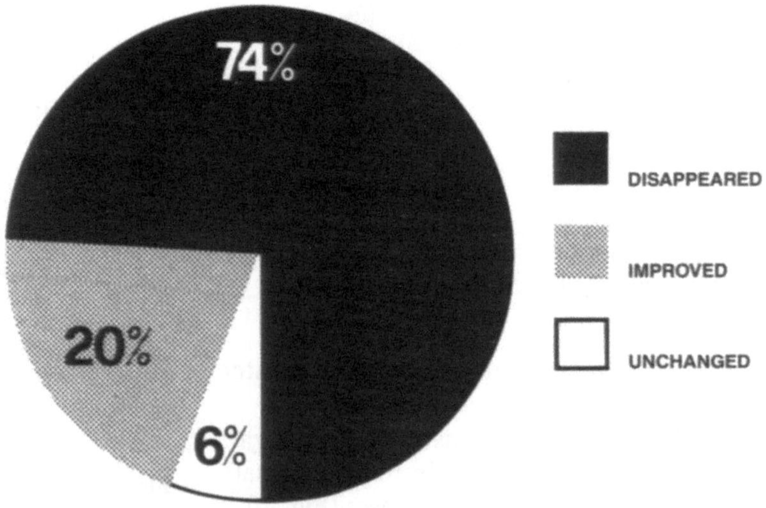

Fig. 10.8 - Effects of surgery on intermittent claudication present preoperatively in 66 out of 97 patients with spinal canal stenosis.

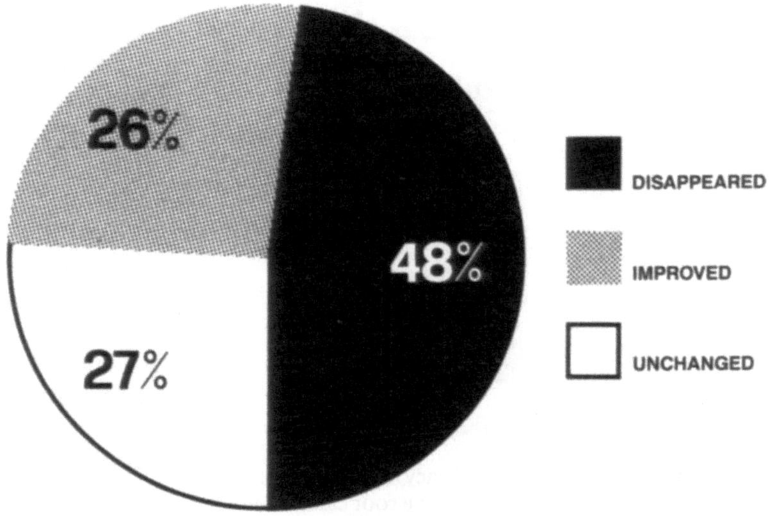

Fig. 10.9 - Effects of surgical treatment on preoperative motor deficits (82 cases) in spinal canal stenosis.

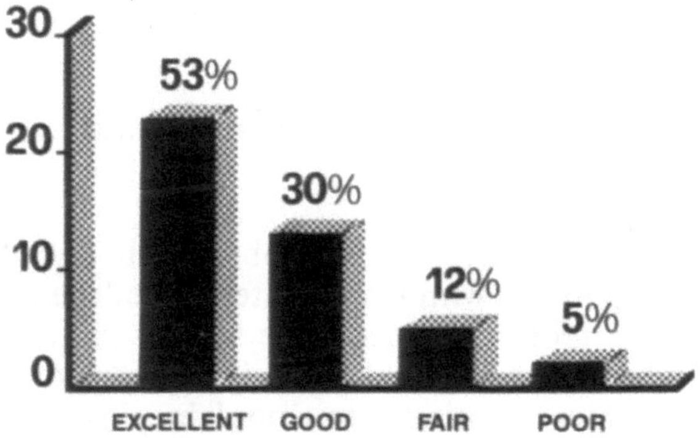

Fig. 10.10 - Overall results of surgical treatment in 43 cases of isolated nerve root canal stenosis.

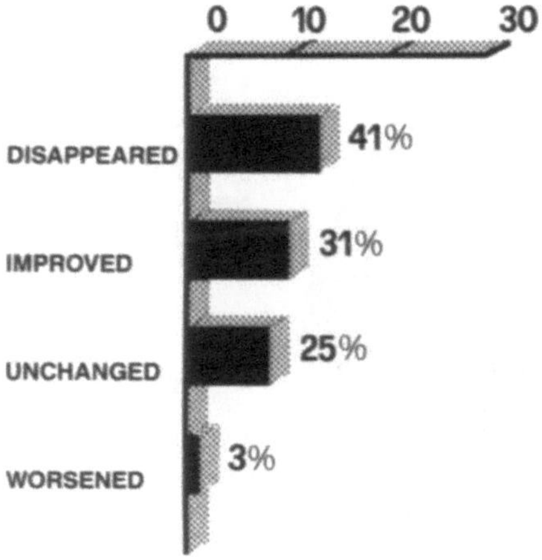

Fig. 10.11 - Therapeutic efficacy of surgery on preoperative low back pain (32 cases) in isolated nerve root canal stenosis.

obtained a satisfactory result, compared with 77% in the 13 patients presenting with mild lumbar spinal stenosis.

Negative myelographic findings in the presence of clinical evidence of nerve root compression did not appear to affect the final result of surgery; however, the proportion of satisfactory results was lower in patients with negative myelographic findings (66%) compared to those in whom myelo-

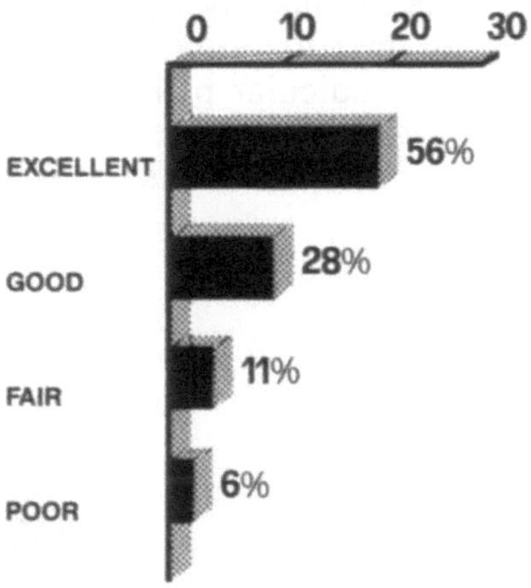
0 10 20 30
EXCELLENT
56%
GOOD
28%
FAIR
11%
POOR
6%

Fig. 10.12 - Effects of surgical treatment on radicular pain at rest (present in 36 cases) in isolated nerve root canal stenosis.

graphy showed evidence of compression of the clinically involved nerve root (88%).

The results, in the three patients who had previously undergone discectomy at the same level and on the same side as the stenosis, were excellent in two cases and good in one.

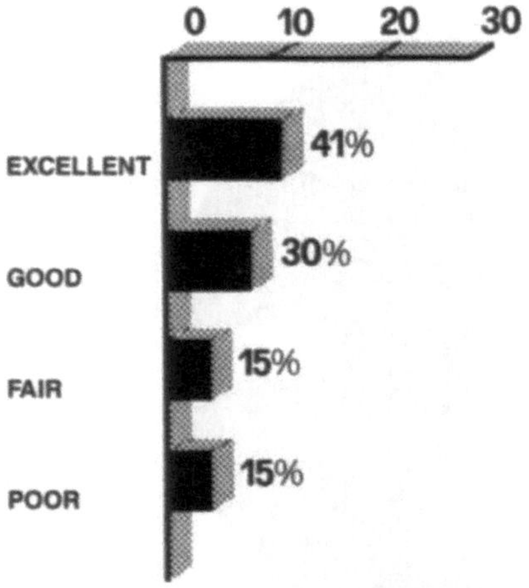

Fig. 10.13 - Therapeutic efficacy of surgery on sensory disturbances in isolated nerve root canal stenosis.

Analytical results

Low-back pain, which was present preoperatively in 32 patients, disappeared or was considerably relieved in 72% of the cases (Fig. 10.11). In no case did back pain increase in severity after surgery.

Radicular pain at rest, which was present preoperatively in 36 patients, disappeared or improved considerably in 84% of the cases (Fig. 10.12). Only two patients, with negative myelographic findings and CT scans of uncertain interpretation, showed no improvement in radicular pain. Of the 6 patients showing little improvement, 3 presented bulging of the annulus fibrosus and the other three mild stenosis of the nerve root canal.

Sensory disturbances disappeared or were considerably relieved in 71% of the cases in which the condition was present preoperatively (Fig.10.13). In two patients, complaining of marked hypoaesthesia in the S_1 dermatome of more than one year's duration, sensory deficit improved only slightly after surgery.

Intermittent claudication, which was present preoperatively in 18 patients, persisted in only one case (Fig. 10.14).

Motor deficits disappeared or improved significantly in 25 (86%) of the 29 patients with preoperative muscle weakness (Fig. 10. 15). The latter was mild or moderate (muscle power 3 or 4) in 23 cases and severe (muscle power 2) in two. The preoperative motor deficit was severe in two of the four cases in which it remained unchanged.

Isolated stenosis of the intervertebral foramen

Excellent results were obtained in one of the patients with isolated stenosis of the intervertebral foramen. The second patient, who had a bilateral stenosis of the neuroforamen, continued to complain of radicular pain and paresthesiae with prolonged walking (fair result).

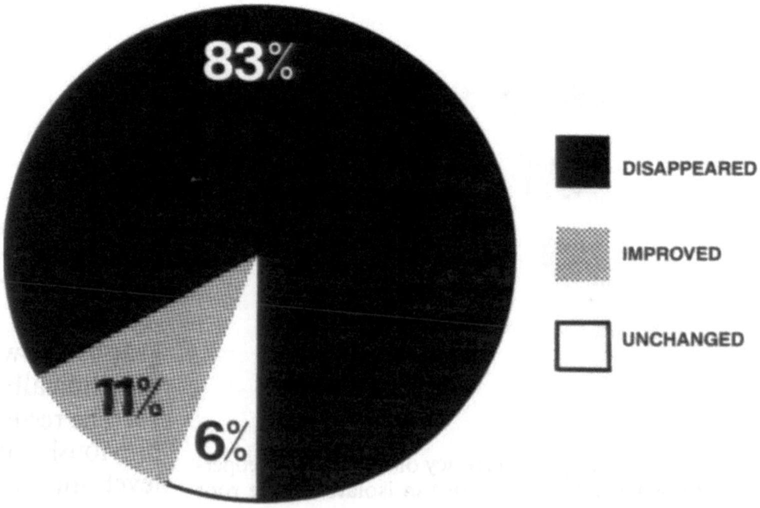

Fig. 10.14 - Effects of surgical treatment on intermittent claudication (18 cases) in nerve root canal stenosis.

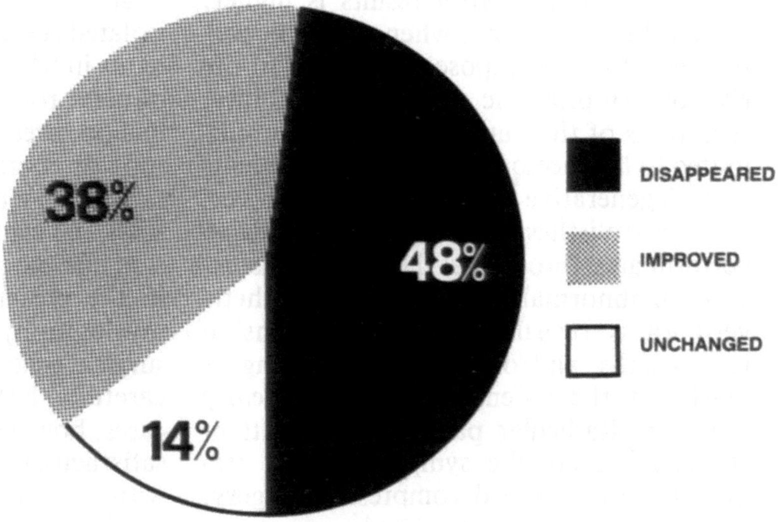

Fig. 10.15 - Therapeutic effect of surgery on preoperative motor deficits (29 cases), in patients with isolated nerve root canal stenosis.

Clinical symptoms and signs after surgery

Spinal canal stenosis

A 69-year-old woman with degenerative spondylolisthesis of the fourth lumbar vertebra and complete myelographic block started to complain, after decompressive laminectomy which completely relieved the radicular symptoms, of rectal tenesmus and severe constipation, apparently not related to any organic bowel disease; symptoms persisted unchanged at two-year follow-up. In one patient, preoperative sensory loss increased and in another patient hypoaesthesia developed in preoperatively unaffected dermatomes; in both cases, sensory disturbances disappeared after a few months. Two patients showed an increase in a preexisting motor deficit (see page 214).

Nerve root canal stenosis

In one patient with bilateral L_4-L_5 stenosis and unilateral radicular symptoms, submitted to bilateral laminotomy and discectomy, preoperative symptoms disappeared after surgery, but a continuous radicular syndrome developed in the preoperatively asymptomatic lower limb. Symptoms which appeared after surgery improved, but did not completely disappear, following repeat operation in which the symptomatic nerve root was exposed along the entire intraspinal course. One patient with marked retrolisthesis of L_4 who had submitted to bilateral laminotomy and monolateral discectomy showed an increase in the posterior vertebral displacement after surgery and six months later suddenly developed paraplegia, which did not improve despite an extensive bilateral laminectomy. Four patients developed a motor deficit after surgery or presented an increase in severity of a preexistent muscle weakness.

CONCLUSIONS

The results of surgical treatment are satisfactory in a large proportion of patients with stenosis of the spinal canal. The greater the degree of compression of the nervous structures, the better the chances of obtaining a satisfactory outcome, provided that the motor deficits, when present, are not extremely severe and long-standing. In these cases, a significant improvement or complete relief of symptoms, but no or only partial recovery of the motor deficits, may be expected. In those patients in whom myelograms show evidence of a mild compression of the dural sac and spinal nerve roots not associated with motor deficits, the decision to proceed with decompressive surgery should be carefully evaluated, since, in these cases, the probability of unsatisfactory results is higher. Bilateral laminectomy, when correctly performed, does not expose the patient to the risk of symptomatic vertebral instability, regardless of the number of vertebrae submitted to laminectomy. However, in patients with degenerative spondylolisthesis or vertebral retrolisthesis, it may be advisable to perform an arthrodesis at the level of olisthesis if an abnormal mobility of the olisthetic vertebra is revealed by flexion-extension radiographs and/or vertebral slipping is marked or the patient is in middle, or early old, age. Radicular pain and intermittent claudication are the symptoms most frequently improved by decompressive surgery. In patients previously operated upon at vertebral levels different from those affected by stenosis, the chances of satisfactory results are similar to those in patients who have not previously undergone surgical treatment, whereas repeat surgery at a stenotic level offers fewer possibilities of determining a satisfactory improvement of the clinical symptoms and signs.

A high proportion of satisfactory results is also obtained with surgical treatment in isolated stenosis of the nerve root canal. Patients in whom myelography shows evidence of nerve root compression and clinical examination reveals a motor deficit of the involved root or roots, have the highest chances of satisfactory outcome. When clinical symptoms and signs indicate a radicular compression attributable to nerve root canal stenosis in the presence of normal findings upon myelography or CT scan, the indication for surgical treatment should be considered very carefully, but not excluded *a priori*. In these cases, however, the probability of obtaining satisfactory results is lower than in patients with positive findings on CT scan and/or myelography. As in spinal canal stenosis, radicular pain at rest and intermittent claudication are the most frequently improved peripheral symptoms; sensory and motor deficits, if severe preoperatively, may, on the other hand, not improve.

The increase in a sensory or motor deficit after surgery is a rare but not exceptional occurrence, particularly if the preoperative deficit is severe and the patient is in old age.

REFERENCES

ALEXANDER E.: Significance of the small lumbar spinal canal: cauda equina compression syndromes due to spondylosis. Part 5: achondroplasia. *J. Neurosurg.* **31:** 513, 1969.

BOCCANERA L., PELLICCIONI S., LAUS M.: Stenosis of the lumbar vertebral canal. A study of 25 cases operated on. *Italian Journal of Orthopaedics and Traumatology* **10:** 227, 1984.

CAUCHOIX J., BENOIST M., CHASSAING V.: Degenerative spondylolistesis. *Clin. Orthop.* **115:** 122-129, 1976.

CHOUDHURY A.R., TAYLOR J.C.: Occult lumbar spinal stenosis. *J. Neurol. Neurosurg. Psych.* **40:** 506, 1977.

DALE B.E., ROWE D.E.: Degenerative spondylolisthesis. Its surgical management. *Spine* **10:** 668-672, 1985.

DICK P.: Intermittent cauda equina compression syndrome. Its recognition and treatment. *Spine* **2:** 75, 1977.

EPSTEIN J.A., EPSTEIN B.S., ROSENTHAL A.D., CARRAS R., LEVINE L.S.: Sciatica caused by nerve root entrapment in the lateral recess: the superior facet syndrome. *J. Neurosurg.* **36:** 584, 1972.

EPSTEIN N.E., EPSTEIN J.A., CARRAS R., LEVINE L.S.: Degenerative spondylolisthesis with an intact neural arch: a review of 60 cases with analysis of clinical findings and the development of surgical management. *Neurosurgery* **13:** 555, 1983.

FEFFER H.L., WIESEL S.W., CUCKLER J.M., ROTHMAN R.H.: Degenerative spondylolisthesis. To fuse or not to fuse. *Spine*, **10:** 287, 1985.

GETTY C.J.M.: Lumbar spinal stenosis. The clinical spectrum and the results of operation. *J. Bone and Joint Surg.* **62-B:** 481, 1980.

HANLEY H.E.: Decompression and distraction-derotation arthrodesis for degenerative spondylolisthesis. *Spine* **11:** 269, 1986.

HASUE M., KIDA H., INOUE K., AWANO N.: Lumbar spinal stenosis. A clinical study of symptoms and therapeutic results. *Intern. Orthop.* (SICOT) **1:** 133, 1977.

JONES R.A.C., THOMSON H.G.: The narrow lumbar canal, a clinical and radiological review. *J. Bone and Joint Surg.* **50-B:** 595, 1968.

LEE C.K., HANSEN H.T., WEISS A.B.: Developmental lumbar spinal stenosis. Pathology and surgical treatment. *Spine* **3:** 246, 1978.

PAINE K.W.E.: Results of decompression for lumbar spinal stenosis. *Clin. Orthop.* **175:** 96, 1976.

PORTER R.W., HIBBERT C.: Calcitonin treatment for neurogenic claudication. *Spine* **8:** 585, 1983.

PORTER R.W., HIBBERT C., EVANS C.: The natural history of root entrapment syndrome. *Spine* **9:** 418, 1984.

REYNOLDS J.B., WILTSE L.L.: Surgical treatment of degenerative spondylolisthesis. *Spine* **4:** 148, 1979.

ROSENBERG N.J.: Degenerative spondylolisthesis. Surgical treatment. *Clin. Orthop.* **117:** 112, 1976.

SAN MARTINO A., D'ANDRIA F.M., SAN MARTINO C.: The surgical treatment of nerve root compression caused by scoliosis of the lumbar spine. *Spine* **8:** 261, 1983.

SCAPINELLI R.: Sindromi da stenosi del canale vertebrale lombare (Presentazione di 29 casi, di cui 17 operati). *La Clin. Ortop.* **24:** 79, 1973.

SURIN V., HEDELIN E., SMITH L.: Degenerative lumbar spinal stenosis. Results of operative treatment. *Acta Orthop. Scand.* **53:** 79, 1982.

TENG P., PAPATEODOROU C.: Myelographic findings in spondylosis of the lumbar spine. *Br. J. Radiology* **36:** 122, 1963.

TILE M., MCNEIL S.R., ZARINS R.K., PENNAL G.F., GARSIDE H.: Spinal stenosis. Results of treatment. *Clin. Orthop.* **115:** 184, 1976.

TSUJI H., TAMAKI T., ITOH T., YAMADA H., MOTOE T., TATEZAKI S., NOGUCHI T., TAKANO H. Redundant nerve roots in patients with degenerative lumbar spinal stenosis. *Spine* **10:** 72, 1985.

VENNER R.M., CROCK H.V.: Clinical studies of isolated disc resorption in the lumbar spine. *J. Bone and Joint Surg.* **63-B:** 491, 1981.

VERBIEST H.: Results of surgical treatment of idiopathic developmental stenosis of the lumbar vertebral canal. A review of twenty-seven years' experience. *J. Bone and Joint Surg.* **59-B:** 181, 1977.

SUBJECT INDEX

Achondroplasia 75
—, aetiopathogenesis 75
—, physiopathology 75
Achondroplastic stenosis 64, 87
Adamkiewicz, artery of, 43
Aetiopathogenesis 75-85
—, aetiopathogenetic factors
——, achondroplasia 75
——, developmental narrowing of the spinal canal 75-76
——, spondylotic changes 76-83
———, degenerative spondylolisthesis 79-83
———, facet joints 77-78
———, intervertebral disc 76-77
———, vertebral body 78
——, traumas 83-84
—, pathogenetic mechanism
——, in degenerative stenosis 84-85
———, single level stenosis 84-85
———, multilevel stenosis 85
——, in primary stenosis 84
———, single level stenosis 84
———, multilevel stenosis 84
Anaesthesia
—, general 189, 191
——, hypotensive 191
—, spinal 189
Angioma 113
Anterior spinal artery 43, 44
Arachnoiditis 207
Arterovenous aneurism 113
Arteriography 115
Articular processes, see also Facet joints
—, anatomy 21, 22
—, computerized tomography 154-155
—, degenerative changes 84, 85, 89, 91, 93, 94, 119-120
——, in degenerative spondylolisthesis 80, 81, 82, 83, 94, 95
—, facetectomy 181, 182, 183, 204, 205
—, radiography 119, 120, 121
—, subluxation 77, 85
Bilateral laminectomy
—, complications 181, 182, 183
——, extravertebral 214
——, intraoperative 212, 213
——, postoperative 213, 214
——, vertebral 212-214
—, extent of decompression
——, longitudinal 180, 181
——, transverse 181
—, indications 148, 152, 177, 187, 189
—, surgical technique 198-208
——, control of deep haemorrhage 206-207
——, disinsertion of paraspinal muscles 199-202
——, exploration of intervertebral discs and spinal nerve roots 205-206
——, opening of dural sac 207
———, complications 207
———, indications 207
———, surgical technique 207
——, opening of spinal canal 202-205
——, osteophytectomy 206
——, prevention of epidural scar formation 207-208
——, skin incision 198-199
——, superficial haemostasis 198-199
——, wound closure 208
Blood supply
—, intrinsic vasculature of the caudal nerve roots 47
—, of the spinal cord and cauda equina 43-47
Bracing 174

Calcitonin 173, 174
—, result of treatment 218
Cauda equina
—, anatomy 37-38
—, arachnoiditis of the cauda 207
Caudal neurinomas 112
Cervical stenosis 113
Classification of lumbar spinal stenosis 54, 55-56
—, isolated stenosis of the nerve root canal
——, combined 65
——, primary 65

——, secondary 65
—, spinal canal stenosis
——, combined 64-65
——, mixed 65
——, primary 61, 62, 64
———, congenital 61, 62
———, developmental 64
——, secondary 64
—, stenosis of the intervertebral foramen 65-66
Computerized tomography
—, articular processes 154-155
—, diagnostic accuracy 163, 166, 168, 169
—, dural sac 155-156
——, area 155-156
——, dimensions 155
——, morphology 156
—, in nerve root canal stenosis 156, 158, 161
—, in spinal canal stenosis 154-156
—, in stenosis of the intervertebral foramen 162
—, intervertebral disc 155
—, intervertebral foramen 162
—, ligamenta flava 155
—, limits 163, 166, 168, 169
—, myelo-CT 169-171
—, nerve root canal 156, 158, 161
—, vertebral body osteophytes 155
—, vertebral canal 154-155
——, midsagittal diameter 154
Conservative treatment 173-174
—, bracing 174
—, drug therapy 173-174
—, physiotherapy 174
—, results 218-219
——, review of the literature 218-219
Constrictive epidural fibrosis, 55
see also Epidural scar
Conus medullaris 37, 38
Corticosteroids 173
Cryomicrotomy 87

Definition of lumbar spinal stenosis 50-53
—, Arnoldi 50
—, Eisenstein 50
—, Kirkaldy-Willis 50
—, Verbiest 49, 50
Degenerative spondylolisthesis 78-83
—, historical review 17, 18
—, incidence 78, 79
—, myelography 142, 143
—, pathogenesis 79, 80, 81, 82
—, pathomorphology 94-95
—, planning of surgery 187, 189
——, indications to vertebral fusion 187, 189
—, radiography 121
—, vertebral instability 81, 82, 187, 189
Diameters of spinal canal
—, interarticular 64
—, interpedicular 26, 28, 29
—, midsagittal 124, 154
——, caudal 26, 27
——, cranial 26, 27
——, in achondroplasia 64, 75
——, in developmental stenosis 64
—, oblique sagittal 128
—, transverse 123
——, in achondroplasia 75
Disc prolapse 50, 51, 53
—, bilateral disc herniation 131, 132
—, differential diagnosis 110-111
—, foraminal disc herniation 146
—, thoracic disc herniation 113
Discectomy
—, complications 183
—, indications 148, 152, 153, 154, 189, 205, 206, 210
Discography
—, indications 148, 152, 153
—, technique 153, 154
Drug therapy 173-174
Dural sac
—, anatomy 38
—, area 155-156
—, dimensions 138, 155
—, intraoperative tears 212, 213
——, extradural cyst 213
——, fistula 213
—, morphology 156
—, opening at surgery 207
——, indications 207
——, technique 207

Electromyography 125-126
Epidemiology 67-74
—, age 68
—, familiarity 69-73
—, incidence 67
—, occupation 68-69
—, physical characteristics 68
—, sex 67-68
Epidural scar 55
—, prevention 207-208
Epidural tissue 97-98
Epidural veins 98
Epidural venous plexus 98

Epineurium 39, 112
Extradural cavernous telangiectasia 113
Extradural cyst 213

Facet joints, see also Articular processes
—, articular space 119
—, degenerative changes 77-78, 84, 85
——, for traumas in torsion 84
——, in degenerative spondylolisthesis 80, 81, 82, 83
Facetectomy
—, partial 181, 182, 183
——, complications 181, 183
——, surgical technique 204
—, total 183
——, complications 181, 183
——, surgical technique 204, 205
Fascia lata 213
Fibrous stenosis, see also Epidural scar 55
Filum terminale 38

Gangliosides 173

H reflex 126
Haemangioblastoma 113
Hemilaminectomy, see also Laminotomy
Hypotensive anaesthesia 191

Incidence of lumbar spinal stenosis 67
Inferior articular processes
—, hypertrophy 89, 91, 93, 94, 119
Interapophysolaminar space 117-119
Interarticular diameter 64
Interlaminar angle 117
Intermittent claudication
—, lumbo-radicular
——, classification
———, algic 102
———, asthenic 102
———, paraesthetic 102
——, differential diagnosis 113-115
——, incidence 110
——, pathogenesis 111
———, compressive theory 111, 112
————, postural pseudoclaudication 112
———, ischaemic theory 112, 113
———, theory of stagnant anoxia 112
—, medullary 113
—, pseudoclaudication due to joint disorders 115
—, vascular 113-115
Interpedicular diameter 26, 28, 29
Interpedicular distance 123
Interspinous ligament
—, excision 178, 202
—, in degenerative spondylolisthesis 80
Intervertebral disc
—, degenerative changes 76-77, 77, 78
——, in degenerative spondylolisthesis 80, 81, 82
——, in degenerative stenosis 84, 85, 89
—, functional changes 42
—, in primary stenosis 84, 87
——, in achondroplastic stenosis 87
—, intraoperative exploration 205-206, 210
Intervertebral foramen
—, anatomy 35-37
—, functional changes 42
—, in degenerative spondylolisthesis 82, 83, 94
—, in degenerative stenosis 85, 89, 91, 92, 94
—, in primary stenosis 89
—, radiography 121-123
Intestinal ileus 214
Isthmic spondylolisthesis 53, 54, 123

Jones and Thomson's spinal index 124-125

Kyphosis 142

Laminae
—, anatomy 22, 24
—, radiography
——, interlaminar angle 117
——, length 117, 119
——, orientation 117, 119
—, thickening 93
Laminotomy
—, complications, see Bilateral laminectomy
—, indications 148, 152, 177, 178, 187, 189
—, longitudinal extent of decompression 180, 181
——, transverse 181
—, surgical technique 209-211
——, microsurgery 211-212
Lateral recesses 24
—, width 29-30
Ligamenta flava
—, excision
——, in bilateral laminectomy 203, 204, 205
——, in laminotomy 210
———, in microsurgery 213
—, functional changes 42
—, ossification 119, 155
—, shortening 93, 94
—, thickening 87, 94, 155
—, transverse narrowing 93
Lumbo-radicular syndrome
—, combined 102, 110

—, continuous 101-102, 110
——, acute syndrome 101
——, chronic syndrome 101, 102
—, intermittent, 102-110
see also Intermittent lumbo-radicular claudication
Lumbosacral fascia 213

Magnetic resonance imaging 171
—, in isolated nerve root canal stenosis 171
—, in spinal canal stenosis 171
—, in stenosis of the intervertebral foramen 171
Medullary arteries 44, 45, 46
Midsagittal diameter 124, 154
—, caudal 26, 27
—, cranial 26, 27
—, in achondroplasia 75
—, in developmental stenosis 64
Morquio's disease 64
Myelo-CT 169-171
Myelography
—, block images 132-133
——, moniliform appearance 137
—, diagnostic accuracy 163, 166, 168
—, dyshomogenous distribution of
the contrast medium 135
—, functional myelography 129, 138-139
—, hour-glass deformation 131-132, 141, 142, 143
—, indentations 130-131
——, anterior 130
——, lateral 130
——, posterior 131
—, in nerve root canal stenosis 139, 143, 144
—, in spinal canal stenosis 140-143
—, in stenosis of the intervertebral foramen 146
—, limits 128
—, nerve roots
——, redundancy 135
——, translucencies 133-134
—, nerve root sheaths
——, myelographic abnormalities 135-136
—, single level stenosis 137
——, multilevel stenosis 137-138
—, technical details 128-129
—, uniform narrowing of the dural sac 129-130
——, generalized 130
——, segmental 130

Nerve root canal
—, anatomy 32, 33, 35
——, distal part 33, 35
——, proximal part 33
—, dynamic changes 94
—, pathomorphology
——, in degenerative spondylolisthesis 82, 83, 94
——, in degenerative stenosis 89, 91, 92, 94
——, in primary stenosis 87
Nerve root sheaths
—, anatomy 38, 39
—, myelographic changes 135-136
—, pial sheaths
——, fascicular pial sheath 38
——, inflammation 98, 112
——, radicular pial sheath 38
——, thickening 99, 112
Neurilemma 39

Oblique sagittal diameter of spinal canal 128
Osteophytes
—, of the articular processes 91, 92, 119, 154, 155, 156, 158
—, of the vertebral body 78, 85, 89
——, computerized tomography 155
——, excision 206
——, pathogenetic mechanisms 78
——, radiography 121, 123

Paget's disease 173
Pedicles
—, anatomy 21
—, length
——, in achondroplasia 75, 87
——, in primary stenosis 87
——, radiography 120-121
Perimedullary venous network 44
—, anterior lateral veins 44
——, posterior 44
—, anterior median vein 44
——, posterior 44
Perinevrium 112
Peripheral arterial pulses 113, 114
Physiotherapy 174
Posterior recess 24, 26
Posterior spinal arteries 43, 44
Preoperative radiography 196, 197
Pseudoclaudication
—, due to joint disorders in the
lower limb 115
—, postural 111
Pseudospondylolisthesis, see Degenerative spondylolisthesis
Pseudostenosis 53, 55
—, fibrous stenosis 55
—, isthmic spondylolisthesis 55
—, vertebral tumours 55

Radicular arteries 43, 44, 45, 46, 47
—, collateral 47
—, distal 45, 46
—, main 47
—, proximal 45, 46
Radicular syndrome, see Lumbo-radicular syndrome
Radicular veins 44, 46, 47, 99, 112
—, distal 46
—, proximal 46
Radiculography, see Myelography
Radiography
—, facet joints
——, articular space 119
——, degenerative changes 119-120
——, orientation 119
—, interapophysolaminar space 117-119
—, interlaminar angle 117
—, interpedicular distance 123
—, intervertebral foramina 121-123
——, sagittal dimensions 121, 122
——, vertical dimensions 121, 122, 123
—, Jones and Thomson's spinal index 124
—, length of pedicles 120-121
—, length of the laminae 117, 119
—, midsagittal diameter 124
—, osteophytes 123
—, preoperative radiography 196, 197
—, vertebral body
——, anterolisthesis 121
——, posterior marginal osteophytes 121
——, retrolisthesis 121
—, Vogue's width index 118, 119
Retrolisthesis 121

Scoliosis 141, 142
Somatosensory evoked potentials 126-127
Spinal cord 37, 38
—, blood supply 43-47
Spinal nerve roots
—, anatomy 37-42
——, extradural course 39, 41, 42
——, intradural course 38, 98
—, blood supply 43-47
—, exploration of spinal nerve roots 205-206, 210
—, functional changes 42
—, redundancy 98, 135, 207
—, translucencies 133-134
Spinous process
—, resection 178, 202, 203, 205
Squatting position 129, 139
Stagnant anoxia 112
Stenosis
—, absolute 175, 177
—, achondroplastic 64, 75, 87
—, cervical 113
—, dynamic 94
—, fibrous, see also Epidural scar 55
—, multilevel stenosis
——, myelography 137-138
——, pathogenesis 84, 85
—, single level stenosis
——, myelography 137
——, pathogenesis 84, 85
—, thoracic 113
Superior articular processes
—, hypertrophy 91, 92, 156, 158
—, osteophytosis 91, 92, 119, 120, 156, 158
Surgical treatment
—, complications
——, extravertebral 214
———, deep venous thrombosis 214
———, intestinal ileus 214
———, urinary retention 214
——, vertebral 181, 212-214
———, nerve root deficits 213, 214
———, spinal cord complications 213, 214
———, tears of the dural sac 212, 213
————, extradural cyst 213
————, fistula 213
—, contraindications 174, 175
—, indications 174
——, to vertebral fusion 181-183, 183, 185, 187
———, in degenerative spondylolisthesis 187, 189
—, patient positioning 191, 193, 194
—, planning of surgery
——, in degenerative spondylolisthesis 187, 189
——, in isolated stenosis of nerve root canal 189
——, in spinal canal stenosis 175-181
—, postoperative treatment 212
—, preoperative identification of spinal levels 194, 196, 198
—, results
——, in degenerative spondylolisthesis
———, author's series 224, 226
———, review of the literature 220-221
——, in isolated stenosis of the intervertebral foramen
———, author's series 221-223, 230
——, in isolated stenosis of the nerve root canal 232
———, author's series 221, 222, 223
————, analytical results 230
————, clinical symptoms and signs after surgery 231
————, overall results 228-229

———, review of the literature 221
——, in spinal canal stenosis 231, 232
———, author's series 221
—————, analytical results 224-228
—————, clinical symptoms and signs after surgery 231
—————, overall results 223-224
———, review of the literature 219-220
—, surgical technique
——, bilateral laminectomy 198-208
——, laminotomy 209-211
———, microsurgery 211-212
——, vertebral fusion 208-209

Thoracic spinal stenosis 113
Tomography
—, multidirectional 125
Transverse axial tomography 18
Transverse diameter 123
—, in achondroplasia 75
Traumas 83-84

Ultrasonography 127-128

Vasa corona 43, 45
Venous thrombosis 214
Verbiest
—, classification of lumbar spinal stenosis 18
——, absolute 18
——, mixed 18
——, relative 18
—, definition of lumbar stenosis 49
—, stenosimeter 18
Vertebral body
—, anatomy 21
—, developmental abnormality 75, 87, 121, 122
—, marginal osteophytes 78, 85, 89, 121, 123
——, pathogenetic mechanisms 78
Vertebral canal
—, anatomy 31-32, 33
——, central spinal canal 33
———, intervertebral portion 31, 32
—————, pedicular 31
—————, subpedicular 31, 32
——, nerve root canal 32, 33, 35
—, dimensions
——, interpedicular distance 123
——, Jones and Thomson's index 124-125
——, midsagittal diameter 124, 128
——, oblique sagittal diameter 128
——, transverse diameter 123
—, functional changes 42, 94, 102
—, hour-glass deformation 87, 131-132, 141, 142, 143
—, pathomorphology
——, in degenerative spondylolisthesis 82, 83, 94, 95
——, in degenerative stenosis 89-95
——, in primary stenosis 87
Vertebral foramen
—, anatomy 21-26
—, dimensions 26-29
——, interpedicular diameter 26, 28, 29
——, midsagittal diameter 26, 27, 28, 29
———, caudal 26, 27
———, cranial 26, 27
—, lateral recesses 24
——, width 29-30
—, morphology
——, ovoidal 24
——, round 24
——, trefoil-shaped 24
——, triangular 24
—, posterior recess 24, 25
Vertebral fusion 181, 187, 189
—, indications 183-187, 204, 206
——, in degenerative spondylolisthesis 187-189
—, postoperative treatment 212
—, results
——, author's series 226
——, review of the literature 221
—, surgical technique 208-209
Vertebral instability 77, 81, 82, 84
—, iatrogenic instability 178, 181, 182, 183
—, in degenerative spondylolisthesis 81, 82, 187, 189
—, in planning of surgery 176, 178
——, indications to vertebral fusion 183, 185, 187, 187-189
Vertebral tumours 55
Vogue's width index 118, 119

MIX
Papier aus verantwortungsvollen Quellen
Paper from responsible sources
FSC® C105338

If you have any concerns about our products,
you can contact us on
ProductSafety@springernature.com

In case Publisher is established outside the EU,
the EU authorized representative is:
Springer Nature Customer Service Center GmbH
Europaplatz 3, 69115 Heidelberg, Germany

Printed by Libri Plureos GmbH
in Hamburg, Germany